My Brain Matters

The NeuroMetabolic Solution

My Brain Matters

The NeuroMetabolic Solution

How to Have More Brain Power
for Your Loved Ones and Yourself

Dr. Joe DiDuro

with ELIZABETH GUDRAIS

AWAKEN VILLAGE
PRESS

This is a work of nonfiction. Any resemblance to persons living or dead should be plainly apparent to them and those who know them, especially in instances where the author has used their real names. The events described herein are all true from the author's perspective.

The content of this book is intended for educational purposes only and is not to be taken as medical advice. The information in this book should not replace, supersede, or interrupt the reader's relationship with a physician, naturopath, chiropractor, and/or licensed mental health professional. Please pursue personalized advice from a health care professional to create a care plan that addresses your individual concerns, especially when it comes to medication and supplements.

Editing by Awaken Village Press
Cover design by Daniel Huenergardt
Author photo by Shhiendl Thanisha Griffiths Norman
Illustrations by Daniel Huenergardt

ISBN 978-1-7356582-2-3 (paperback)
ISBN 978-1-7356582-3-0 (ebook)
ISBN 978-1-957408-08-8 (hardcover)

Library of Congress Control Number: 2021918872

Published by Awaken Village Press
Sioux Falls, South Dakota, U.S.A.
www.awakenvillagepress.com

To

my loving Parents

to whom

I owe so much

I

dedicate

this

Book

This is the same dedication my father used for his book when he wrote a memoir titled *Me, Myself and I* in 1939 at age fourteen.

PRAISE FOR
MY BRAIN MATTERS

"As someone with a sleep optimization company, I believe that you cannot do that job effectively without understanding the latest science around the brain and photobiomodulation. This book (and all of Dr. Joe DiDuro's work) has been critical for me and for the people I serve in aiding their brain and bodily health—and, by extension, their sleep. Read this book, and most importantly, implement the things that Dr. DiDuro shares, and it will change your life."

—Mollie Eastman, host of the "Sleep Is a Skill" podcast

"Much of my career has been dedicated to researching photobiomodulation, establishing and substantiating the transformative benefits of this therapy for human health—and yet, even though we've known about some of the benefits for decades, most people have never heard of photobiomodulation. This book will help to change that. More people need to learn about how photobiomodulation can increase brain power and overall vitality. *My Brain Matters* will help them do just that, laying out the research piece by piece so that readers can see how safe and effective this therapy is. The book also discusses a broader range of lifestyle factors for brain health—essential reading for everyone, given the widespread incidence of brain injury and neurodegenerative conditions, as well as the ways that the everyday stress of life affects brain health for all of us."

—Michael R. Hamblin, Ph.D., Distinguished Visiting Professor,
Laser Research Centre (University of Johannesburg, South Africa)
and Editor-in-Chief, *Photobiomodulation,
Photomedicine, and Laser Surgery*

"*My Brain Matters* is an insightful and well-researched guide for anyone looking for ways to maintain brain health after a dementia diagnosis or brain injury or who is caring for a loved one with neurodegeneration—or is simply looking for ways to increase brain power to lead an optimized life. Dr. Joe takes you on a journey with him through his own family life and the insights gained from his long career as a chiropractor, research clinician, and photobiomodulation expert, bringing to life this cutting-edge therapy and providing hope and practical, implementable tips and recommendations—as well as the scientific background to be able to understand how light therapies can be integrated into a healthy lifestyle for optimal effect. I loved his idea of monitoring progress with a 'joy score' and found myself totally engrossed in the section on the glymphatic system, the 'waste removal' of the brain. The book also contains excellent advice on additional measures to optimize any brain-centered therapy—including hydration, exercise, diet, and supplement recommendations. This is a scientific text written in clear, easy-to-understand English that details the frontier therapy that is photobiomodulation. Easily accessible to the beginner and an excellent resource for medical professionals and those already in the field. Read this book and learn from an expert who truly walks the walk as well as he talks the talk."

—Sarah Turner, founder of CeraThrive, host of the "Rebel Scientist" podcast, and brain photobiomodulation expert

"Brilliantly written! I loved the analogies and metaphors the book used to make science accessible. Dr. Joe does a fantastic job of explaining complex subjects in an easy-to-understand manner. I've not seen anything like this before. When I'm reading it, it feels like I'm having a conversation with myself. The book helped me to consolidate my own knowledge and understanding. I love the concept of a 'recipe' to enhance our health as well—very memorable and approachable. Just awesome!"

—Karim J. Delgado, CEO and head of product research and development, Brain Mechanics

"As a physician for the past fifty years, I've seen my share of healing modalities, including pharmaceuticals, non-inflammatory diets, detoxification, mind/body interactions, nutritional supports, and grounding, to mention a few. I myself have had great success, especially in the management of heart failure, with metabolic cardiology—which, like photobiomodulation, drives ATP in a preferential direction, thus assisting cellular rescue, repair, and rejuvenation. Although I was aware of photobiomodulation years ago, I never deeply studied the merits or realized the enormous benefits of it until I reviewed Dr. DiDuro's book. Let's be clear: The alarming increase in neurodegenerative afflictions and Alzheimer's disease in the world today requires a valid remedy that demonstrates superior results without side effects or risk. Especially given the polluted environment humans are living in, this book provides hope for healing the greatest threat to our civilization: mental decline. Although every health professional *must* read this book, the content will be meaningful to anyone who personally wants to upgrade the clarity of their brain, mind, and perhaps even intuition. Highly recommended!"

—Stephen Sinatra, M.D., cardiologist and
co-author of *Get Grounded, Get Well*

"As a physician, I think this book is excellent. It's about restoring function, developing resiliency, and reversing cognitive decline in people suffering from neurodegenerative diseases. The information is clear and concise, and the book is well-researched. I would recommend it to anyone suffering from a neurodegenerative disease or to their caregivers."

—Willem Gielen, M.D., cardiologist and internal medicine
liaison for psychiatric hospital patients; medical director,
Corsano Health; chief product officer, CardioMood

"Whether you are a newbie or geek when it comes to light therapy, *My Brain Matters* is a great read. The combination of Joe's personal story and scientific details makes this book easily digestible. Put this book on the must-read list for anyone interested in brain health, healing, and recovery—and don't forget the photobiomodulation aficionados!"

—Bastian Groiss, CEO and cofounder, Circadian Ltd. (home of the app "Circadian: Your Natural Rhythm")

"This book drew me in, and I instantly fell in love with the clear, straightforward prose. I found myself taking notes on literally every page, as the book contains a great deal of information I have not seen anywhere else before. This effort by Dr. DiDuro to collect and disseminate knowledge about photobiomodulation, as well as the **PRONEURO** program, will appeal to academics and laypeople alike. If you believe in a holistic and science-based approach to healing the brain, this is the book for you. It holds a wealth of scientific information, but perhaps more importantly, it focuses on empowering us each to take charge of our health. As the book notes, there is quite a long lag time between the time a research finding is published and the time it becomes common practice or is recommended by your physician. *My Brain Matters* not only presents vital research that should have long since made its way into our everyday lives, it encourages each of us to engage with new scientific research and practice critical thinking rather than treating someone else's advice (whether it's that of our family doctor or a social media influencer) as gospel. In addition, the book empowers readers to believe that healing is possible and gives them the steps to move in that direction, providing the hope that is such a crucial ingredient in recovering from brain injury."

—Rico Petrini, former Division I college football player, CTE survivor, brain injury recovery advocate, and cofounder of 4CTE by CTE (a California nonprofit)

"It's extremely well written. I really like the **PRONEURO** approach. It's really comprehensive and logical. Overall, two thumbs up!! I'm excited for it to be available to the masses."

"The balance between a medical adventure novel and the real science coming with it is fantastic!"

"Humans have long dreamed of immortality. In the twentieth century, we extended lifespan, but what is the value of extending the period of physical and cognitive decline from forty-five years of age until a painful death at age seventy-five? The goal in the twenty-first century is to extend *healthspan,* so we live a healthy, active, and fulfilling existence past a hundred years of age. The science and technology to achieve this exists in the world today. For those ready and willing to apply the new principles of longevity, aging is no longer something to fear but an opportunity. This book by Dr. Joe DiDuro is a guidepost for anyone seeking to follow the path of super-longevity. If you apply the ideas contained within, you will definitely live a longer and better life. It's the path less traveled but one filled with joy and new possibilities—and you only need to step on the path to find where it leads."

"At the turn of the twenty-first century, modern medicine still believed brain and nerve injuries were equivalent to cell death and impending tissue necrosis, with no chance of recovery. To all our benefit, in the last decade this myth has been debunked. In *My Brain Matters*, Dr. Joe DiDuro delves into how we can create (and recreate) a healthy nervous system, pulling together knowledge from scientific research and alternative medicine disciplines to elucidate ways to accurately evaluate and treat the underlying brain pathology. Dr. Joe bases his approach on a thorough understanding of the cell—and, specifically, mitochondria—using photobiomodulation as the bedrock of his treatment options. With a pharmaceutical approach to treating dementia yielding lackluster results at best, we must look to lifestyle factors for preventing this devastating condition. This book takes a deep dive into the evidence in multiple areas of health-promoting behaviors that can help restore the body to a healthy state of balance (homeostasis). Having practiced medicine for nearly thirty years, from medical school through residencies and fellowship and on to clinical practice, I've heard it said umpteen times that the brain is the last frontier. The nervous system is so intricate and extensive it's no wonder that scientists haven't fully figured it out. In this book, Dr. Joe has shown me he's a kindred spirit who finds fascination in exploring that frontier. I envision Dr. Joe as a modern-day Captain Kirk, conquering the final frontier (the central nervous system) and 'boldly going where no man has gone before.' This insightful book may soon become a household name; for the overall well-being of our species, I can only hope that it will."

—Kipp A. Van Camp, D.O., diagnostic and interventional
radiologist performing regenerative medical research and
neurodegenerative alternative treatments since 2011

"I have followed with great interest the health and medical applications of lasers since being introduced to them by my late husband, Theodore Maiman, inventor of the first laser. If I were to rely upon only one book for my health, it'd be *My Brain Matters*. Dr. Joe DiDuro is an important visionary leading the way in photobiomodulation backed up by his own research and that of other world-class technological laser scientists. He reveals in accessible language revolutionary advances for our health and well-being now using light-emitting diodes (LEDs). His book is comprehensive and deeply informative."

—Kathleen Maiman, widow of laser inventor Theodore Maiman

"Knowledge is knowing a fact; wisdom is knowing what to do with that fact."

– B. J. Palmer

FOREWORD

The human brain is one of the most complex, advanced, and daunting organic life structures to exist in all of nature. Containing some one hundred billion individual cells, each connected by and conducting electrical signals through ten thousand dendritic connections, it remains our body's most astronomically complex structure. Because of this complexity, disorders of the brain have befuddled many a neurologist, psychiatrist, and psychologist for centuries. For many clinicians, brain disorders remain a giant "black box" of mystery. Most attempts at treating brain disorders have amounted to little more than sticking band-aids on symptoms of the problem without ever really understanding the underlying mechanisms that caused the problem. Meanwhile, over the centuries, science has been slowly peeling back the layers on the "onion" of this mysteriously complex vital organ—and fortunately, the pace of growth in this understanding has been accelerating in recent decades.

Among these scientific advancements, modern X-ray technology, computed tomography (CT) images, and magnetic resonance imaging (MRI) scans have helped identify and evaluate basic anatomical and structural abnormalities seen in certain brain disorders. Diffusion tensor imaging (DTI) has enabled us to look at the anatomy of individual functional axonal circuits. Magnetic resonance spectroscopy (MRS) and functional MRI (fMRI) technology have allowed us to visualize the specific functional circuits that serve specific brain functions, such as attention, memory, sensation, and speech. Metabolic imaging techniques such as positron emission tomography (PET), single-photon emission computed tomography (SPECT), and magnetic resonance spectroscopy increase our understanding by orders of magnitude by allowing us to observe the basic underlying cellular processes associated with various brain functions and diseases.

Over the course of a long career in medicine, I became increasingly interested in how brain imaging can help us visualize brain injury and observe healing—as well as the role photobiomodulation can play in helping to achieve healing. (If that's an unfamiliar term for you at this point, it definitely won't be by the end of this book.) In 2019, I published a landmark study that used SPECT imaging to visualize the disruptions in cellular metabolism that were causing traumatic brain injury patients' continuing symptoms—a type of damage that, because it is not visible on CT or MRI scans, some doctors believed to be "all in a patient's head" (figuratively, not literally). Because of this expertise, I have been called on to testify as an expert witness in more than 150 court proceedings to date, helping judges and juries understand what they are seeing in SPECT images presented as evidence of a plaintiff's brain injury. In these trials, I see firsthand how debilitating brain injury can be—but I also see how it offers a sense of hope when someone can better understand their own brain through imaging and know that they're not imagining the symptoms they're experiencing.

In *My Brain Matters*, my friend and colleague Dr. DiDuro (or Dr. Joe, as most people call him) contributes to "peeling the onion" by comprehensively reviewing the latest medical literature and translating it to help build understanding of what contributes to brain disease as well as how to prevent it and even foster healing. Drawing on recent advancements in knowledge about the cellular basis of many common brain problems, Dr. Joe provides up-to-date research data on how to keep our brains healthy. His **PRONEURO** program, which is detailed in this book, incorporates cutting-edge information from scientific studies on non-pharmacological interventions such as photobiomodulation, nutrition, exercise, heart rate variability monitoring, and other brain-based therapeutic modalities that have the power to not only repair brain problems at the cellular level but also slow down the aging process to promote brain health.

Our brains reflect our knowledge, our personality, and our spirit. Dr. Joe's thoroughly researched brain-based strategies have the potential not only to improve your own brain-related issues but to keep your brain healthy for a very long time. It's not often enough that brain science is explained in a way that allows a lay reader to put to use—and that's exactly what Dr. Joe has done in this fantastic voyage through the human brain, what ails it, and what heals it. His work is a great contribution to our field.

S. Gregory Hipskind, M.D., Ph.D.
Founder and President, Brain Injury Consulting LLC
Expert in nuclear and behavioral neurology
Consulting physician to CereHealth Corp.
Certified Brain Injury Specialist (2010)
Certified Polychromatic Light Technologies Instructor (2018)

GLOSSARY OF TERMS

I've made every effort to thoroughly and clearly define these terms when each one is first introduced in the book, but I understand that your memory may still need refreshing. This section of the book is intended as a resource for you to turn back to when you need to remind yourself of what a given term means. Please don't feel the need to memorize this list—or even read it—right now, before you've read any of the rest of the book's content. That's a lot to process all at once, and I want you to take it step by step! Go ahead and turn to the introduction and dive in; just know that this list is here when you need it.

abscopal effects: indirect, or off-target, effects (in the context of this book, referring to the effects of photobiomodulation on parts of the body other than the spot where light was applied)

adenosine triphosphate (ATP): an energy molecule found in all life forms on earth, and the final product of the mitochondria's energy production processes

adrenaline (also known as epinephrine): a hormone secreted by the adrenal glands in increased amounts under conditions of stress, and which drives sympathetic activation by increasing heart rate and respiratory rate and directing energy away from digestion to the muscles for the fight-or-flight response

allele: a variant form of a gene; for example, each human has two alleles for eye color (one from their mother and one from their father), with the dominant allele determining the person's visible eye color

allostatic load: the cumulative burden of chronic stress and life events, measured through a composite index of multiple indicators; this measure can be influenced both for the worse (e.g., by chronic stressors or damaging infections) and for the better (with modalities that help the body to heal, recover, and regenerate)

amino acids: organic compounds that are sometimes called the building blocks of life; there are twenty-two that appear in the human genetic code, and which, in different combinations, make up peptides and proteins

amygdala: a part of the brain primarily involved in the processing of emotions and memories associated with fear

amyloid beta: a peptide that accumulates in the brain to form the plaques that are a hallmark of Alzheimer's disease

apoptosis: cell death that occurs when cells are marked for destruction after they have been damaged beyond repair

astrocyte: a large, star-shaped type of glial cell that holds nerve cells in place; more numerous in the body than neurons, these cells tile the entire central nervous system

autonomic nervous system: the branch of the nervous system that controls involuntary functions like heartbeat, vasodilation, breathing, and digestion (as opposed to the *somatic nervous system*, which is under our conscious control)

autophagy: the body's "reduce, reuse, recycle" process in which the body cleans out the usable materials in cells that have been marked for destruction

biofeedback: using electronic monitoring to track a normally automatic bodily function for the purpose of training yourself to acquire voluntary control of that function (as with biofeedback breathing to influence heart rate variability)

biogenesis: the synthesis of new life (often used in this book in the context of *mitochondrial biogenesis*, i.e., the creation of new mitochondria)

biomarker: a quality of a living organism that can be measured as an indicator of some phenomenon (e.g., a fever is a biomarker of infection)

brain-derived neurotrophic factor (BDNF): a protein that helps to maintain existing neurons and encourage the growth of new neurons and synapses and whose deficiency is a contributing factor in Alzheimer's disease; an essential molecule for neuroplasticity

cell danger response: changes in the cell (in response to a chemical, physical, or microbial threat) entailing defenses such as stiffer cell membranes and releasing antiviral and antimicrobial substances to kill invaders as well as epigenetic features

central nervous system: the brain and spinal cord

chromophore: a molecule that absorbs a particular wavelength of light (e.g., cytochrome c oxidase with near-infrared light)

chromosomes: bundles of tightly coiled DNA that contain our entire genetic blueprint and are located within the nucleus of almost every cell in our bodies

cortisol: a steroid hormone that originates in the adrenal glands and manages bodily processes including metabolism, immune response, and inflammation; a key player in the fight-or-flight response

cytochrome c oxidase: an enzyme found in the mitochondria; the final enzyme in the electron transport chain (Complex IV)

cytokines: small proteins with a function of signaling between cells

deoxyribonucleic acid (DNA): the genetic material contained within almost all the cells of our bodies; essentially, the blueprint or set of instructions that is unique to each human

dopamine: a neurotransmitter that plays a role in many body functions, including the reward system that is hijacked by addictive substances; the breakdown of dopamine production is a key feature of Parkinson's disease

dysautonomia: dysfunction of the autonomic nervous system

electron transport chain: a multi-step process that takes place along the inner membranes of mitochondria and drives the synthesis of ATP

enzyme: proteins that act as biological catalysts by accelerating chemical reactions (e.g., ATP synthase, which catalyzes the synthesis of ATP from ADP and phosphate)

epigenetics: the role played by modification of gene expression (e.g., by environmental factors) rather than by the genetic code itself

excitotoxicity: neuronal damage or death caused by excessive stimulation/activation (i.e., excessive levels of excitatory neurotransmitters)

glial cells: the cells of the central nervous system other than neurons

glymphatic system: the brain's system for waste clearance

heart rate variability (HRV): a measure of the variation in time between heartbeats (an indicator of nervous system balance and how active the parasympathetic nervous system is)

hippocampus: a part of the brain that plays a key role in learning and memory

homeostasis: a state of equilibrium or balance to which the body constantly seeks to return

hormesis: adaptation to a substance or phenomenon, such that the body increases its capacity to handle that substance or phenomenon up to a certain limit, beyond which the substance becomes toxic or has an inhibitory rather than stimulatory effect (in a biphasic dose-dependent response)

hormones: chemical messengers of the body's endocrine system; examples include cortisol, insulin, estrogen, and adrenaline, among others (some, but not all, neurotransmitters are also hormones)

hyperperfusion: excessive blood flow (e.g., when capillaries are damaged because the body cannot adequately regulate blood pressure)

hypoperfusion: reduced blood flow (in the context of this book, specifically, inadequate supply of oxygenated blood, typically to the brain or a specific brain region)

hypothalamus: a part of the brain that produces hormones that regulate bodily functions including temperature, heart rate, and hunger

hypothalamus-pituitary-adrenal (HPA) axis: a system connecting the hypothalamus and pituitary gland (in the brain) with the adrenal glands; as the brain responds to stress signals in the environment, a fight-or-flight response travels to the adrenals via corticotropin-releasing hormone, which cues the release of the stress hormone cortisol

hypoxic: low in oxygen

in vitro: in this context, a research study that takes place outside of a living organism (e.g., with cells cultured in a petri dish)

in vivo: refers to a study conducted with living subjects (but is often used specifically to refer to studies in non-human animals)

infarction: tissue injury or death due to inadequate blood supply (i.e., after prolonged ischemia)

interstitial: between cells (as in *interstitial fluid* or *interstitial space*)

ischemia: decreased blood flow to a tissue resulting in hypoxic conditions

limbic system: a collection of brain structures involved in processing emotion and memory, including the hypothalamus, thalamus, hippocampus, and amygdala

lipids: fatty compounds that perform a variety of functions in the body, including making up cell membranes; a common example is *blood lipids* such as cholesterol

macrophage: a type of white blood cell that surrounds and kills microorganisms, removes dead cells, and stimulates the action of other immune system cells

mild cognitive impairment (MCI): a condition involving difficulties with memory and cognition less severe than dementia, but which indicates that someone is at high risk of developing dementia; diagnosed with the help of neurological and cognitive tests as well as an interview to determine the patient's own perception of how much the condition affects the activities of daily life

mesenchymal stem cell: a cell with the ability to develop into many different cell types

meta-analysis: a type of review article that conducts its own statistical analysis on the results of multiple studies

microbiome: the community of microorganisms living together in a particular environment (e.g., gut bacteria)

microglia: immune cells of the central nervous system

mindfulness: the practice of being aware of one's surroundings and senses in the present moment (as opposed to worrying about the future or numbing one's awareness with technology); yoga, meditation, and breathwork are examples of practices that incorporate mindfulness

mitochondria: organelles that generate ATP and are found in most types of cells in the body

mitokines: molecules that perform a signaling function to indicate levels of mitochondrial energy status and function or dysfunction

mitophagy: autophagy for mitochondria; a mitochondrial quality control mechanism that marks weak or damaged mitochondria for destruction

neurogenesis: the creation of new neurons

neuroinflammation: an inflammatory response within the brain or spinal cord

neurometabolic: relating to the energy systems of the brain and central nervous system

neurons: the central nervous system cells that transmit information to other nerve cells, muscles, or glands

neuropathy: nerve damage leading to pain, weakness, numbness, or tingling (often used as shorthand for a specific type of neuropathy, *peripheral neuropathy*, which affects nerves in the limbs)

neuroplasticity: the ability of the brain to form and reorganize synaptic connections, especially in response to learning or experience or following an injury

neurotoxin: a substance that is destructive to the cells of the nervous system

neurotransmitter: a signaling molecule secreted by a neuron to affect another cell across a synapse; examples include dopamine, serotonin, norepinephrine, and gamma-aminobutyric acid (GABA)

nitric oxide: a compound in the body that causes the blood vessels to relax and dilate; also acts as a retrograde neurotransmitter, creating a feedback loop in the brain

norepinephrine (also known as noradrenaline): a neurotransmitter and hormone that affects heart rate and blood pressure, constricting blood vessels and increasing alertness, attention, and physiological arousal

organelle: a small structure within a cell (such as a mitochondrion) that is surrounded by a membrane and has a specific function

oxidative stress: cell and tissue damage that results when reactive oxygen species outnumber antioxidants in the body or a part of it

parasympathetic nervous system: a network of nerves that relaxes the body after periods of stress or danger; the branch of the autonomic nervous system in charge of the rest-and-digest response

peptide: a short chain of amino acids (as distinct from a long chain of amino acids, which is called a protein)

peripheral nervous system: the network of nerves that runs throughout the head, neck, and body (outside of the central nervous system)

photobiomodulation: using light to trigger photochemical reactions in a living being

pituitary gland: an endocrine organ in the brain that makes hormones that regulate many bodily processes, including reproduction, growth, and metabolism; as part of the HPA axis, the pituitary gland releases a hormone that stimulates the adrenal glands

prefrontal cortex: a brain region that plays a central role in decision-making, complex cognition, and moderating social behavior

reactive oxygen species: a type of unstable molecule that contains oxygen and plays a key role in oxidative stress and inflammation

review article: a type of scientific study that, rather than conducting original research, collects and synthesizes the results of multiple other related studies

serotonin: a neurotransmitter and hormone produced in the brain and gut whose presence is linked to feelings of well-being and whose deficiency is linked to depression

sympathetic nervous system: the branch of the autonomic nervous system that's responsible for the fight-or-flight response in stressful or dangerous conditions

synapse: a gap between two neurons, across which nerve impulses are relayed by neurotransmitters

tau: a type of protein predominantly found in the brain, and which forms tangles that are a signature of Alzheimer's disease

telomere: a region of DNA found at the end of a chromosome, and whose length is thought to be a marker of biological age

traumatic brain injury (TBI): an injury to the brain caused by an outside force, usually a blow to the head (e.g., in a sports injury or a car accident)

vagus nerve: the main nerve of the parasympathetic nervous system, extending from the brainstem down to the abdomen

vascular: relating to the blood vessels

vasodilation: widening of the blood vessels

CONTENTS

INTRODUCTION

"I did then what I knew how to do. Now that I know better, I do better."

—Maya Angelou

I like to say that I've been a brainiac for a long time—but despite how it might sound, I'm not bragging about my intellect when I say that. A bit to the contrary, in fact. I know a lot about the brain now, but my fascination with learning about it was prompted, in part, when I realized just how far short of its potential my own brain was falling.

In my younger days, when I treated patients in my chiropractic practice, I was always intrigued by the brain and the nervous system. Even though my chiropractic training had given me deep and detailed knowledge of anatomy and physiology as well as the nervous system, I desired to learn even more—and so I pursued a specialization in chiropractic neurology and a master's degree in clinical research. I was a brainiac in the sense of being obsessed with learning about the brain and understanding how it functions best. Think about it—the three pounds of Jello-like material inside your skull is the most complex thing in the entire universe. Doesn't it just blow your mind (pun intended) that the number of neurons in the human brain is about the same as the number of stars in the Milky Way?

When my own mother began to struggle with Alzheimer's disease, suddenly the professional became very personal. I saw firsthand the suffering the disease causes, and this led me to create my **PRONEURO** approach and develop the light devices I offer for sale on my website. In reading this book, you'll not only learn *how* to practice the **PRONEURO** approach—including everything I've learned in testing it with my coaching clients over the last several years—but also learn *why* it works. I hope you'll find the science as fascinating as I do, and I'll do my best to make it entertaining. By the time you're done reading, my hope is that you'll be a brainiac too—both in the sense of loving to learn about the brain *and* in the sense of having increased your brain power.

Whether you picked up this book to learn how to take better care of your own brain or to help someone you love, I want to tell you that *there is hope*. Recent scientific research—much of which is outlined in this book—is demonstrating that the human brain and nervous system have an incredible ability to heal.

If you are reading this book in hopes of helping a loved one, I want to acknowledge this act of care and concern you are undertaking. I know from direct experience that being a caregiver for someone with a neurodegenerative condition can be incredibly draining—and heartbreaking as you watch the person you once knew recede from you. The advice in this book can help slow the decline and even reverse neurodegeneration.

But I want to make one other point very clearly. By the time neurodegeneration interferes with the functions of daily life, the problem is grave and the need to do something about it urgently clear—but the damage and decline actually begin long before the symptoms are readily apparent. The earlier you begin to address the symptoms of cognitive decline, the better your chances of reversing it or at least stopping it in its tracks.

For best results, you'd begin to make lifestyle changes with the earliest warning signs—long before a diagnosis of Alzheimer's or dementia. In fact, in an ideal world, we'd all practice the lifestyle habits outlined in this book regardless of symptoms or risk factors. The truth is that we are all at risk. That's right: If you are living and breathing, you are at risk of neurodegeneration.

This may seem like hyperbole, but I'm not merely making the statement for shock value. The factors predisposing people to neurodegeneration are not limited to a select few among us; rather, these risk factors affect just about *all* of us. If this truth feels alarming, I would encourage you to receive it as a call to take action and practice what you learn from reading this book.

When people speak of risk factors for Alzheimer's, they tend to place too much emphasis on genetic markers. They view genes as destiny.

If you have the genes, you're on an unstoppable march toward disease and debility—or so the line of thinking goes, but I beg to differ. While genes certainly play a role, I'm not sure why we are so quick to disregard the role environment plays. Our environment, in the form of behaviors and lifestyle factors, plays an enormous role in determining whether genes express themselves early, late, or not at all.

I believe—and will make the argument in this book—that most of us go in and out of periods of cognitive decline throughout our lives. Here, a minor head injury; there, a very stressful period of life that interferes with our sleep cycles. Multiple seemingly minor incidents can add up over the course of a lifetime to a kind of "brain damage" that predisposes us to cognitive decline and dementia.

And it's not just disparate, easily identifiable incidents that cause the damage. The standard modern lifestyle is setting us up for neurodegeneration. If we're going to bed too late and getting too much screen time at night, this can interfere with sleep quality—and thus with the body's ability to heal itself while we sleep. If we're constantly anxious and tense and don't know how to relax, then we're not allowing our bodies to fully activate their healing capabilities. If we lead a sedentary lifestyle and we don't move enough, we're losing out on the body's innate capacity to heal because we are not sufficiently stimulating the circulatory system, which plays a crucial role in healing (among other benefits of exercise). If we're not taking in key nutrients that enhance the brain's power to heal, our nutrition can also contribute to suboptimal brain function.

Plain and simple, the way we live is setting us up for brain damage—but the fact that it's so common doesn't mean we have to accept it. This brain damage can be healed and it can be reversed.

If you picked up this book to help a loved one, you might be wondering why I'm telling you all this. You might be thinking, "Just get to the point. How can I help my (mother/father/aunt/uncle/spouse) who has Alzheimer's?" Keep reading, and you'll certainly learn practical tips you can use to help them. But what you learn in this book also has the potential to help our entire society and the entire human species if we spread the word far and wide that we can all improve our brain health and protect ourselves against cognitive decline by changing our lifestyles.

There's one other reason I'm telling you all this—and that is that caregivers are at risk of cognitive decline themselves. The act of caregiving is so intensely stressful that it can (and often does) cause the caregiver's health to take a nosedive. Even if you are reading this book primarily to learn what you can do to help a loved one, I would encourage you to take the recommendations to heart and start practicing them in your own life. You will be a better caregiver and a healthier person for it—and you may even break the cycle by stopping your own neurodegeneration and avoiding having to lean on someone else as a caregiver in your older years, or at least delaying the onset of disease.

When it comes to the cardiovascular system, we have largely accepted as conventional wisdom that it requires routine maintenance if we want it to work well throughout our life course. Although actually following this advice may be another matter entirely, most of us accept as truth that we need to exercise and eat a heart-healthy diet if we want to avoid hypertension and heart disease. My vision is that one day, it will be just as widely accepted that our brains, too, can be primed for a long and healthy life through routine maintenance.

In the course of developing the **PRONEURO** approach as a manual for this routine maintenance, I noticed my own personality changing as I practiced these lifestyle habits—and I came to realize that things I thought were personality traits were actually symptoms of brain damage. There was a time when it felt like I was experiencing failure after failure, with relationships and business ventures slipping through my fingers like sand. I wonder if these things might have gone differently if I'd been practicing the **PRONEURO** approach back then. I have some regrets—but mostly I feel tremendously relieved to understand now that I'm not a jerk and I'm not impossible to get along with. I just had a damaged brain that needed healing.

Today, I don't have the quick temper that I used to. I have more patience, and as I approach senior citizen status, my memory is better than ever—and has improved noticeably in the last decade. It's nothing short of a miracle—but it's a miracle that everyone has access to if they take the advice in this book.

The **PRONEURO** approach holds the keys to restoring function, building resiliency, and reversing cognitive decline for people with neuro-degenerative conditions, regardless of the stage of progression. Moreover, as you'll see with the evidence presented in this book, the **PRONEURO** approach can also be massively beneficial for mental health issues such as depression, anxiety, and post-traumatic stress disorder. It can even be combined with the treatments typically used in the mental health field (such as pharmaceuticals and cognitive behavioral therapy) for faster and fuller recovery. What's more, mental health conditions are usually treated as something altogether separate from cognitive decline—but as you'll see in this book, there's quite a bit of overlap, and the two categories of brain disorders share some underlying causes and contributing factors. My hope is that this book can contribute to the breaking down of silos toward a collaborative rather than competitive approach for all who care about brain health.

Chronic, subclinical neurodegeneration can be healed—and so can Alzheimer's. In this book, I'll show you how I arrived at this con-clusion and all my discoveries along the way. I'm not just asking you to take my word for it. There are too many unsubstantiated claims out there and too many people claiming to know what they are talking about but merely spreading myths and misunderstandings. This book is as much about taking charge of your own health as it is about the brain. *My Brain Matters*, and so does yours.

I don't want to be a guru. I don't want you to give me power over your health and your brain. I want you to recognize the power *you* have over your own health and share this message with the people you love. This book is a call for you to take personal responsibility for caring for your brain. To give you a reason to trust me and take my advice, I'll be sharing with you all the science that shaped my recommendations.

As you go through the book, you'll encounter some parts that contain dense and detailed explorations of scientific research, but I'll always do my best to break it down into terms that are easily grasped by a non-scientist. Besides raising awareness of how we can all improve our brain health, increasing people's scientific literacy and comfort is another goal of this book. I don't expect that you'll necessarily go and read academic journal articles for fun after this, but I do want you to know that those journals aren't as intimidating as they seem. You can learn a lot from reading an abstract (that is, an article summary/overview) and looking up a few key terms that might not be familiar.

From the time scientific research identifies a finding that should be broadly adopted, it takes an average of seventeen years for it to be broadly adopted by the medical community and widely put into practice.[1] Let that sink in—*seventeen years.*

There are a variety of reasons for this. After finishing medical school, physicians may not keep up to date on the latest published results in their field, or they may simply have trouble changing how they operate. (Old habits die hard.) It takes time for health insurance systems to change their payment structures and, thus, what they incentivize.

Regardless of the reasons, you can shrink this time lag by taking matters into your own hands. Just as I'm asking you not to hand your power over to me, I'm asking you not to hand it over entirely to your doctor. Don't rely on their advice during your annual check-up to determine the actions you take to maintain your health and vitality. Your doctor's opinion may be an informed one, but it is not the only one. Learn as much as you can about how to best take care of your own health—because *your brain matters.*

It was once conventional wisdom that type 2 diabetes was not reversible, but in the last decade, researchers have discovered that with certain lifestyle changes, in some cases the condition can indeed be reversed and people can safely come off of their medications.[2] In the same way, the conventional wisdom about Alzheimer's disease is wrong. There is a growing and irrefutable body of evidence that Alzheimer's can be reversed. It is not just about slowing the decline and therefore living a longer life with abysmal quality of life. Many people still assume that once someone is diagnosed with Alzheimer's, their cognitive decline is an inevitable progression—but that's simply not the case. Just like diabetes, we are seeing: Yes, it is reversible.

If you're doubtful about the claim I just made, keep reading. I'll show you all the evidence so you can decide for yourself. Like I said, I don't want to be your guru—instead, I want to be your guide. The power to create lifelong vitality lies within you. The sooner we can each take responsibility for the care and maintenance of our brains, the sooner we can turn around the sickness that is leading to so much suffering and loss. But if you want unconventional results, you might have to follow an unconventional route. The standard American lifestyle (which is increasingly the standard lifestyle everywhere) will not get you there.

This book has three sections. In the first, you'll learn all about the healing power of photobiomodulation, the practice that uses the light device I mentioned above. (Don't worry, I've included plenty of references so you can check out the evidence for yourself.) In the second section, you'll learn about how both acute and chronic trauma impact our brains and how we can create the conditions for healing. The third section focuses on the aging brain and the cognitive decline we have come to accept—and why it doesn't have to be that way.

In each section, the scientific findings are woven into my own story of how I came to ask these questions—or, really, how they appeared in front of me. My life has been one long series of signs guiding me to create this approach and put it into this book so you can read it. Each section also contains a "recipe"—part of the **PRONEURO** approach, broken down into specific practices you can easily implement in your life.

To borrow a metaphor from my colleagues Dale Bredesen and David Perlmutter, who also speak and write about the possibility of reversing cognitive decline, there is no silver bullet—my approach is more similar to silver buckshot. No one behavior solves the problem on its own, but if you combine multiple behaviors that each make a small impact on their own, they add up to a larger collective impact.

Each letter of **PRONEURO** stands for one area:

> **Photobiomodulation**
>
> **Repair/Regrow/Regain**
>
> **Optimize**
>
> **Nourish**
>
> **Exercise**
>
> **Unwind/Unstress**
>
> **Restore**
>
> **Oneness**

If you address all eight of these areas, you will be incredibly well prepared for resiliency from life's stressors and healing from the damage they can do to your brain. But eight distinct lifestyle domains means a lot of habits to change all at once, and that could easily become overwhelming. So, in this book, I also offer my suggestions for how to prioritize—make the highest-impact changes first or go for the "low-hanging fruit" that feels easily achievable—and only make additional changes once your first new habits are solidified.

By the way, it's not all about discipline and leading a monastic lifestyle. Joy, fun, and play are all incredibly beneficial for your health—and we want you to experience more of that, too, by the time you're done reading this book!

When my publisher asked me who this book is for, I couldn't help but say it's for everyone. There's no point in "niching down" with this message because, truly, everyone alive today needs to hear it. This book may be my story, but every one of us will come face to face with the issues I address. Perhaps more specifically, though, this book is for anyone who's ready to take charge of their own brain health or to help a loved one struggling with cognitive decline or the aftermath of a traumatic brain injury. Incidentally, there is a growing body of evidence that the lingering symptoms of COVID-19 infection, known as "long COVID," have a neurological component, so the **PRONEURO** approach will grow even more important as humanity grapples with the aftermath of the pandemic.

So, let's get into it. Let me take you on a journey of how I learned to take better care of my brain and how you can take better care of yours.

SECTION ONE

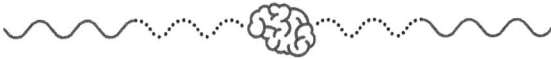

Let There Be Light

CHAPTER ONE

Follow Your Intuition

"When you come to the fork in the road, take it."

—Yogi Berra

I don't have a memory problem anymore. And so I can tell you exactly where we were when a series of conversations happened that would determine my life path.

We were having dinner at a picnic table in a quiet neighborhood in Missoula, Montana. It was August 1982, and my parents had come to retrieve me from college, fearing that my '73 Jeep Commando wouldn't survive the return trip. The prior January, we'd made the cross-country trip together, but the Jeep's breakdown in Erie, Pennsylvania, had cost us one miserably cold night waiting for the repairs. We weren't going to make that mistake again; my parents had driven their brand-new Cadillac as a backup vehicle, and we had some tours in mind as we made the trip back home to upstate New York at a more leisurely pace.

Over that picnic dinner in Missoula, we discussed my plans for my future. I'd arrived at the University of Montana intending to major in chemistry but, after taking a class on the works of local Montana writers, ended up graduating with a double major (chemistry and creative writing). The discussion got heated, exceeding the normal decibel level for polite conversation—even for an Italian-American family—as I tried to explain to my dad why I wanted to be a writer. I've always had an instinct to follow my joy and trust that it will all work out and gel together somehow—but my dad didn't see it that way. A little concerned we'd be reported for violating the local noise ordinance, I suggested we not linger over dinner but instead get started on the long drive we had ahead of us. As we drove off down Chestnut Street, leaving the small house I'd been renting in the rearview mirror, little did I know that this trip would play a pivotal role in determining the course of my life and career.

My first writing class had been an intoxicating experience that left me wanting more. In my prior academic training, I'd learned that compound A plus compound B gives the reaction to form compound C in a sequence that was predictable, straightforward, and always the same. (And if it wasn't, you knew there must be a confounding variable you were missing—but regardless, it could somehow be explained by logic.) In the writing class, on the other hand, as we discussed Camus or Shakespeare, I'd share my opinion of what the author meant—an opinion I held with complete certainty—only to hear in the next moment that my classmates had interpreted the passage entirely differently. Coming from the black-and-white world of science, I felt like I was discovering a world in full color.

My dad wanted the best for me, but in his mind, that meant choosing a career field that would be a reliable source of income and provide me with a comfortable life. That night in Missoula, my pleas to let me follow my passion were getting me nowhere, so I decided to table the topic. Our trip had just begun, and we needed to be able to tolerate being in the same car with each other.

I picked it up again the next day over breakfast, looking out over picturesque bluffs from the Prince of Wales Hotel in Waterton, Alberta. Maybe my dad didn't quite understand the appeal writing held for me, I thought, so I tried to explain it calmly and clearly. Still, he was having none of it. "No" was his response, again. (My father was a man of few words. He believed that his decisions should stand on their own and he shouldn't need to explain himself.) Rather than rattle the chandeliers of this historic lodge with another family "discussion," I put it aside once more. We were headed out for a tour of Glacier National Park, and I wanted us all to have a good time.

Driving across the Badlands of North Dakota a couple days later, as I watched the heat rise in waves off the road, a new idea rose into my consciousness in a similar fashion. It was just Mom and me in the air-conditioned Cadillac—Dad was driving the Jeep up ahead—and even though I should have been comfortable, I was feeling a bit carsick. Mom was trying to fill me in on everything that had happened back in our home-town during my nine months away in Montana, but every time she would start talking, her foot would ease up on the gas. Maybe it was the rhyth-mic motion of acceleration and deceleration like rocking a baby to sleep, maybe it was my strong inner knowing—but suddenly I couldn't keep it to myself. I blurted out: "Mom, I'm going to be a chiropractor."

This was a plan I knew my father would approve of, and it was one that excited me too—almost as much as being a writer. At that moment, I saw two paths diverging. I had arrived at a fork in the road and had cho-sen the path that wasn't what I preferred. Still, this was a close second and an area where I was eager to deepen my education. What I didn't know then was that I would get another chance to be a writer. At that moment, I thought a door was closing—yet, here I am writing this book.

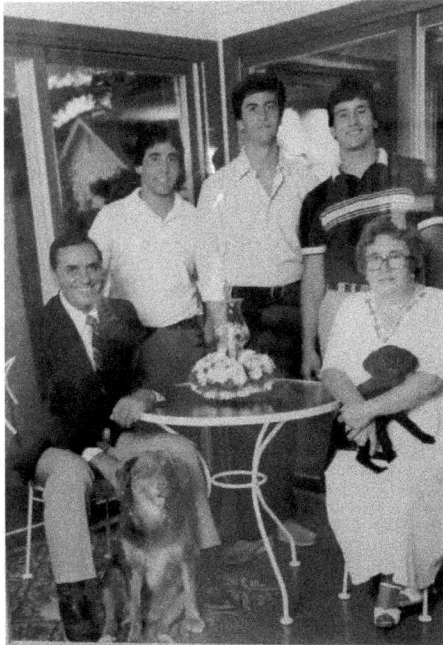

My father, my brother Matthew, my brother John, myself, and my mother on the back porch of my parents' house in Geneva, New York, in the spring of 1979 with two of the family pets. This is the same porch where, forty years later, I began work in earnest on this book.

15

If something in life is meant for us, it will keep coming back around. When we ignore a calling, it only gets louder. This is what I've learned on the meandering path of life. Second chances do exist, and they appear in ways we could never predict. I tell you this to give you a sense of hope and peace about your own fork-in-the-road moments and because I find it profoundly beautiful how choices I made seemingly at random (or so it felt at the time) have combined into a cohesive picture and life story that only I could live and only I can tell.

You might suspect by now that I am not the average Joe—and you would be right. Instead of following a well-worn career path and paying my dues to get to a predetermined destination, I've forged my own path. I've never been afraid to follow where my curiosity leads, even if it might appear eccentric to others.

I have no shortage of degrees—after my bachelor's degree in chemistry and creative writing, I added on advanced degrees in chiropractic neurology and a master's degree in clinical research. But for some people, those aren't the *right* degrees. For whatever reason, many medical doctors don't view chiropractors as "real" medical professionals, and this closed-minded view has stood in the way of my collaborating with certain researchers. But I actually believe my knowledge of several different fields—and my ability to consider problems and solutions from multiple perspectives—makes me stronger as a scientist, researcher, and doctor. If somebody else doesn't see it that way, then I guess they aren't someone I was meant to work with. It took me some time to get over taking it personally when people didn't feel I was qualified to be their healer, enter their university, join their group, or collaborate with them. From where I sit today, I know that my unique blend of knowledge and experience gives me a perspective no one else has.

I'm telling you all this because my winding and meandering life story brought me to the practice I have today, coaching people to increase their brain power and creating devices to help them do so. At each step along the way, it wasn't necessarily clear where the path was leading, but it all makes sense looking back. I hope you'll enjoy learning about the science a little more if you understand what led me to ask these questions and seek these answers. Plus, I know you'll remember what you learn better if it's embedded within stories. That's just how the human mind works.

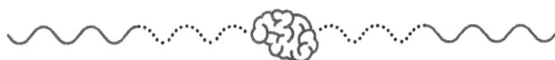

I grew up in the Finger Lakes region of upstate New York—beautiful wine country and the heart of the once-powerful Iroquois Nation (whose descendants in the U.S. and Canada numbered about 125,000 according to a 2010 census). My mother was a teacher and school librarian, and my father was a small business owner who operated a local shoe store. My parents paid for me to go to Hobart College—located in my hometown of Geneva, literally down the street from where I went to high school—so I didn't really question it. Initially I was focused on athletics more than academics—I was excited to play for Hobart's NCAA division–winning lacrosse team—but I enrolled in the hardest courses available. I figured it was an expensive school, and my parents had better get their money's worth.

My drive to succeed in this environment faltered after I saw some of my classmates cheating on a test in our advanced-level chemistry class. These were supposed to be our future doctors and scientists. Patients would place trust in them for the rest of their professional lives, yet they took this responsibility so lightly as to scoff at the concept of integrity? When I reported what I'd seen to the professor, I expected him to be indignant, but he focused more on my reaction than on what I'd seen them doing. This was when I realized that just because someone has a fancy credential or an expensive diploma does not mean they are honest or good at what they do.

My professor's response did not reassure me about the integrity of this particular class of future doctors, but he did tell me one helpful thing during that encounter. He said, "Joe, you've gotta get out of Geneva." He knew there was a much bigger world for me to discover than the one I'd seen so far and that my world would expand once I got away from all of these classmates who were big fish in a small pond.

Adrift in the conversation and feeling disillusioned about the world, I latched on to an idea that would at least bring me pleasure. I loved to hunt, and I'd seen photographs of the biggest whitetail deer on record being shot in Montana. "I was thinking about going to Montana for the summer," I blurted out as the idea jumped into my mind. The words were barely out of my mouth before the professor replied back enthusiastically, practically shouting: "Go to school in Montana!" In that serendipitous moment, it was settled.

I had another meeting just after that with my academic advisor. We were supposed to be discussing the requirements to complete my junior year and move on to become a senior, but I couldn't focus on the topic at hand. "Do you know any places to go to school in Montana?" I blurted out, interrupting him mid-sentence. That professor happened to be a scholar of Native American studies, and he recommended the University of Montana based on its excellent program in that field. This appealed to me too: I had developed an interest verging on obsession after studying the Iroquois people in fourth grade, and I was thirsty to learn more. Great hunting *and* an eminent Native American studies program? I was sold.

Now, picture this: My first day as a Montana Grizzly, the two guys in the room across from me in the dorm, Kenny and Roy, were wise-cracking kids from my home state of New York (Long Island, to be precise). Naturally, we became fast friends.

I enrolled in the advanced chemistry classes that made sense for my intended major, but just for fun (or so I thought at the time) took a class called "Local Montana Writers." And thanks to the tip from my professor back home, I looked up the legendary Joseph Epes Brown and got the chance to study Native American culture with him.

One day, I went with Kenny from Long Island over to his girlfriend's house, and she had a small paperback book out on the coffee table. The cover said "Palmer College of Chiropractic Handbook." I picked it up for a closer look, thinking, *They have schools for this?* Perhaps at that moment, the seed was planted that would lead to my dramatic announcement while speeding (or lurching) across North Dakota in the car with my mother.

The notion of a chiropractic career came up again in an interview I did for one of my writing classes. (See what I mean about patterns and life bringing things back around?) The assignment was to do an interview, so

I called up Gene Wensel, who, along with his twin brother, was one of the greatest whitetail deer hunters in North America at the time. I figured, why not combine two of my interests and use the writing assignment to learn more about one of my idols in the world of hunting? Gene invited me to interview him at his house, and when I got there, he invited me into his trophy room (with dozens of pairs of massive whitetail deer antlers mounted on the wall) for the interview. Natural art, Gene called these wall ornaments. He also told me the antlers were never the same from year to year because he would change them out after each hunting season. Not all the antlers came from animals he had hunted; in fact, most of them were "shed" antlers, discarded at the end of the mating season. These antlers are considered rare and hard to find and can indicate the best hunting locations based on antler size. I was stunned and even more in awe of my interview subject.

He and I got to talking, and as we were flipping through his deer hunting photo album, he was telling me a little bit about the people in the pictures and mentioned that several of them were chiropractors. He shared that he and his brother were also chiropractors, Gene practicing in Hamilton and his brother in Whitefish. This sounded like a life I wanted, and although I didn't make that connection at the time, it was another reference filed away in my brain.

All these signals were percolating in my mind on the drive through North Dakota after my dad had said no to writing as a career possibility. With my parents' blessing, I switched from pre-med to complete my prerequisites for chiropractic college (plus the requirements for a double major in creative writing) and graduated from the State University of New York at Buffalo in 1983. In the fall, I enrolled at Palmer College, the same institution whose catalog I'd seen on the coffee table that day.

Located in Davenport, Iowa, the school is named for its founder, the Canadian magnetic healer Daniel David Palmer. It was the first dedicated school for chiropractors, and in a sense, Palmer himself discovered many of the founding principles of chiropractic healing. Palmer's first chiropractic adjustment, performed in 1896, restored a person's hearing. Even though in today's culture, people are most likely to think of going to the chiropractor as something you do for back pain, from the very beginning, the field had loftier aspirations for the power of what it could do in the human body. That first adjustment had an effect on the nervous system such that interference was removed and function was restored—and clearly that adjustment had an impact on not just the patient's skeleton but also his brain. (Incidentally, my first published research paper was on a similar topic. I attempted to replicate Dr. Palmer's methods and success-fully restored hearing in fifteen consecutive patients.)[3]

By the time I entered chiropractic school, I was already getting some good practice in following the signs life set out for me, having followed my love for hunting and my interest in Native American culture to Montana and then having followed the different mentions of a chiropractic career that came into my awareness. Now, as I settled in for my first semester of the program, here was another one: Among my classmates was Dr. Riccardo Poggetti, a gynecologist from Italy who wanted to add chiro-practic skills and knowledge to his practice.

Just like Kenny and Roy from Long Island, Riccardo (who would become a good friend) seemed familiar right away. His Italian-infused English reminded me of my immigrant grandparents. I had read about the STATIC S.P.A. system of chiropractic clinics that had been set up throughout Italy after World War II and were one of the first institu-tions to produce solid, peer-reviewed research on chiropractic care. I was already interested in traveling to Italy to connect with my heritage and learn about the chiropractic system there. The more time I spent with Riccardo, the stronger that impulse became.

It took some time, but eventually I found a way to follow this sign. By 1994, I'd spent a decade building a thriving chiropractic practice back in Geneva, New York. My uncle and cousin took a trip to Italy, and when they returned, we got together so they could show us a VHS tape of their memories from their trip. I remember so clearly seeing, on that grainy video, a stone building in Civitaluparella (our ancestral village in Abruzzo) with the letters DVRO (a variation on our family name) carved in the keystone block of stone above the doorframe. In that moment, I had a sense of deep knowing, just like on the drive through North Dakota. In this case, the message was: *I will see that for myself.*

Shortly after that, I found myself in the vice-consul's office, applying for an Italian passport and answering questions about my ancestry. My brother was about to graduate from chiropractic college in Marietta, Georgia, and instead of building up his practice from scratch as I had done, he was prepared to step in and take over my practice in Geneva while I moved to Italy. I moved my wife and children there for what was supposed to be a one-year sabbatical, but we ended up staying for ten.

In New York, I'd lain awake at night praying for a chiropractic college to open near us—that's how much I yearned to be part of a research and teaching environment. Now in Italy, I finally had access to an academic community and that sense of being immersed in learning. It was actually illegal for chiropractors to practice in Italy, but practicing under the table on a cash-only basis had its advantages. Maybe I shouldn't admit this, but practicing in an unregulated environment gave us tremendous freedom in our research. We were still guided by ethics and our consciences, but there were far fewer hoops to jump through.

During this time in Italy, I got a sneak peek of what would be the next chapter of my career when I traveled to Amsterdam to see a lecture by Dr. Ted Carrick. I knew Dr. Carrick's name because I'd heard him speak at Palmer College back when I was a student. Whereas chiropractic practice was—and still is, to a large extent—thought to be about the body, he was talking about the brain. This made complete sense to me, and I didn't understand why everyone in my field wasn't framing the problems and solutions in these terms. But Dr. Carrick was ahead of his time. He understood that any problem with the nervous system is a problem with the brain—that there is no distinction.

Dr. Carrick's lecture was about electromyography (EMG), which uses electrodes and needles to assess the health of the muscles and the nerves that control them by measuring electrical signals. Intrigued by this line of research, I got an EMG machine to use with my patients. (Remember when I said chiropractic care was unregulated? As long as I was convinced of this technology's potential to help my patients and that it wouldn't hurt them, there was nobody whose approval I had to get before starting to use it. We had a full neurophysiologic lab in our office; something new, something high-tech, something from America was a great selling point to get people in the door. Socialized medicine was limited in scope, and patients were looking for results. Chiropractic care was thriving in Italy because people would gladly pay cash if you could help them get better.)

Since I essentially had to teach myself how to use the EMG machine, a medical doctor friend of mine connected me with the noted Italian neurologist Dr. Giampetro Zanetti. An expert on amyotrophic lateral sclerosis (ALS, also known as Lou Gehrig's disease), Dr. Zanetti was then at the University of Verona. I spent two years making the hour-long drive back and forth from Vicenza, where I lived and practiced, to Verona. It didn't take me long to learn how to use the machine, but once I made the connection with Dr. Zanetti, I wanted to make the most of the chance to work with this renowned expert. His skill with the EMG machine was nothing short of magical. He pointed out that each muscle fiber had a different sound, and he could play them like a fine violin—that's how sophisticated his technique was.

In observing Dr. Zanetti with his patients, I came to see that his perspective on nervous system diseases and disorders was very different from mine. Patients would come to see him from all over northern Italy. He would cross his arms over his chest and tell them they had six months to live. He rarely hinted at any kind of a solution. Dr. Zanetti was an extremely talented guy—he could tell by the sound the needle made as it passed through the layers of skin, fascia, and muscle precisely which motor neuron disease a patient had. But he and I had completely different perspectives. His patients had many of the same conditions as the people coming to me for chiropractic care. I didn't think in terms of how close my patients were to the end of life. My focus was on improving the life they had left.

Back in my office after learning from Dr. Zanetti how he used the EMG machine, I had a somewhat different idea of how I would use it. I knew I could not stick a needle into a patient like Dr. Zanetti did. It was simply too risky in a country where it was illegal for me even to put my hands on a patient. Instead, I wanted to use the machine to measure outcomes for my patients. Using a measurement known as evoked potential, I could measure how well a patient's nervous system was working. My idea, sparked during Dr. Carrick's lecture, was to develop an exam that could be used in chiropractic care along the lines of the exams neurologists use with their patients. In a neurologic exam, the doctor taps a hammer on the patient's knee and measures the results: Is the knee jerk reflex crisp, sluggish, or absent entirely? Similarly, the EMG machine could be used to deliver a specific square wave pulse of electricity. What if we could use an electrode to deliver a pin prick–like pain sensation on a different part of the body to measure the strength of the nerve signals relayed across a given distance? (Stick with me, and remember that this is all leading up to my current work and the information I'll share with you about how we can make the nervous system—of which the brain is a part—work better.)

A few journal articles had been published using existing EMG machines in this "off-label" way, but my friend Gian Domenico Dalla Bona and I built and patented a device specifically designed to measure nervous system activity—the strength and efficiency of the signals. This machine would enable us to measure the progress our patients were making in terms of their nervous systems working better. (This device later became the subject of my thesis for my master's degree; eventually, even the luminary Dr. Zanetti acknowledged that the equipment and method Gian Domenico and I developed was a valuable innovation that improved on prior research and measurement capabilities of pain evoked potentials.)

In the process of validating that our machine worked, I realized that collecting research data was one thing, but writing it up in a way that it would be accepted by scientific journals was another matter entirely. I wanted to learn how to approach scientific questions with that level of rigor, so I applied to the Ph.D. program in neurology at the University of Padua—which, by the way, is the second-oldest university in Europe (after the University of Bologna) and was where Galileo lectured and taught. Considered the father of observational astronomy, the father of modern physics, and even the father of modern science altogether, Galileo also taught geometry, mechanics, and astronomy at the University of Padua. In those days, you didn't have to pick just one sub-specialty and get pigeonholed to do only that for the rest of your life. He also was a renegade of his time, insisting that the Earth revolved around the sun instead of the other way around. Can you see why I feel some solidarity with the guy? Anyway, I passed the written and oral entrance exams for that Ph.D. program, but once again life had other plans for me.

One day our chiropractic office in Vicenza had a visit from the *carabinieri*. There was no way to hide it—I'd been caught red-handed practicing in an unlicensed profession. I knew what this meant—several of my fellow chiropractors around Italy had been shut down recently—and I was on my cell phone to the Association of Italian Chiropractors, begging them for advice on what to do in between calls pleading with the investigators: *Think of my kids. Think of my wife. Think of my patients! Please don't shut me down.*

In the end, the investigators left without taking action. They had seen all my equipment, including a full rehab gym, a full neuropathology setup, and a medically licensed anesthesiologist conducting acupuncture, and concluded, "With all this stuff, you must be helping somebody." I got more than a few new gray hairs that day.

I was allowed to continue practicing, but I started to fear that Italy was going to be a dead end for my career. In addition to problems with the *carabinieri*, I was also facing the fact that the Ph.D. program didn't want to recognize my chiropractic degree. The prerequisite for the program was either an M.D. or a master's degree in a relevant field, and technically I didn't have either.

I saw the writing on the wall and instead decided to return to the U.S. and pursue a master's degree in clinical research. I knew I needed to strengthen my scientific writing skills and deepen my knowledge of quantitative and statistical methods, so I went back to the Palmer Center for Chiropractic Research. On the twenty-year anniversary of my graduating from chiropractic college, I walked across the same stage to receive my master's degree. My thesis presented the data and methods I had used to demonstrate that my patented device collected nervous system activity measurements that were accurate, reliable, and replicable.

Going into the last year of my master's program in Iowa, I was trying to figure out what exactly I was supposed to do with a master's degree in clinical research without a place to perform research. I saw a potential home for myself in the neurology lab of Dr. William R. Kennedy at the University of Minnesota. He was a bit of a maverick himself, focusing on a very understudied organ in neurology: the skin. In the 1970s, Dr. Kennedy developed a technique for counting the individual nerve fibers, thus demonstrating that neuropathy was an observable physiological condition and not just perception—and that it was a systemic disease that affected the entire legs and arms (as well as the organs), not just the fingers and toes. Once considered a fool by his colleagues, he went on to receive numerous awards, including the Lifetime Achievement Award from the American Association of Electrodiagnostic Medicine and being named a "Giant of Neurology" by the American Academy of Neurology Foundation.

I drove through a winter storm and settled into a hotel room the night before my big meeting at Dr. Kennedy's lab. I awoke the next morning to a crisp, clear blue sky and two feet of fresh snow. To add a bit of pressure to the morning, there was none in my right front tire—but as God would have it, a friendly bystander helped me change it, and I was off to the U of M campus. After parking, I navigated the network of underground tunnels that connected the buildings—a genius addition to a campus that's no stranger to heavy snowfall. Dr. Kennedy waited for me at the end of a long, wide, windowless corridor. As I approached to greet him, I confronted the reality that this dark, dismal environment—infused with the distinct smell of mice—was not something I could see as my professional home for the next decade or more of my life.

For a time, I became an expert in adverse outcomes of chiropractic patients, such as when patients experience a stroke after a chiropractic adjustment. Although quite rare, this potential outcome understandably evokes fear due to its severity, and in my research, I was able to identify risk factors so chiropractors can use extra caution with the patients whose risk is highest. I visited university medical centers all over Europe and discussed stroke risk factors with eminent physicians. What that work revealed—that differences in the vascular system from one person to another can increase the risk of certain adverse health outcomes—would become important to my later work for totally different reasons.

In 2006, I moved to Arizona (where I didn't have to worry about snowstorms and spending the whole winter traveling via underground tunnels) to work with my friend Dr. Chris Colloca, one of the most celebrated chiropractic researchers and device manufacturers of our time. He was my brother's classmate in chiropractic college and a "local dude" (according to me), hailing from upstate New York—Oswego in his case. Before we even met, he stayed at my lake house in Geneva when he sat for the New York State Chiropractic Board Exam. I finally met him in 2001 when we both presented our research at the World Federation of Chiropractic Biennial Congress in Paris (and he and his team received the award for best research paper). Our connection continued when I invited him to Italy to host a training for my colleagues about neuromechanical adjustment and his mechanical adjusting instrument. The year I graduated with my master's degree was the first year in the entire history of the National Institutes of Health that the institution's research funding was cut. This left me high and dry on the research job I had hoped for, and I accepted Dr. C's invitation to work in his office in Phoenix.

There, I began using what was then called low-level light therapy (now called photobiomodulation) to treat neuropathy patients. That's when, at last, all these separate interests of mine began to come together into a cohesive picture, and I realized not a single thing I'd done along the way had gone to waste. It all had a purpose.

My work in New York, my work in Italy, my research training, my work with Dr. C—it all came together into the work I'm doing now and the insights I'm sharing in this book. Thinking back to that lecture in Amsterdam with Dr. Carrick and my light-bulb moment of realizing chiropractors can only do so much with the body and really need to be working on the brain—that moment changed the direction of my career. That lecture brought into my conscious awareness an idea I had grasped intuitively because of my work with neuropathy patients. From my studies of Native American cultures, I had learned about an approach to healing centered on eliminating interference. Modern Western medicine tends to put the power in the hands of the doctor, while chiropractic care places the power to heal where I believe it belongs—with the patient. This ability to heal and the view of healing as the elimination of interference form the cornerstone of my **PRONEURO** approach. Scientific research is illuminating more and more (with new papers published every week, to the point that the references will be out of date by the time you read this) the incredible extent to which the brain his able to heal, repair, and regenerate—especially under the right conditions.

Caring for my mother through the late stages of Alzheimer's disease and seeing the toll it took on her companion and caregiver made it clear to me that this is a crisis—and that we urgently need to get this information into more people's hands. I came to see that everything I'd been working on for my entire professional life had been guiding me toward helping her and informing the work I'm doing today—including writing this book for you. Although the road might have had a lot of twists and turns, and seemingly even some detours, no effort was in vain.

Here's one more piece of advice in addition to all the other recommendations I'll give you in this book: Your intuition is your greatest power. Follow the signs life places before you because you never know where they might lead. Even if it doesn't make sense to you now, eventually it will.

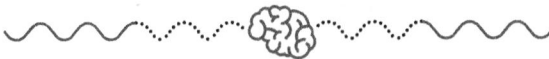

An unorthodox career path can have the downside of branding you as an outsider. Being the point of the spear is not an easy task; like Galileo, those who advocate for new ideas and unconventional viewpoints are often scorned. But throughout my life, I've inhabited the archetype of the outsider, pushing the envelope in various ways. It's required me to have a great deal of faith in myself to keep pushing forward, explaining myself to those with an open mind to listen while knowing not everyone will give me the time of day, and that's okay. The skepticism I've encountered has challenged me to develop and refine my theories further and to test them thoroughly to make sure they're up to snuff.

At this point in my life story, I think you can see why my motto is "Always forward, never straight"—but that's exactly how it was meant to be. If I had taken a well-defined, predictable path in my career (the one that felt so comfortingly certain back when I was a naive chemistry major), I wouldn't be here today, writing a book about recovery from neurodegenerative conditions.

I'm actually glad I didn't pursue my one-time career plan of attending medical school; conventional medicine thinks only about treating the symptoms of disease, not about addressing the root causes. By working outside of the medical establishment, I can integrate multiple perspectives that are relevant and, dare I say, necessary. For example, medical school includes almost zero training in nutrition, despite the crucial role our diet plays in preventing disease and even managing many of the conditions medical doctors are supposed to be treating.

It's unfortunate that conventional medicine too often ignores lifestyle factors that can help people avoid drugs and surgery—or even can help them recover *alongside* drugs and surgery. With a less narrow-minded approach, the medical system could work better for every patient, improving quality of life and saving the time and expense of needing additional care. We would be much better off if holistic, naturopathic, integrative, and functional medicine (and chiropractic care, for that matter) were considered complementary modalities rather than branded as "alternative" medicine—a term that, at best, implies these modalities are "beside the point" and, at worst, discards them as snake oil.

This is where the rigor of my scientific research training gives me an advantage. Generally speaking, the scarcity of scientific evaluation in so-called "alternative medicine" fields doesn't help the situation. People who bring a scientific approach to holistic medicine can help bridge the gap to benefit everyone, and this is exactly the need I hoped to help fill by pursuing my master's degree even while I continued to see patients as a chiropractor. Solid research that substantiates the benefits of nat-ural remedies, in the form of randomized controlled trials published in peer-reviewed journals, will help the ones that are effective gain accep-tance in the medical field. What's more, this type of research also helps to protect people from the charlatans and quack treatments that are out there. When we subject more of these treatments to the scientific method, we discover which ones actually work and which ones don't. We should never shy away from this process. Knowledge is power—in this case, the power to heal ourselves.

Hesitation to apply the scientific method to traditional practices sometimes stems from the fear that those practices won't pass the test. Still, in, many cases, research trials have validated ancient wisdom in fas-cinating ways. Even if we've always known something to be true, there's value in understanding *why* it works. And as we validate the effectiveness of herbal remedies that have been in use for millennia, we can abandon the ones that turned out not to work—or we can come to understand that their value may lie in another factor. (For example, if a massage ther-apist applies herbal ointment to your back for pain relief, does the benefit come from the herbs in the ointment or from the healing power of touch? The scientific method can help differentiate between these two hypothe-ses to discern the healing power's true source. And if the treatment makes you feel better because of the touch and not the herbs, you can still get the treatment!)

Before we close out this chapter and start diving into the science of brain health, one final note on being a maverick: For the record, chiroprac-tors are not just imagining the scorn that's directed at them. In the 1970s, Chester Wilk and several of his fellow chiropractors brought a federal antitrust lawsuit against the American Medical Association (AMA) for labeling chiropractors as "unscientific practitioners" and our work as an "unscientific cult" and forbidding AMA member physicians from asso-ciating with chiropractors. In 1987, after a judge ruled in favor of the plaintiffs based on evidence presented in court showing how chiroprac-tors actually helped people, the AMA was forced to change its principles to state that member physicians "shall be free to choose whom to serve, with whom to associate, and the environment in which to provide medical services."[4] Although some medical doctors still hold the views that got the AMA in legal trouble in the first place, I prefer to call people in rather than call people out and to work with the physicians who are open to taking a broader view that includes other modalities with the potential to help their patients.

Fortunately, it seems that at least in some corners of the medical field, doctors are becoming more open to alternative therapies and taking a broad view of what's best for the patient rather than limiting their scope to drugs and surgery—but there are still plenty of counterexamples where they ignore treatments that could greatly benefit their patients. Overhauling the health care system to focus on wellness and better reflect holistic knowledge about what benefits human health is an enormously complex task. Until that happens (if it ever does), it's in each of our hands to take responsibility for our own health care. We cannot keep handing it over to doctors who are more focused on "sick care." True health care is what happens every day of our lives in between the occasional office visits.

I have a vision that one day we might achieve a truly holistic system in which common practice and incentives line up with what's actually best for human health—rather than being driven by the egos of researchers, the profit motives of companies, the politics of academic institutions, and other factors that serve as barriers between knowing the best course of action and following it. And I'm idealistic enough to hope that this book might play some small part in making that vision a reality.

CHAPTER TWO

Mitochondria: The Power Plant for the Body—and the Brain

"The energy of the mind is the essence of life."

—Aristotle

I f your eyes started to glaze over the moment you saw this chapter title, don't close the book or skip ahead—hear me out. It might be tempting to move straight to the next chapter, where I'll start to share my "recipe" for optimal brain health. But understanding the science is part of taking ownership of your health.

Even though you know a lot about me and my background from Chapter One, I want to encourage you not to just trust me blindly. Instead, I would love it if, in the course of reading this book, you'd become more of a maverick, too. Always ask questions. Don't take anything at face value. Your health is too important for you to hand away your power that way.

So, with this chapter, by outlining the scientific evidence behind my recommendations, I'm telling you why you can trust the **PRONEURO** approach—just like teachers would ask you to "show your work" on a math test to make sure you understood the method and didn't just guess the correct answer. As much as I hope you'll learn about science by reading this book, that's only part of the point. It's not just about the content—it's about the approach.

If you hate taking tests or you didn't do that well in school, biology terms and talking about test taking and story problems might make you break out in a cold sweat. I get it. Many of us have endured traumatic experiences, either in our younger years or more recently, that made us feel stupid and incapable of understanding technical terms or a complicated topic. But this book is as much about rewiring that damaged self-concept and approach to learning as it is about the mitochondria and the nervous system.

You already know that it takes a long time (seventeen years!) for research to find its way into medical practice and that, when it comes to your health, the buck stops with you—not your doctor. So, part of the purpose of this book is to help you feel more comfortable going to the primary source and digging into the science yourself.

In this book, I do my best to explain all the concepts in terms that don't require specialized technical knowledge—and also use analogies to make the concepts easier to understand by relating them to something familiar. But I'm not going to dumb it down or ask you to "just take my word for it." One of my favorite quotes is, "If you kill the dragon, bring back a piece." In other words, always have proof.

Once you're done reading this book, I hope you'll help spread the knowledge within it—and that, when you do, you'll share not just *what* you learned but *why* it's true. My twofold goal is to equip you with knowledge and to embolden you to seek more knowledge on your own. The endnotes at the back of the book are a great place to start. Pick a topic that particularly intrigues you to learn more. When you click through to the reference, there may be some related papers linked from that page. Let yourself go down the "rabbit hole" for a bit and see what you can learn. Science's progress is unceasing, and I guarantee you that as you hold this book in your hands, there are already papers that have come out since its publication that further expand on or qualify the knowledge contained here.

In a world of dueling health claims, people's opinions about the best approach may be tainted by a conflict of interest, selective blindness to conflicting information, or sheer ignorance. Don't just throw up your hands and say you don't know whom to believe. You're smart enough to dig deeper and figure out the truth. In some cases, both sides may be right, and as you learn more, oversimplified claims will give way to a more nuanced understanding—and you're smart enough to figure that out, too.

KEEPING THE LAMPS LIT

Now that we've established why I'm telling you all about the mitochondria, let me connect one more set of dots for you. *Mitochondria are the key to brain health, and there is no physical health separate from brain health.*

As you'll see in the next chapter, the first letter of the **PRONEURO** approach, photobiomodulation, gets its power from the effect it has on the mitochondria—but really, the *entire* **PRONEURO** approach is about the mitochondria. By helping the mitochondria work better, we help the brain work better. All eight steps in the approach are geared toward improving mitochondrial function. Many of them also have other benefits, but the mitochondrial impact is key.

To understand why and how the **PRONEURO** approach works, first, it's important to understand the vital role played in our health and well-being by tiny structures called mitochondria that reside in almost every cell of our bodies.

Mitochondria are the power plants of our cells. There are only a few cell types (red blood cells, for example) that do not have them. Our mitochondria convert energy from food (in the form of glucose, or blood sugar) into a molecule called adenosine triphosphate, or ATP. In short, your mitochondria take the hamburger and French fries you eat for lunch and turn them into hair, skin, and muscle (i.e., bodily tissues)—but also the hormones and neurotransmitters that fuel every bodily process. The food we eat is not usable as energy until our bodies carry out the process of converting energy from food into ATP, and this process takes place in the mitochondria. Without ATP or the mitochondria, we wouldn't have the juice for any bodily process—organ function, muscle movement, brain activity—to work properly.

Let's back up one step. Just what *are* the mitochondria, anyway? They are categorized as subcellular organelles—that is, structures within a cell. There is evidence that mitochondria were once bacteria living on the outside, but about 2.7 billion years ago, they were taken inside the cell and gave the organism a survival advantage—so much of an advantage, in fact, that all animals alive today (and even plants and fungi) have mitochondria. Only single-celled organisms known as prokaryotes (a category that includes bacteria) lack mitochondria. Similar to the way chlorophyll is activated by light so plants can make energy, our mitochondria are photosensitive and can make more energy when light is applied. At that point in the evolutionary timeline, bringing mitochondria inside the body allowed for the evolution of larger and more complex life forms because these tiny subcellular organelles facilitated the production of larger volumes of energy.

Mitochondria have their own DNA, which each of us gets from our mother—so however efficient your mother's body was at making energy, by default, yours will probably be roughly the same. But environmental factors also play a role, and there are things you can do to ramp mitochondrial function up or down. A healthy mitochondrion is shaped like a capsule, with an outer membrane that can be more or less porous depending on the surrounding conditions and an inner membrane containing the mitochondrial DNA and an enzyme called ATP synthase. (When mitochondria become unhealthy, they can resemble doughnuts and can even explode entirely—but more on that later.)

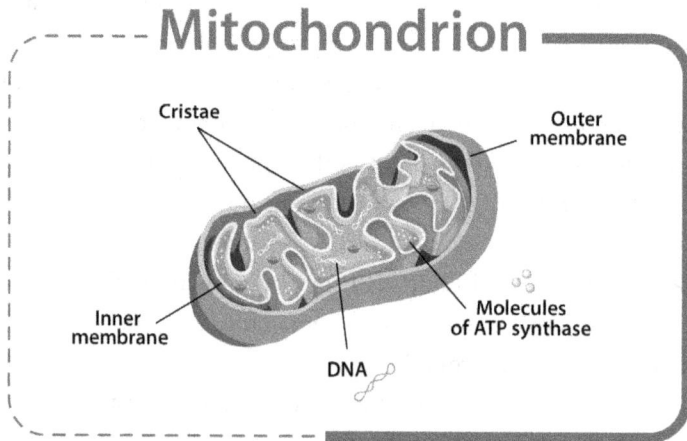

Mitochondrion

Cristae

Outer membrane

Inner membrane

Molecules of ATP synthase

DNA

Within the inner membranes of the mitochondria, adenosine triphosphate, or ATP, is generated when ATP synthase attaches to adenosine diphosphate, or ADP. The folds in the inner membrane, called cristae, increase the membrane's surface area to maximize the number of particles that can be pushed across the membrane to generate energy as a result of the Krebs cycle.

You might have heard about mitochondrial disorders, and I want to note that these are a special case where the statement above about inheriting your overall energy level from your mother doesn't always apply. Mitochondrial disorders can be caused by a variety of factors. One of these is the DNA within cells' nuclei: Mitochondrial disorders can result when someone has two recessive genes for the trait (just like Gregor Mendel's pea plants, which you probably learned about in high school biology). In this case, when one child has a disorder, their siblings have a twenty-five percent chance of also being born with it. On the other hand, if the disorder is caused by mitochondrial DNA, the person's siblings have a *one hundred percent* chance of also being born with it since mitochondrial DNA is passed down from the mother. (In these cases, although both siblings have the disorder, their symptoms can differ in severity due to something called epigenetics, which you'll learn about in the next chapter.) Mitochondrial disorders can also result from replication errors in mitochondrial DNA (in which case siblings would not be affected) and from certain medications and other toxic substances (in which case the cause is not genetic at all, although genetic factors may influence a person's vulnerability or innate protection levels).

From observations of people with mitochondrial disorders, we can see the devastating consequences when the mitochondria are severely impaired. Depending on which types of cells within the body have non-working mitochondria, the complications can be anything from hearing and vision impairments to impaired liver or kidney function, from seizures and strokes to problems with cardiac function. Essentially, whatever organ or system has impaired mitochondria will be held back from functioning properly. But even within what we consider normal mitochondrial function, there is a range. What we consider normal may not be optimal.

The mitochondria are part of an exquisitely interconnected system that, when things are working properly, has ingenious ways of regulating itself. When our cells are not getting the fuel they need, they produce an enzyme called AMP-activated protein kinase, or AMPK. This serves as a signal that the body needs to ramp up energy production, which it does through mitochondrial biogenesis (that is, producing new mitochondria).

In addition to producing energy, the mitochondria take part in a complex signaling process with implications throughout the body. These signals are like the lamplighter of olden days, walking through the streets and lighting the lamps as he goes. If the lamps are lit, we know there is fuel. When the mitochondria are working well and energy is plentiful, the signals tell our bodies it's safe—but if they're not working well and energy is scarce, our bodies will get the signal to shut down non-essential functions. Fertility may take a dive; wounds may take longer to heal. At least in smaller, simpler organisms, research has shown that mitochondrial function can influence longevity not just of the cell but of the entire organism.[5]

There are two ways the body can get more energy, or ATP: (1) increasing mitochondrial density (through mitochondrial biogenesis) and (2) improving the efficiency of the mitochondria you have. Your mitochondria work best when the weak ones are "culled from the herd" through apoptosis, or cell death. It wasn't until relatively recently (the 1990s) that scientists discovered that the mitochondria play a key role in initiating apoptosis throughout the body, releasing proteins that either activate enzymes or neutralize the substances that inhibit enzymes.[6]

It may seem counterintuitive, but in order for our bodies to operate at their best, the process of cell death needs to be working at *its* best. Cell death isn't always a bad thing; in fact, our health depends partly on our bodies' ability to detect cells that aren't working properly and kill them off. This is part of normal, natural cell turnover and regeneration—but it's a process that becomes slower and less efficient with aging. When apoptosis doesn't work as well as it once did, the effects range from slower tissue healing to cancer (in which malignant cells proliferate faster than the body's ability to detect them and root them out). In fact, some types of cancer treatment take advantage of this exact process, inducing mitochondrial apoptosis for the cancerous cells. And apoptosis doesn't work correctly in the body unless the mitochondria are working correctly.[7]

So, the mitochondria play a role in apoptosis for all types of cells— but apoptosis of the mitochondria themselves is also important. Just like the larger organisms they are part of (e.g., humans), mitochondria get a bit tired and worn out as they get older. If you have a bunch of old, poorly functioning mitochondria hanging around, using up the inputs but not creating enough output, you won't be able to generate the energy you need. Better to kill off these "slackers" so the inputs can go to the cells and organelles that will use them more efficiently.

The mitochondria are extraordinarily dynamic, changing shape and changing location easily and frequently. One of the ways this happens is with fusion and fission. Two mitochondria can temporarily fuse together into one organelle to allow for the transfer of genetic material, enzymes, and metabolites. When this process is working well, it helps to counteract the effect of mutations—which occur with mitochondrial DNA just as they do with other DNA and RNA in the body.

Fission, meanwhile, occurs in the usual sense of cell division—one cell (or, in this case, organelle) dividing into two to reproduce. But in a different kind of fission, instead of dividing into two identical organelles, a parent mitochondrion divides into one strong and one weak daughter mitochondrion. The weaker one is then eliminated by the body in a process called *autophagy*—essentially, the consumption of dead cells and organelles to recycle their usable components and remove the rest in a kind of reduce-reuse-recycle process within the body. This type of fission results in a kind of mitochondrial "quality control" so that only the strongest survive.[8]

You might have noticed the word *neurometabolic* in the title of this book and be wondering what I mean by that. Typically when you hear the phrase *metabolic disorders*, it refers to how the body regulates blood sugar levels, produces insulin, and stores fat. I'd like to propose a different definition of metabolic disorders, referring to the level of the cell metabolism—and it all comes back to the mitochondria. When they're not working well, we don't have the energy we need for life. The lamplighter can't light the lamps if there's no fuel. The body has ways of compensating when there is a fuel shortage—for example, eliminating the lamps that aren't working properly through fission and fusion and constructing more lamps through mitochondrial biogenesis. But these

Fission and Fusion Enhance Mitochondrial Function

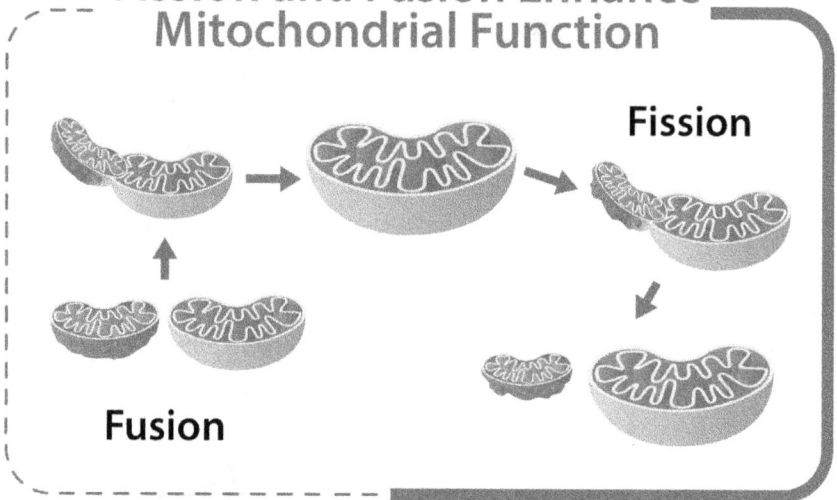

In mitochondrial fusion, two mitochondria temporarily become a single organelle. After fusing together to allow for the transfer of genetic material, enzymes, and metabolites, the "parent" mitochondrion becomes two "daughters" again—but when it splits, it divides into one stronger and one weaker mitochondrion. This results in a kind of mitochondrial "quality control" in which the usable materials are salvaged before weak or damaged mitochondria are marked for targeted destruction.

processes, too, require energy. For many humans, these lamp construction and maintenance systems aren't working well either. When we feel sluggish and our cells don't have the energy they need for life, this is what I consider a metabolic disorder—and when those conditions affect the brain, this is a *neurometabolic* disorder.

There is also evidence that mitochondria play a key role in fertility[9]—a process that requires plenty of energy, if ever there was one. Scientists have observed how mitochondrial function influences the processes of egg maturation, fertilization, and early development of the embryo.[10] Current research is investigating whether the ability of the mitochondria to generate energy is part of what determines whether an embryo is viable. In addition, researchers are testing experimental therapies for infertility that involve improving mitochondrial function or combining one woman's genetic material with a donor egg from a woman with stronger mitochondrial function. Mitochondrial function also influences fertility levels in men: It affects sperm motility and how sperm interact with an egg, among other factors.[11]

Fortunately, there are steps we can take to help the mitochondria work better. One of those steps is photobiomodulation. In the next chapter, I'm going to walk you through the evidence for why and how it works. But before we get there, let me tell you the story of how two of my paths of inquiry—neuropathy and light therapy—converged to lead me to working with the mitochondria. Seemingly random or unrelated interests were leading me, in ways I never could have predicted, to be right here sharing this information with you.

RUNNING A SPRINT BUT GETTING NOWHERE

In my time as a practicing chiropractor, I came to realize that neuropathy was an underlying issue for the reasons many of my patients came to me—and this was one of the reasons I became fascinated with the brain. When people develop nerve damage (usually in their feet) from diabetes, the use of statins, or chemotherapy, it means the brain isn't getting the feedback it needs—and this leads to problems with balance. The way the medical field studies these topics tends to create artificial divisions—a problem with the brain or a problem with the peripheral nerves—but viewing it this way loses sight of important connections. Simply put, *there is only one nervous system*. A problem with the nerves in the feet *is* a problem with the brain.

You'll never find neuropathy on a death certificate, but falls are one of the most common causes of death for senior citizens. By causing people to lose sensation in the feet, toes, and legs, neuropathy causes falls. The brain doesn't receive feedback from the feet, and people literally can't feel the ground they are walking on. What's more, even when people don't die from the fall itself, many go on to die from pneumonia in the hospital or other complications that never would have happened had they not fallen and become unable to walk on their own. Because neuropathy is a consequence of both chemotherapy and type 2 diabetes, it's a condition that affects large numbers of people (more than twenty million in the U.S. alone, according to the National Institutes of Health).

My desire to help patients with neuropathy led me to learn more about the healing power of light. Around the same time I moved to Arizona, a scientist named Gary Bennett from McGill University in Canada was investigating the relationship between mitochondria and neuropathy. In 2005, as a Pain Research Forum article recounts,[12] Bennett's research group was studying rats, looking to learn more about how chemotherapy causes neuropathy. They expected to find lesions on the affected nerves, and when there were no lesions to be seen, they decided to use quantitative electron microscopy, a technique that would allow them to count all the individual nerve fibers.

During the process of counting the fibers, one of the researchers noticed something was wrong with the mitochondria in the affected nerves. "Some were swollen, some had vacuoles, and some had a disrupted membrane and looked like they'd blown up," Bennett later explained. When the rats were left to recover and their pain disappeared, so did the abnormal-looking mitochondria.

Once his team had identified a potential issue with the mitochondria, they designed another experiment with rats to test the suspected link between energy production (i.e., the essential function of mitochondria) and neuropathy. The results confirmed their theory: Exposure to chemotherapy drugs (specifically, paclitaxel and oxaliplatin) led to a steep decline in energy production within the neurons. In other words, the mitochondria weren't working, and *this* was what was causing the neuropathy. This experiment confirmed that it was not just a structural issue (which they'd seen in their earlier experiment with the swollen mitochondria riddled with holes) but also a metabolic issue. Without sufficient ATP to power the sodium/potassium pump in each neuron, the nerve fiber's axons would depolarize, leading to spontaneous discharge. The nerve was failing at its usual touch/pain signaling function and was instead producing sensory input (nerve pain) independent of any stimulus.

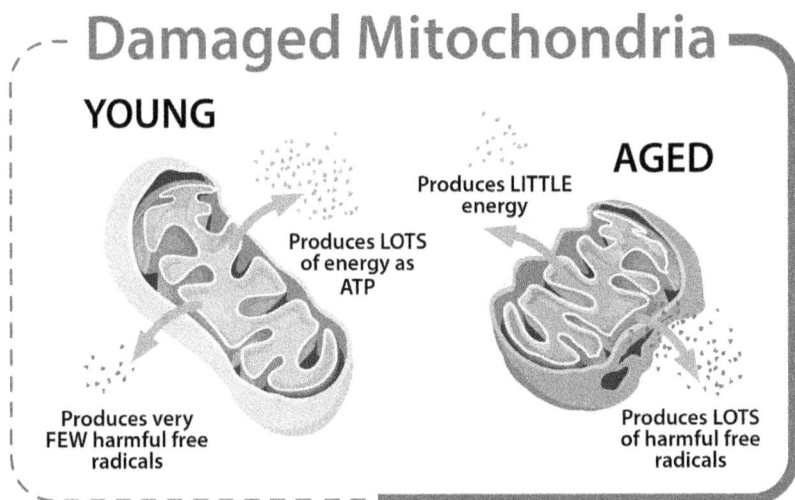

Damaged Mitochondria

YOUNG

AGED

Produces LITTLE
energy

Produces LOTS
of energy as
ATP

Produces very
FEW harmful free
radicals

Produces LOTS
of harmful free
radicals

Aged mitochondria produce less ATP and emit inflammation-promoting free radicals. Thus, it is important that the body is able to either repair damaged mitochondria or target them for destruction via mitophagy; an overload of sluggish, damaged mitochondria leads to a state of chronic inflammation.

The same research team found that administering known mitochondrial poisons worsened nerve pain and spontaneous nerve discharge in rats that had received the chemotherapy drugs, further confirming the role mitochondria play in neuropathy. Along the same lines, they showed that two drugs with known protective effects for mitochondria worked to prevent or reverse neuropathy in the rats that had received the chemotherapy drugs. In other words, the drugs that we know help mitochondria also proved to help neuropathy, lending even more credence to the chain of evidence linking neuropathy, nerve damage, and mitochondrial function. Essentially, they tested their findings in multiple ways to confirm the link. I won't go into as much detail about the research process for most of the findings I cite in this book. However, I think this story sheds light on just how thoroughly scientists test their hypotheses to rule out possible alternative explanations. The timeline for updating our collective understanding of a given problem through the peer-reviewed research process can feel painfully slow, but when it works the way it's supposed to, the results are solid, clear, and reliable—at least until new advancements in knowledge call for another revision of the conventional wisdom.

I met Dr. Bennett in person in 2010 at a neuropathy summit for physicians held at the Hilton in Washington, D.C., where I was the only chiropractor in attendance (an outsider as usual). I heard Dr. Bennett's presentation and was fascinated that he had developed a method of measuring mitochondrial function as it relates to neuropathy. After his talk, I followed him outside, and as we discussed his research, I remember him lighting a cigarette, then taking a puff and pointing to a spot a few feet from where we were standing. "There's the spot where President Reagan was shot" in the 1981 assassination attempt, he informed me. (Since Reagan was the most famous president diagnosed with dementia, I consider that fact relevant to this book. In fact, as the influential Alzheimer's researcher Jack de la Torre speculates in his book *Alzheimer's Turning Point*, brain injury resulting from blood loss after the shooting may have contributed to Reagan's cognitive decline, making an impact that unfolded over the following decades through the mechanisms outlined in Sections Two and Three of this book.)

Thanks to Dr. Bennett's research, we know that the mitochondria play a crucial role in nerve damage and nerve regeneration. It follows that when we help the mitochondria work better, we can reverse neuropathy, prevent falls, and ultimately save lives. As solid as these research findings are, why haven't they been widely adopted? As you'll see in the next chapter, photobiomodulation is an extremely effective method of helping the mitochondria work better. Moreover, it is safe, non-invasive, and inexpensive—so why would it not be used preventively with cancer patients who are undergoing chemotherapy and therefore at risk for neuropathy? I don't really know the answer, other than to say oncologists focus on helping their patients survive, and they don't always give as much thought as they could to the patient's quality of life after finishing treatment. Neuropathy "treatment" too often focuses on medicating away the pain when we could instead be regenerating the nerve fibers.[13] Until we can count on physicians to reliably add this to treatment plans, it's up to each of us to share it with people we love.

In case you're wondering what such a lengthy discussion of neuropathy is doing in a book about the brain, remember that it's all one nervous system. When you amputate someone's finger, the parts of the brain that were connected to that finger start to deteriorate. Skin biopsies taken from neuropathy patients show reduced intraepidermal nerve fiber density—meaning the nerves on the surface of the skin have died and retracted. Neuropathy and cognitive decline are both neurodegenerative issues. The symptoms are different, but they are both problems with the nervous system.

It's all one nervous system—but the distinction between central and peripheral, which we all learned in high-school biology, comes from a time before scientists really understood this and persists today. A loss of feeling in the foot begins in the brain; when it comes to the nervous system, it makes no sense to consider these two parts of the body as separate. When a finger or a limb is amputated, you can observe physical changes in the parts of the brain that process movement and sensation for the missing body part. Conversely, in neuropathy patients, we've seen from biopsies that the nerve fibers are less dense in the affected area. In one case, a loss of a body part leads to changes in the nervous system; in the other, changes in the nervous system lead to a loss of sensation. People might think about the nervous system as something amorphous and undefinable (although, given my experience as a chiropractor, I've never felt that way)—but it's very clearly and concretely observable. If you feel pain in your left foot, you aren't actually feeling it in your foot. You're feeling it in the part of the brain that relates to your left foot.

INFLAMMATION SOUNDS THE ALARM

When the mitochondria are damaged, it can set in motion a vicious cycle, like having broken lamps all over town and insufficient staff to remove or repair them. This is partly why it's so important to interrupt that vicious cycle and convert it into a virtuous cycle by helping the mitochondria work better.

As Gary Bennett's team saw in their rats with neuropathy, the initial damage to the mitochondria not only impaired their ability to produce ATP; it also led to the formation and discharge of molecules known as *reactive oxygen species*, which can further impair mitochondria and attack other parts of the cell.

In order to understand the importance of these reactive oxygen species, we first need to talk about inflammation. Just like apoptosis, inflammation in the body is not inherently good or bad; rather, it needs to be properly calibrated to happen under the right conditions.

You may be familiar with the health claims on food and supplement labels declaring that they reduce inflammation. That's because most of us generally have *too much* inflammation in our bodies. It's not that we want to get the level down to zero, though. That would indicate that our immune systems don't work at all! Rather, what we are aiming to achieve is a healthy balance: an inflammatory response that is triggered in the right volume at the right time and then quiets down once it's done its job.

Acute inflammation is the positive (right on time, right on target) kind of inflammation. The body's response to a minor cut is a clear and simple example of this. When the skin's protective barrier is breached and the tissue is damaged, your body mounts a response—including increased blood flow and directing white blood cells to the area—to repair the tissue and prevent infection. The response is strongest right away; as the cut heals, the swelling and redness fade and your skin returns to normal—a wonderful example of the body's innate healing power. Acute inflammation is a healthy response that serves a valuable purpose. Without it, the cut would heal more slowly, and you might get an infection that spreads throughout your body.

Chronic inflammation, on the other hand, is inflammation run amok. It can come on in a variety of different ways, and it can manifest in a variety of different ways. For example, chronic inflammation can result from acute inflammation that doesn't fade as it should once the threat of infection and the need for repair have passed. But chronic inflammation can also come on without a known case of acute inflammation—for example, as a result of diet and lifestyle factors that promote inflammation. In some cases, chronic inflammation shows up as a diagnosable autoimmune condition, such as Hashimoto's disease or multiple sclerosis. But even without such a diagnosis, chronic inflammation can linger for long periods—even a lifetime—and set the stage for disease. For example, chronic inflammation is considered a risk factor for cancer; something about the condition makes it a friendlier state for the growth of tumor cells. And there is mounting evidence that depression—once thought to be "all in your head" and not to have a physiological cause—actually results from chronic inflammation[14] or that inflammation is at least a strong contributing factor.[15] In people with depression, higher levels of certain inflammatory cytokines correlate with a higher likelihood of attempting suicide—indicating inflammation may not only drive mood but behavior as well.[16]

So, in the case of the rats' damaged nerves in Dr. Bennett's research lab, the reactive oxygen species acted like a fire alarm, letting the animals' bodies know that damage was occurring so they could initiate processes to clean out the damaged cells and promote healing. But too much inflammation sets off a vicious cycle; unable to heal fast enough to get ahead of the damage that's occurring, the nerves stop working—which is neuropathy.

When a serious event such as a heart attack or significant bodily injury occurs, mitochondrial DNA is also released into the bloodstream—and this, in and of itself, is a powerful promoter of inflammation. This signaling function is known as the *mitokine response*, and it plays an important role, triggering a type of white blood cells called neutrophils to attach to the blood vessel walls—a crucial step in the healing process but not something we want to become a permanent state of affairs.[17]

When the human body is in balance, it's a grand symphony with many different parts playing in intricate harmony—and when the balance is disturbed, one subtle change can have wide-ranging effects. Our bodies have processes for restoring balance until the stress becomes too great and the balance tips toward disease. To stick with the orchestra analogy, this might be when the musicians around you are playing so badly out of time with one another that you can't find the beat at all anymore.

Remember that all-important process of apoptosis and the role mito-chondria play in triggering it? It turns out that this process also influences systemic inflammation levels. When a cell dies, it is ingested by neighboring cells and phagocytes—that is, cells with the specific function of ingesting foreign particles, bacteria, and dead or dying cells. (This is the process of autophagy I mentioned above.) Phagocytes clean up these "troublemakers" before they can contribute to inflammation or infection—but if the mito-chondria aren't signaling properly, the body can't identify and destroy these troublemakers efficiently enough to prevent the inflammation they create. Think of it like a ticketing system that alerts the lamplighters they need to remove and replace the broken lamps. When the system goes down, the repair work won't occur because the notification never arrives.

In the first step of the signaling process that leads to apoptosis, the mitochondrial outer membrane becomes permeable. This triggers the dissipation of the proton gradient created by electron transport, caus-ing the uncoupling of oxidative phosphorylation. When the membrane becomes porous, water travels through, causing the membrane to swell and rupture, resulting in the release of proteins such as cytochrome C, endonuclease G, and apoptosis-inducing factor, triggering a chain reac-tion that leads to cell death.

This grand symphony seems to have the fingerprints of a divine design, and it's a process that's essential for a healthy body. But in some neurodegenerative conditions, such as Alzheimer's and Parkinson's, cell death becomes more rapid and plentiful than the creation of new, healthy cells, ultimately affecting the brain's structure and function.

Taking into account the mitokine response, we can say that mito-chondria not only serve as power plants but also as traffic signals, indi-cating the health status of cells and triggering other processes such as apoptosis. Reactive oxygen species are one of the main ways this signal-ing system works—and if that system isn't properly calibrated, things can quickly go haywire. We want the signaling system inside our bodies to work like a well-marked intersection with traffic lights that are easily

Life Cycle of Mitochondria

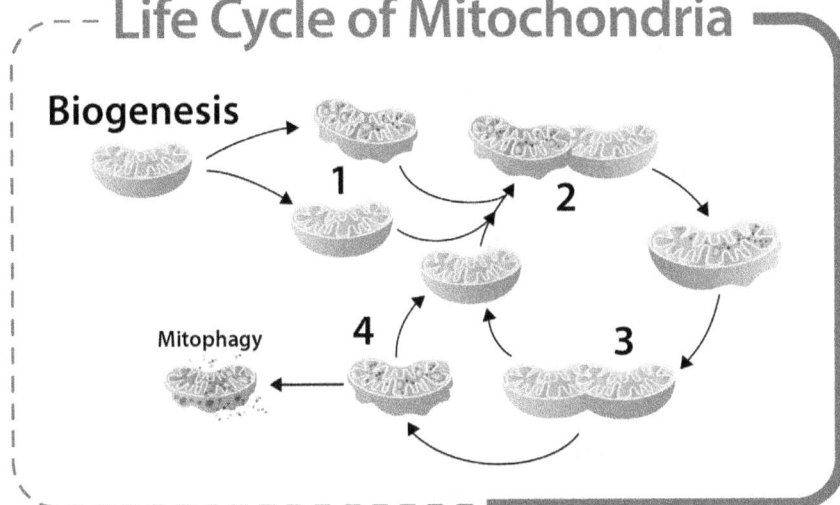

Biogenesis

1

2

Mitophagy 4

3

Mitochondrial biogenesis occurs when new mitochondria are formed; this can happen in response to stress, as the cells respond to energy demand by increasing the number of mitochondria—and, as noted in this book, photo-biomodulation promotes mitochondrial biogenesis. Mitochondria accumulate damage over the course of their lifespan (1); when this happens, a damaged mitochondrion can fuse with a healthier mitochondrion (2). After fusion occurs, usable materials are transferred into the healthier mitochondrion; fission then takes place (3). With the healthier mitochondrion made even more robust, the less healthy one either recovers (4) or is marked for death via mitophagy, the body's reduce-reuse-recycle process for mitochondria.

visible—not like an intersection where the power has been cut, with several vehicles approaching and none of the drivers knowing who has the right of way.

Keeping the mitochondria working well and keeping the body out of chronic inflammation are both keys to vitality and avoiding disease—and the "recipe" in this book, which I'll start to introduce in the next chapter, is designed to help with both.

TOO MUCH OF A GOOD THING

The mitokine (signaling) function of mitochondria might have reminded you of a different word: *cytokine*, which is a kind of protein that engages in cell signaling to modulate the immune response. Cytokines have gotten a lot of press in the context of the *cytokine storm*, which is an outsized immune response in which the body begins to attack its own tissues. This response was common among COVID-19 patients sick enough to require hospitalization. Once it's triggered, the cytokine storm is very difficult to reverse. It's like a fire raging out of control beyond all possibility of containment.

Whether cytokines or mitokines are the messengers in question, a little inflammation helps us, but too much can be harmful and even fatal—a concept known as dose-dependent response. This concept has its origins in the field of toxicology, and that context provides clear examples of its meaning. The question of whether a given substance is poisonous often does not have a simple yes/no answer; rather, the answer depends on the dose. Drink a single beer and your body will be able to metabolize it easily; chug a fifth of vodka and you just might end up in the hospital with alcohol poisoning. With a sufficient dose, even water can be poisonous: Drinking too much water in too short of a time can actually upset the body's electrolyte balance severely enough to result in death.

As with alcohol and water, the concept of a dose-dependent response also applies to exercise. Although we know that exercise, in general, is very good for our health, in excessive amounts, it can actually be deadly. It is possible to push so hard during exercise that muscle fibers rupture, triggering a condition called rhabdomyolysis, which causes damage to the kidneys and also stresses the heart and the liver. The condition can have long-term consequences, such as requiring kidney dialysis, and can even result in death if not treated promptly. Although it can occur in elite athletes or even from manual labor, its incidence has been increasing in recent years, largely due to the trend of "extreme" fitness that urges people to push past their limits rather than listen and rest when their bodies show signs of overexertion.[18] Of course, we shouldn't let the possibility of

Biphasic Curve of Dose-Dependent Response

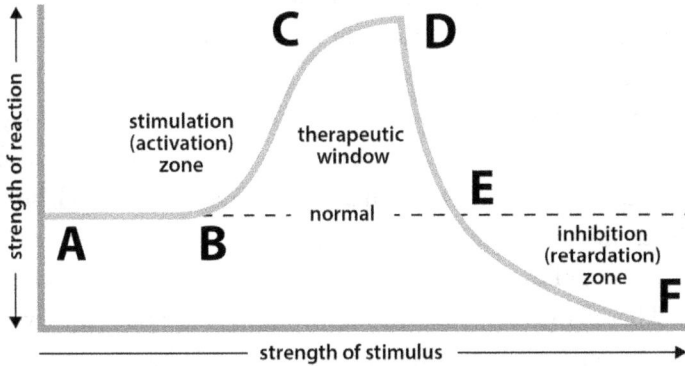

In a dose-dependent response, a therapeutic substance or practice begins to have an effect at point B, raising the desired output from baseline (A) to a more beneficial level (C). Beyond that point, increasing the dose of the substance or practice has no additional beneficial effect, and at a certain point (D) becomes detrimental rather than beneficial, causing the level of the desired output to fall. If the therapy's strength or dose continues to increase beyond that point, the level of the desired output falls back to the original baseline (E) or even below it (F).

rhabdomyolysis scare us out of exercising at all. We just have to be smart about it. Exercise is good, but exercise in excessive amounts or at excessive intensity levels is not.

Now let's add one more wrinkle to this discussion that will help illustrate an important modifying factor for dose-dependent response. Exercise-induced rhabdomyolysis occurs most often in sedentary or lightly active people who overdo it, taking on a particularly long or intense workout. Whether it's in response to peer pressure, the desire to finish a race, or just bad luck and poor judgment, they push past their bodies' limits and suffer a consequence that's less likely for athletes whose bodies are already conditioned to long, intense workouts.

The rhabdomyolysis example illustrates one of the key concepts in this book: *hormesis*. This term, too, has its roots in toxicology and was first used to describe the way substance abusers require an ever larger dose to get the same high. An alcoholic in the throes of addiction is able to consume amounts of alcohol that would seem unbelievable to most of us and certainly would be poisonous for someone whose body has not adapted to copious alcohol consumption.[19]

In this context, hormesis does not sound like a positive thing, but keep in mind that—setting aside the relationship, health, and life difficulties that accompany addiction—on a purely physiological level, hormesis is an illustration of the human body's extraordinary ability to adapt and survive. This applies to stress just as it does to alcohol and other substances. There is no such thing as a life without stress—and even if it did exist, I would argue that it's not even desirable because it means we are not taking risks or challenging ourselves to grow. A healthy life isn't one in which we avoid stress—it's one in which we practice our ability to adapt to stress and come out stronger for it. I'm not recommending that anybody pursue alcohol dependence, but the concept of hormesis is informative. We hear over and over how detrimental stress is, but what if instead we could accept stress as a fact of life and shift our focus from avoiding stress to optimizing our bodies' ability to *recover* from stress and adapt to it?

Incidentally, reactive oxygen species play a role in how this comes about in the body. For example, hypoxic conditions (when oxygen is low) prompt the mitochondria to release reactive oxygen species, which "turns on" the genes responsible for metabolic adaptation to low oxygen.[20] Extreme stress—such as the amount of available oxygen dropping rapidly when an airplane cabin depressurizes—is too much of a shock to the system, and the body can't adjust fast enough. But under a manageable amount of stress—such as spending a few days at base camp to give your body time to adjust to a higher altitude and less oxygenated air—the body adapts. In an analogy that is also another example of this process, over time, the garden hoe handle becomes smooth and the farmer's hand becomes calloused.

Scientists once thought that reactive oxygen species were responsible for aging through the damage they caused in the body, and therefore the goal would be to either limit the amount of reactive oxygen species produced or to balance them with antioxidants—but a more nuanced understanding has developed as recent findings have complicated the picture.[21] Too much stress overwhelms us, but a little stress is good for us, providing a level of challenge we can rise to. To understand how this plays out in the body, it's useful to know about a concept called *allostatic load*, which refers to the burden of stress and specifically the degree to which that burden challenges or exceeds the body's ability to cope.

It's a concept we all know intuitively through direct experience. For example, when you get less sleep than you need for one night, you feel a little tired, but your body adapts to the situation—but if you get very little sleep for several nights in a row, the exhaustion becomes nearly unbearable. What you are feeling is the allostatic load building up as your body does its best to maintain all the necessary functions under the stressful condition of operating without the rest it needs.

Scientific researchers have successfully isolated biomarkers associated with allostatic load—that is, indicators of exactly how much stress someone's body is under. Among these indicators are the hormones cortisol, adrenaline, norepinephrine, and DHEA; measures of systolic and diastolic blood pressure; and levels of cholesterol and hemoglobin A1c (an indirect indicator, or proxy, for higher-than-normal blood sugar levels).

In short, many of the factors we know jeopardize our long-term health can be summed up with the concept of allostatic load—and if we can reduce our allostatic load, these indicators of poor health will improve. Allostatic load affects everything in the body—from cognitive function to mood, from immune function to digestive function, from heart health to metabolism. Think about it like a computer with too many programs running; there's no bandwidth left for the next program you open. But again, it's not *just* about reducing your allostatic load (although at times, resting and recovering after periods of extreme stress may be necessary); it's also about increasing your capacity. You cannot create more brain power without increasing your bioenergetic capacity, and this means appropriately stressing your system. The goal is not to remove stress altogether but rather to train your body and brain to handle it better.

Allostatic load is a complex measurement resulting from a combination of factors both within and outside our control. These include genetics and the environment in which we grew up but also our own diet and lifestyle habits. Poverty and having experienced discrimination based on race, gender, or sexual orientation stack our deck with a higher allostatic load. So do career-related burnout or work stress, adverse childhood experiences, and recent traumatic life events such as a death in the family. On the other hand, social support and strong family support act as protective factors, as does having a sense of purpose in life. People who exercise regularly have a lower allostatic load, on average; meanwhile, people who report sleeping poorly, drinking alcohol, smoking cigarettes, and eating an unhealthy diet have a higher allostatic load, on average. So, if you focus on intentionally increasing protective factors in your life (which, by the way, describes much of the **PRONEURO** approach), even a high dose of stress is more likely to be tolerable instead of sending you into the dose-dependent response danger zone where too much stress becomes toxic.

At this point, you might have some questions about cause and effect. Are people who are under a lot of stress (and thus have high allostatic load due to external circumstances) more likely to sleep poorly, smoke cigarettes, drink alcohol, and eat junk food? Almost certainly, yes. When a butterfly flaps its wings, this tiny action can set off a chain reaction that grows and spreads—but we also have the power to shut that chain reaction down. We have to take the first step of choosing to change. Then, as we learn how to destress, rest, and create the conditions for our bodies to heal, we can become masters at dealing with stress.

People with higher allostatic load have a higher risk of death, disability, chronic illnesses, psychiatric illnesses, and chronic pain—and, remarkably, this burden of stress and trauma has a physiological signature. People with higher allostatic load have shorter telomeres (a part of our chromosome that gets shorter as we get older—stay tuned for more on that), meaning we can observe, by measuring telomere length, how stress makes us biologically older. One pair of researchers even postulated that the mitochondria have their own allostatic load through which chronic and acute stress can alter mitochondrial function and structure.[22] But don't despair—stress is not a death sentence. We have the power to reduce stress and to heal. Although we can't change the hand of cards we were dealt, the good news is we have a lot of control over how we play that hand—enough to change the outcome of the game.

So, let's talk about the kind of hormesis we want to pursue. A more desirable analogy than that of an alcoholic adapting to their addiction might be that of a sedentary person who embarks on a "Couch to 5K" running program. There's a reason these programs add distance gradually over time. Can you imagine if someone who's used to being completely inactive went out the door on day one of the program and tried to run a 5K? It would be just about impossible, and they might get seriously injured. But over the course of a nine-week training program, it's possible—and not even that difficult.

If you're completely sedentary or have been bed-bound due to illness, going for a slow walk around the block may be more than your body can handle. You'll be out of breath, and your calves will be sore the next day. But the same walk around the block is nothing to an ultra-marathoner. It's hormesis that explains why you can walk a little farther and feel a little less exertion the next day, after your body has had a chance to rest and repair. And it's hormesis that explains how the ultra-marathoner became able to run exceedingly long distances as a result of building up distance gradually through training.

When it comes to exercise, hormesis involves a variety of processes that increase the body's strength and endurance. As the body's limits are tested, it builds back stronger. The heart muscle becomes stronger, and the body gets more efficient at delivering oxygenated blood to the muscles.[23] The efficiency of the recovery process itself also increases as your body learns with experience. Someone who lost muscle mass due to becoming inactive after an injury will have an easier time building back that muscle than someone who is building that same amount of muscle for the first time.

Like alcohol, water, and exercise, stress is a dose-dependent substance. At too high of a level, it can even be fatal. But a little stress makes us stronger. What I'm trying to get you to see is that stress is not inherently a bad thing, and having stress in your life doesn't mean you are doomed to ill health. Our bodies adapt to stress in the same way they adapt to exercise—by becoming more efficient at the processes that restore balance. Part of the reason childhood stress is more likely to have long-term health effects than stress you undergo as an adult is that children have less control over their environment and have not yet developed the emotional skills and behaviors some adults possess to help their bodies adapt to stress and increase their capacity.

Adaptation to stress takes place on the level of the whole organism, and we can also observe it taking place at the cellular level, where our old friends, the mitochondria, play a key role. When our cells are under stress (such as an injury that challenges tissue to heal or exercise that challenges our muscles to work harder), a process is activated involving reactive oxygen species and other mitokines (i.e., signaling molecules). In response, cells increase their production of protective and restorative proteins, including growth factors and antioxidants.[24]

Side note about antioxidants: This is another case where the outcome is dose-dependent. You've probably seen nutrition labels proudly proclaiming that foods are "rich in antioxidants!"—but did you know that most studies of the effects of antioxidants in humans have not shown any beneficial effects on age-related diseases?[25] As it turns out, reactive oxygen species trigger cell death at high levels, but at lower levels, they actually act to promote healthy aging and increase lifespan through adaptation to stress—and antioxidants only interfere with this process.[26]

Our goal, then, should not be to avoid all stress—but rather, to expose ourselves to just the right amount of stress, matching up to our body's ability to handle it and come out stronger—and as we further develop that ability, we increase our capacity to handle stress. In the next chapter, we'll take a look at how that happens.

CHAPTER THREE

The Recipe: Photobiomodulation

"Health is more than the absence of disease."

—Former U.S. Surgeon General
Joycelyn Elders

My initial interest in mitochondria stemmed from a desire to make a difference in the lives of the huge numbers of people living with neuropathy. It just so happens that neurons have triple or quadruple the number of mitochondria found in other types of cells in the body. If mitochondrial function is important to every task our bodies carry out, it's especially important to the operation of the nervous system. However, I soon discovered that improving mitochondrial function had the potential to make an even broader impact on human health.

As you learned in the previous chapter, our mitochondria generate the energy we need for life. They produce signals that let the body know to kill off injured or sluggish cells so there will be more energy left for healthy cells. They play a key role in nerve signaling, such that when they're not working, neuropathy results. In addition, there is evidence that they play a key role in brain function and cognition—a topic we'll explore in greater depth in the second and third sections of this book.

Given all this, you want your mitochondria to be working as well as possible. Throughout this book, I'm introducing you piece by piece to the ingredients in a "recipe" for creating optimal brain health. The foundation for this is getting your mitochondria working better—and for this, the simplest and most powerful step you can take is to incorporate photobiomodulation into your routine.

I made Photobiomodulation the first step in my **PRONEURO** approach because of how easy it is. It's convenient and it doesn't require any major habit change. All you have to do is stick a red and near-infrared light pad on your body while resting or going about your daily activities. The body pad looks like a heating pad with little light-emitting diode (LED) light bulbs on it. There are also intranasal devices whose light probes go up your nose, but a body pad might be a more comfortable place to start if you're new to photobiomodulation. Aside from being safe and effective, this practice is nearly foolproof. Unlike some other health behaviors you might consider adding into your routine, there's pretty much no way you can do this wrong or mess it up.

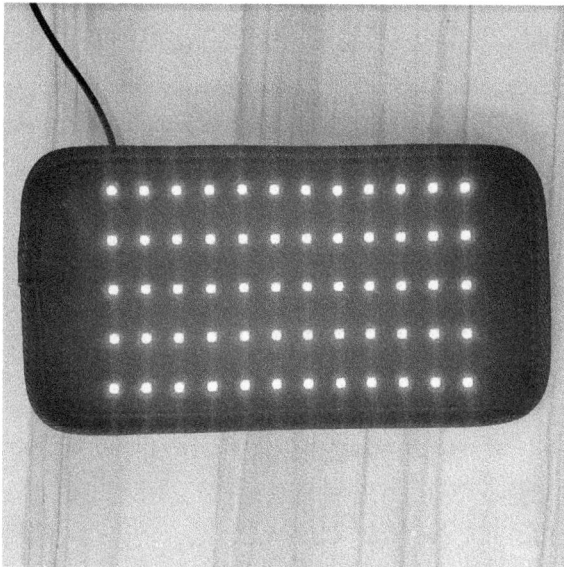

A ProNeuroLight body pad photobiomodulation device

Think of our recipe for brain health like an ice cream sundae. You can't have a sundae without ice cream—and photobiomodulation is our ice cream, the essential bottom layer. The ice cream by itself is pretty great, but when you build on this foundation by adding your favorite toppings, the result is even better. But there's no point in adding the toppings unless you have the ice cream first. Start with photobiomodulation and add on other brain health habits (as outlined later in this book) once you've established your foundation.

ADD LIGHT FOR MORE BRAIN POWER

In 1893, Niels Finsen, a physician from the Faroe Islands, developed a monochromatic red-filtered sunlight irradiation technique that effectively treated skin lesions from smallpox and tuberculosis. This seems to have been the first application of monochromatic photobiomodulation in modern medicine, and Finsen received the Nobel Prize in Physiology or Medicine for it in 1903. Since then, numerous studies have found that red light therapy works to speed up wound healing and reduces pain and inflammation in both animals and humans with burns, surgical incisions, and other wounds[27, 28, 29, 30, 31, 32, 33, 34, 35, 36, 37, 38, 39, 40, 41]—and administration of this powerful therapy has gotten easier as experiments have shown that powerful medical-grade lasers are not needed for photobiomodulation to be effective and, in fact, a simple LED will suffice.[42] Yet somehow, despite copious research validating these effects over the last century, photobiomodulation still has not made its way into the standard best practices for wound care.

Although awareness of the therapeutic use of light is growing, I understand that it might not be familiar to you and might even sound like a scam. It's actually one of the most powerful tools in my toolbox, both for healing and for overall health (since those are one and the same—but more on that later). And it doesn't require much in the way of lifestyle change. You don't need to eat anything different, drink anything different, or change your daily schedule. All you need to do is place an LED pad on your body or an LED helmet on your head while you go about your normal activities. Because it works so well and is such an easy practice to adopt, I made it the first letter of **PRONEURO**—the very first step in my approach. The P stands for Photobiomodulation: *photo* (light), *bio* (living/cell), *modulation* (change)—using the photons of the energy of light, in both visible and invisible wavelengths, to change living cells.

In this book, when we refer to photobiomodulation, we mean the use of red and near-infrared frequencies for their effect on the mitochondria (via cytochrome c oxidase). You may also be familiar with the way sunlight on our skin converts one type of cholesterol into vitamin D_3. This is also a type of photobiomodulation! We have structures within our bodies called *chromophores* that are equipped to capture light. As my colleague and mentor Dr. Gregory Hipskind puts it, "We are truly beings of light."

As I continued to work with photobiomodulation in Arizona, we were seeing patients' conditions improve that they'd been told (and conventional wisdom in medicine generally held) had no possibility of getting better. I became more and more convinced that we had to get the word out about the healing power of photobiomodulation—to the point that I retired from private practice in 2015 to develop my own LED devices and the approach you're reading about in this book.

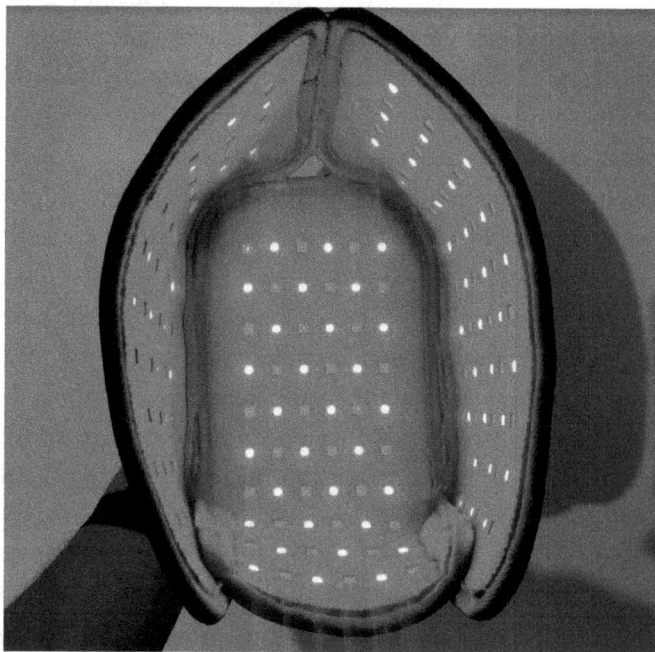

ProNeuroLight's photobiomodulation helmet delivers red and near-infrared light transcranially.

The effect of photobiomodulation on the mitochondria was what initially led me to develop a light helmet. I built the prototype on Christmas Day in 2017. I always try to relax over Christmas, and ironically that's often when I'm the most productive—when I take the time to relax and allow new ideas to come in. My father was a small business owner—he had been a cobbler's apprentice and ran a shoe store in our hometown. I believe I inherited his entrepreneurial spirit as well as the propensity for working with my hands. I remember watching him piece together separate pieces of leather, stitching them on his specialized sewing machine into the finished pairs of shoes displayed in the store window. His level of craftsmanship was truly something to behold, and I'm pretty sure I could feel his hands guiding me as I stitched together the first flexible, full-head transcranial photobiomodulation helmet anyone had ever made (to my knowledge). The helmet was the culmination of my work for the prior decade on nerve regeneration and my desire to help my mom's brain work better. I've since built an entire program to coach people on increasing their brain power, and photobiomodulation is the foundation.

Back in 1986, as I'd been finishing up my chiropractic degree, I'd figured my curiosity would need to be put on hold once I entered clinical practice, so I'd considered entering a Ph.D. program in biomechanics. I'd gone for an interview at the University of Iowa Department of Biomedical Engineering, where they had been working on manufacturing a lumbar disc replacement. At the time, it felt like a good fit—I could see myself designing highly advanced medical devices—but the following week, my wife announced that she was pregnant, and with that, an extended period of study with no income was ruled out. Once again, it seemed like I was choosing one path at the fork in the road; I didn't suspect that thirty years later, I would indeed find myself making medical devices that are making a difference in the health of people worldwide.

Working with collaborators including my brother Matt—a leader and innovator in his own right, bringing the latest science and technology to treat ailments such as neuropathy, restless legs syndrome, sciatica, and whiplash in his chiropractic practice—I first used the light pads with neuropathy patients, sharing the results as patients experienced reduced pain, enhanced sensory function, and improved balance.[43, 44, 45, 46] At the time, nobody thought the nerves could grow back. People laughed at me when I asked about this at conferences. But in my mind, there simply was no other way it could be working. If people were regaining their balance and normal sensation, their nerves had to be regrowing. Nobody had yet shown that this regrowth could happen; furthermore, the medical establishment did not even believe the symptoms of neuropathy were reversible. With contributions from giants such as Dr. Kennedy in Minnesota and Dr. Bennett in Montréal, the tide was starting to turn, and in 2011 I demonstrated in a case study that regeneration of nerve fibers was possible with photobiomodulation.[47] Subsequent research showing that degeneration—and impaired regeneration—of the nerves plays a role in the progression of symptoms in conditions such as Parkinson's disease[48] relies on the techniques for assessing intraepidermal nerve fiber density developed by Kennedy and Bennett—and, of course, on the once controversial observations that neuropathy has a physiological manifestation and that the nerves can regrow.

The personal stories of how we came to do this work can be as interesting as the research evidence itself. One of my favorites comes from my colleague Michael Hamblin, who is now retired from teaching at Harvard Medical School and is considered one of the world's leading researchers on photobiomodulation.

Depending on the intensity, light has the power to kill or to save a cell from death. We are all aware of sunlight's power to burn our skin and our retinas. Ironically, it was through this destructive power of light that Dr. Hamblin first observed one of photobiomodulation's beneficial side effects.

While pursuing his Ph.D. in organic chemistry, Dr. Hamblin was researching porphyrins, a highly pigmented family of molecules that include heme, the pigment in red blood cells, and chlorophyll, the green pigment that allows plants to use light to make energy. In a technique called photodynamic therapy, light applied to the porphyrins causes them to produce reactive oxygen species—a method that can be used in a targeted way to kill cancerous or precancerous cells. To validate the effectiveness of photodynamic therapy, Hamblin needed a control group for his experiment. That control group would receive the light therapy without the porphyrins, allowing the researchers to compare the results in the control group to those in the treatment group.

There was just one problem. Contrary to the researchers' hypothesis, the control group also started experiencing beneficial effects, such as faster healing and enhanced tissue regeneration. The light was helping them, even though it wasn't killing cancer cells. This light-bulb moment (I hope you'll forgive my frequent use of this phrase since it applies both literally and figuratively to the events described in this book) led Dr. Hamblin to dedicate much of the rest of his career to studying the beneficial effects of red and near-infrared light (i.e., photobiomodulation).

Sometimes in the scientific method, your findings don't match your hypothesis. This can be frustrating, but it can also lead to new discoveries. With an open mind and a willingness to travel wherever the path leads, those pesky "confounding factors" can become breakthroughs in scientific knowledge. (Also, I want to reassure you that photobiomodulation is safe with the devices available on the market. The research mentioned here targeted cells for destruction specifically through the use of porphyrins.)

As medical treatments go, photobiomodulation is relatively well understood, and the effects well substantiated. It has been widely studied—because, after all, if we're shining light on people, we first wanted to make sure we weren't doing any harm—and for that reason, there is a wide body of evidence documenting its safety and efficacy. There are no reported serious side effects of photobiomodulation applied to the head (or, for that matter, anywhere else on the body). None. Zero. Zilch. Nothing bad is going to happen. But what about the good? Let's dive in so you can understand why photobiomodulation needs to be part of your self-care routine.

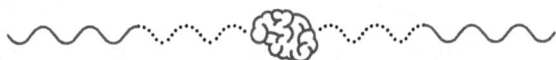

One billion mitochondria would fit within a grain of sand—yet, when adjusted for scale, our mitochondria convert between ten thousand and fifty thousand times more energy per second than the sun.[49] You already know that mitochondria are dynamic, not static—they change shape, fuse with other mitochondria, and run around in the cell to wherever they're needed. This movement is especially apparent in nerve cells simply because of the length of those cells. The nerve that travels from the dorsal root ganglion in your spine down to the tip of your toe is *one single cell* that is dozens of centimeters long (depending on the length of your legs). This is why neuropathy most often happens in the feet. Mitochondria travel an average of three centimeters per day, which is really incredible considering their microscopic size: A single mitochondrion measures less than one micrometer in length. In case tiny units of measurement in the metric system aren't your forté, that means taking a millimeter (already minuscule) and dividing by one thousand. In the course of one day, the average mitochondrion travels *thirty thousand times* its own length. But with the long nerves of the legs, it takes about ten days for a mitochondrion to travel the length of the nerve. For someone whose mitochondria aren't working well, this trip takes longer—and the mitochondria may never get down to the tip of the toe at all, resulting in the numbness that characterizes neuropathy.

As the mitochondria run around inside our cells, they are propelled by little tubules that actually look like feet—and applying light enables them to run faster. Remember that in prehistoric times, mitochondria gave organisms a survival advantage by enabling a higher level of energy production—and this extra power supply comes not just from the energy we take in from food but also from light.

The mitochondria can produce ATP in a few different ways. This flexibility allows our cells to produce energy from different nutrient sources (using glycolysis to convert glucose to ATP or using beta-oxidation to convert lipids to ATP). It also creates a kind of surge capacity, where another method of producing energy can be enlisted if one way isn't working fast enough. (For example, our muscles enlist anaerobic respiration when aerobic respiration is not sufficient to meet energy needs, which are unusually high during intense bouts of exercise—part of the reason this level of intensity can't be sustained for long.)

This is significant because aerobic respiration is much more efficient than anaerobic respiration at producing ATP: One glucose molecule transforms into thirty-four ATP molecules through aerobic respiration versus just two ATP molecules in anaerobic. That's a very good energy bang for the buck!

What's more, when mitochondrial respiration switches from anaerobic glycolysis to aerobic oxidative phosphorylation—a transition that photobiomodulation encourages—it not only increases ATP output but also mobilizes stem cells to migrate toward injury sites in the body where they can repair damage.[50] When I say the healing power of light approaches being magical, I'm really not exaggerating!

In aerobic respiration, protons are pumped across the mitochondrial inner membrane to generate an electrochemical gradient—basically a difference in electrical charge that sets off a series of events known as the citric acid cycle, or the Krebs cycle (after Hans Krebs, who discovered it and received the Nobel Prize in Physiology or Medicine in 1953 for that discovery). The last step in that process, an enzyme called cytochrome c oxidase, is a molecule that acts as a photo-acceptor, harnessing the power of red and near-infrared light to make energy.

There are three components to how photobiomodulation increases ATP synthesis:

1. It stimulates cytochrome c oxidase, thus enhancing cellular respiration and metabolism.
2. It dissociates nitric oxide, increasing the proton gradient—that is, creating a higher concentration of protons outside the inner membrane of the mitochondria than inside the membrane— which also drives ATP synthesis.
3. It converts glycolysis to oxidative phosphorylation, a much more efficient method of producing ATP.

Electron Transport Chain

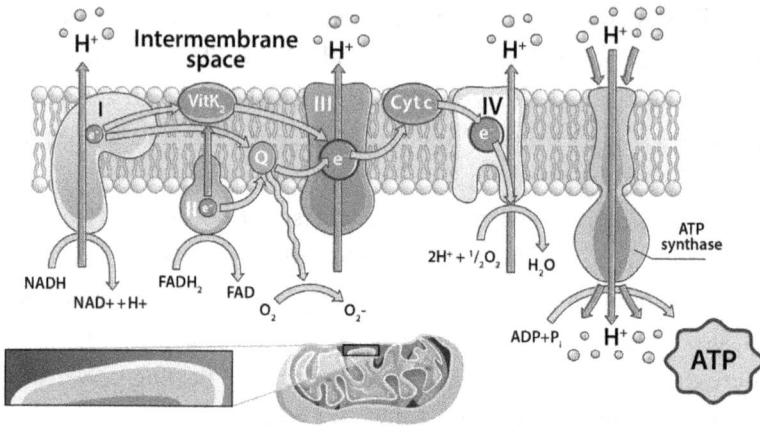

The electron transport chain is a process that takes place along the inner membranes of mitochondria, creating an electrochemical gradient—that is, a discrepancy in electrical charge inside and outside the membrane—that drives the synthesis of ATP. In complex I, NADH (a coenzyme form of vitamin B_3) sends a hydrogen ion across the membrane and becomes NAD+ (also a coenzyme, or an organic compound that assists enzymes in activating to carry out their functions in the body). In complex II, the coenzyme $FADH_2$ becomes FAD with the help of vitamin K_2; the two hydrogen ions continue along to complex III (known as the Q cycle due to the involvement of ubiquinone, or coenzyme Q), where oxygen molecules become negatively charged, priming them to combine with hydrogen molecules (with the help of cytochrome c) in complex IV and form molecules of water (H_2O). In the final step, hydrogen ions that have been pumped across the membrane cross back in to transform ADP and inorganic phosphate (P_i) into ATP.

Think of this process like a machine that spits out pieces of candy. All the ingredients are there in abundance, and if the machine is able to spin faster, it spits out more candy. This is what happens when your mitochondria can spit out more ATP—just like candy, it will give you more energy, and you won't even get a sugar crash afterward.

Absorption of red and near-infrared light by the mitochondria also increases the mitochondrial membrane potential, setting it up to produce more ATP in future cycles.

As it turns out, although cytochrome c oxidase plays a key role, photobiomodulation increases ATP even under experimental conditions where cytochrome c oxidase is not present. This led researchers to discover another mechanism of action: Photobiomodulation also reduces the viscosity of the water inside mitochondria—causing the "molecular rotor" to spin faster and produce more ATP. The special properties of water on intracellular membranes mean these changes take place without excessive heating of the surrounding tissue[51]—an important factor to note since heating of tissue, if it occurred, could cause other less desirable effects and because it is one more way photobiomodulation seems tailored to work with our biology to produce the desired effect without creating less advantageous side effects.

The specific frequencies of red and near-infrared light used for photobiomodulation have been shown to influence levels of reactive oxygen species.[52] Remember the autophagy process, in which the body breaks down worn-out cells to reuse the components and conserve energy for use by healthier cells? Reactive oxygen species are one of the markers the body uses to identify these cells—but applying light affects the levels of these markers in ways that promote survival (or, in some cases, efficient removal and "cleaning" of the cells that are too damaged to survive). We know that oxidative stress occurs when there's an imbalance between the production of reactive oxygen species and the body's ability to counteract their effects—so it would seem that antioxidants would be a simple solution, right? Not so fast... Even though oxidative stress has been linked to conditions including depression, traumatic brain injury, cardiovascular disease, and Alzheimer's disease, the solution is not as simple as administering antioxidants. In fact, clinical trials of antioxidant supplementation have largely led to disappointing results. Here's where the so-called Goldilocks effect of photobiomodulation (referring to the desired porridge temperature in the tale of Goldilocks and the Three Bears—not too hot and not too cold, but *juuuust* right) comes in. Photobiomodulation appears to help regulate reactive oxygen species to optimal levels rather than uniformly increasing or decreasing them.[53] It prompts a temporary increase in reactive oxygen species, which prompts the body to activate an antioxidant defense.[54] With light, we can turn a tired cell into a reenergized one.

In addition to the mechanisms outlined above, when light in the red and near-infrared range of the electromagnetic spectrum is applied to the mitochondria, it prompts the release of metabolically active calcium, touching off a process that activates transcription factors and gene expression.[55] By virtue of this effect, photobiomodulation plays a role in what's called *epigenetics*.

Think of your DNA like an instruction book—it's complete as written, but not all the instructions in the book will necessarily be carried out during your lifetime. A specific gene or combination of genes may put you at risk for a certain disease, but your environment and lifestyle (including allostatic load) will help to determine whether those genes ever express themselves or if, instead, they stay silent. Scientists believe this is part of how traumatic experiences can have a ripple effect for subsequent generations. There's no doubt that emotional habits and patterns of behavior are passed down through learning and traditions—but in a separate process, the "instruction book" that is passed down in the form of genetic material is different when it was created under traumatic conditions, and the effect persists for at least two generations.

To sum up: Genes are not destiny. Your environment (including your own behavior) can influence whether particular genes are expressed or not. In addition, your environment (including your own behavior) can influence how your genetic material gets passed on to your descendants. Epigenetics as a field only developed during the second half of the twentieth century, and the degree to which environment influences genetic expression is still underemphasized in my opinion.

Here's one more tidbit that may not have been in your high school biology textbook: Your DNA does not stay exactly the same from birth to death. Remember telomeres, the cellular markers of aging mentioned in the previous chapter during the discussion of allostatic load? Telomeres are bits of DNA that sit at the end of each of your chromosomes like a cap. Like rings on a tree, your telomeres show your body's age—but some people have unusually short telomeres for their age, while others have unusually long telomeres (and thus are more youthful on a cellular level). Critically short telomeres are a risk factor for cancer and other diseases typically associated with aging.[56] Telomere shortening also seems to inhibit the body's innate ability to soothe and reduce pain signals—making this a risk factor for chronic pain.[57]

Here, too, photobiomodulation is, in a sense, a quick fix. It causes a type of protein binding interaction that is known to impact gene expression and to have a protective effect on the telomeres.[58] So, if you've had traumatic experiences or environmental risk factors that contribute to allostatic load, your cells may appear older than your actual age—but some time with your light pad or helmet can help. What's more, this protein binding interaction has effects beyond the cells that are directly treated with the light—so light applied to one part of the body can have effects in other spots or even bodywide.[59]

One study found that photobiomodulation significantly increased the concentration of cytochrome c oxidase and oxygenated hemoglobin in the area of the body where a light probe was applied, providing further evidence for the role of cytochrome c oxidase and also a mechanism by which photobiomodulation's effects can extend beyond the treated area to affect the whole body (sometimes referred to as the *abscopal effect,* meaning indirect or system-wide effect—the word *abscopal* literally means "off-target").[60]

Although abscopal effects have been observed for some time (and we'll cite many of those papers as we go along), how exactly they work is not completely understood. Proposed mechanisms included immune and inflammatory signaling effects, influencing mitochondrial function in circulating platelets, and a type of stem cell activity that we'll explore later in the book.[61] Scientists recently added a new mechanism to these hypotheses with the discovery of so-called *cell-free mitochondria,* which circulate in the bloodstream independent of any particular cell type.[62, 63] "The recent discovery of respiratory-competent cell-free mitochondria that are circulating in the blood of normal individuals might offer an explanation for how the beneficial effects of light that is incident on the body can be transmitted to distant organs including the brain,"[64] Michael

Hamblin and collaborator Farzad Salehpour (who also contributed to the pre-publication scientific review of this book) wrote in a 2020 paper. In fact, the authors suggest this indirect effect might be more important than direct effects when it comes to photobiomodulation of the head and brain due to the limited ability of light to reach beyond the outermost regions of the brain.

One study assessed the role of photobiomodulation in helping people recover from intense exercise. The researchers found the formation of "giant mitochondria" with unusually high respiratory rates, creating unusually high volumes of energy. They also observed local increases in circulation, accelerated tissue regeneration, and upregulated angiogenesis (formation of new blood vessels).[65] Although photobiomodulation has wide-ranging effects, many of them start with the effects on the mitochondria—which, in turn, have wide-ranging effects throughout the body.

Another reason photobiomodulation is so important is that it addresses the side effects of two of the most widely prescribed classes of medication. Statins—a class of drugs prescribed for lowering cholesterol, taken by more than 200 million people around the world—are poisonous to the mitochondria and drastically increase your chances of developing neuropathy. Proton pump inhibitors, which are widely prescribed for heartburn, also affect mitochondrial function,[66] reduce nitric oxide production,[67] and damage the endothelial cells that line the blood vessels[68]— all mechanisms that may factor into the drugs' association with increased dementia risk.[69]

What's even more fascinating is that there is some evidence mitochondrial dysfunction may contribute to psychiatric disorders, including depression, anxiety, bipolar disorder, borderline personality disorder, schizophrenia, and psychosis—and therefore photobiomodulation might be especially helpful for patients at risk for the onset of these conditions. What's more, many psychotropic medications interfere with mitochondrial function—so photobiomodulation may offer a way to help balance the detrimental side effects of these medications.[70, 71]

Investigating potential alternative explanations to rule them out is an important part of the scientific method for validating the efficacy of treatments. One study tested whether photobiomodulation might be creating its effects through the heat it generates rather than the light itself. To test this, the study gave some subjects a treatment that felt like photobiomodulation but omitted the light—essentially just applying a heating pad to their foreheads. The rest of the study subjects received actual photobiomodulation treatment, with the heat generated by the red and near-infrared light that was applied. As expected, the heating pad alone did not affect cytochrome c oxidase—but it's good that they ruled out this potential explanation since it would be rather embarrassing to build a company around selling light pads and light helmets if a heating pad would be just as effective![72]

From 1967 to 2019, a total of 63 *in vitro* studies examined photobiomodulation's effects on cells in a lab environment (i.e., outside of a living organism).[73] These studies helped establish the treatment's overall safety and the best dose of photobiomodulation to optimize the desired response. They also demonstrated that photobiomodulation makes neurons more resistant to damage in the presence of neurotoxins—a pretty amazing discovery since toxins are a major factor in neurodegeneration and the development of disease. (Photobiomodulation can save cells and bring them back from the brink of death. This was discovered by researchers who found that cells treated with the neurotoxin rotenone resisted death when treated with light—a "light-bulb moment" in more ways than one![74])

Over the last half-century, researchers have applied photobiomodulation to everything from cell cultures to pretty much every living creature on the planet.[75] Studies in live animals have provided some additional insight into photobiomodulation's mechanisms of action. The safety of putting LEDs or laser light on the head has been validated with studies in pigs and mice (with a similar ratio of skull thickness to brain size as humans have). Studies with human cadavers have also allowed observation of how deep the light penetrates the brain and how much it heats up the brain tissue, providing further evidence for the treatment's safety.

Since the initial confirmation of safety, additional studies have demonstrated photobiomodulation's neuroprotective effects, including increased synaptogenesis (i.e., it improves the brain's ability to form new connections), increased angiogenesis (formation of new blood vessels), increased blood flow, reduced inflammation, increased antioxidant activity, reduced apoptosis (indicating the cells are staying healthier longer instead of being killed off due to aging and degeneration), an increase in neuron progenitor cells (the precursors to new neurons), increased activity of neurotrophic factors (molecules that support neurons' growth and survival), and reduced neuron excitotoxicity (a type of neuronal cell death that is seen in dementia, among other neurological disorders).

One fascinating study found that applying low levels of red and near-infrared light appear to cause more M2 (anti-inflammatory) macrophages to be produced and fewer M1 (pro-inflammatory) macrophages to be converted to M2 (anti-inflammatory) macrophages.[76] A *macrophage* is a cell that detects and destroys bacteria, viruses, and other invaders as part of our immune system. The two types of macrophages work together to signal the onset of inflammation when the body begins to fight infection and promote the resolution of inflammation once the infection has been conquered, thus playing a key role in regulating inflammation in both the upward and the downward direction. As healing progresses and reducing inflammation becomes a priority, photobiomodulation could thus be used to aid in this process.[77]

Also in the time period 1967–2019, a total of 83 *in vivo* (animal) studies were published specifically on photobiomodulation applied to the brain.[78] The findings have identified many promising applications for photobiomodulation: It protects against brain injury in cases of hypoxia (conditions of low or no oxygen) and improves long-term functional outcomes in cases of cerebral ischemia (when tissues are deprived of oxygenated blood) by increasing the expression of so-called neurotrophic factors that support the growth and survival of neurons. Photobiomodulation protects neurons in the hippocampus, a brain region that is critical for memory, from secondary damage in cases of traumatic brain injury. In studies of animals with induced Parkinson's disease, photobiomodulation was shown to improve motor function (in a study with monkeys) and to ameliorate dopaminergic cell loss (in studies with rodents). In studies of animals with induced Alzheimer's disease, photobiomodulation was also shown to improve spatial and episodic memory and to protect the hippocampus from neuronal cell death induced by amyloid beta (a peptide that builds up in the brains of people with Alzheimer's). We'll get into much more detail about the brain, brain injury, and neurodegeneration—and regeneration—later in the book, but for now, I just want to make the point that photobiomodulation has been shown to be both safe and beneficial.

Some of the lasting damage from a heart attack results from cell death. The resulting scar tissue impairs heart function—but research has shown that photobiomodulation can be used to limit the damage and help cells survive, leading to reductions in both inflammation and scarring and increases in tissue repair.[79] Studies in mice also found that photobiomodulation could help prevent the formation and progression of abdominal aortic aneurysm[80, 81]—a leading cause of death in older people, as the main blood vessel that delivers blood throughout the body swells and then bursts.

In a study of diabetic rats, photobiomodulation showed promise in helping increase collagen production and accelerate wound healing via its effects on mitochondrial dynamics.[82] Assuming this same mechanism works for humans (which we can assume it does, given the established benefit for wound healing in humans), imagine the impact that could result from including photobiomodulation in the protocol for diabetes care and perhaps protecting people from one of the symptoms that can make the condition life-threatening (namely, wounds that get infected because they don't heal). And that's without even considering the effects photobiomodulation has on other downstream effects of diabetes, such as neuropathy![83] (Incidentally, photobiomodulation has been shown in many more studies than just my own to accelerate the regeneration of peripheral nerves after they are damaged[84]—just one more way the treatment can help diabetics and anyone else suffering from neuropathy.) Based on results from animal studies, photobiomodulation also has the potential to promote integration and viability of skin grafts.[85]

Multiple studies have now found benefits from using photobiomodulation to treat depression symptoms,[86, 87, 88, 89, 90, 91, 92] and the Massachusetts General Hospital Guide to Depression now includes a section on photobiomodulation for the treatment of depression.[93] One intriguing study showed that photobiomodulation helped people with depression shift their focus away from fixating on negative stimuli.[94] In a study of rats exposed to chronic stress, photobiomodulation was more effective at staving off symptoms of depression than Citalopram (an antidepressant drug in the selective serotonin reuptake inhibitor, or SSRI, category).[95] (Incidentally, a study in mice found that photobiomodulation carries out its depression-fighting effects in part by influencing serotonin levels.[96])

Small studies in humans have found lessening of autism symptoms with photobiomodulation treatment.[97, 98, 99, 100] Studies in mice have connected autism symptoms with a phenomenon called the cell danger response, which you'll learn about later in the book. Administering a medication that normalizes mitochondrial metabolism had the effect of reducing autism symptoms in the mice,[101, 102] and the drug is being investigated for use in humans. Meanwhile, since the drug exerts its influence via the mitochondria, it makes sense that photobiomodulation would help as well.

One of the most fascinating studies regarding photobiomodulation and wound healing is one that helped establish the existence of abscopal effects: Subjects agreed to have minor wounds created on both of their forearms, and then to receive either real or placebo photobiomodulation treatments on one arm. The treatment group's wounds healed faster than those of the placebo group—on both arms, not just the arm where photobiomodulation was applied.[103] The treatment has also shown promise in treating carpal tunnel syndrome,[104] sexual dysfunction,[105] post-traumatic stress disorder (PTSD),[106] anxiety,[107, 108] and bipolar disorder;[109, 110] for preventing sunburn after exposure to the ultraviolet rays that would typically cause it;[111] for preventing lymphedema in breast cancer patients after mastectomy;[112, 113, 114] and for managing cravings in recovery from opioid addiction.[115, 116] Researchers in Japan are studying photobiomodulation's ability to help women overcome fertility challenges;[117, 118, 119, 120] a separate body of research has found benefits for male factor infertility.[121, 122, 123, 124, 125, 126, 127] At least one study in humans has found the potential for photobiomodulation to help ease phobias such as claustrophobia and fear of public speaking.[128] A team of researchers in China noted its potential for treating diseases of the eye, such as optic nerve trauma, retinal injury, and macular degeneration.[129] Additional studies on the success of photobiomodulation as a treatment for headaches, insomnia, depression, mild cognitive impairment, and Alzheimer's disease, among other conditions, were published in Chinese-language journals twenty years ago or more. Only recently have researchers begun to work across the language barrier, recognizing and building on the solid foundation of research substantiating the benefits of photobiomodulation.[130]

Photobiomodulation's health benefits are on par with exercise—without having to actually exercise.[131] (For more on what exactly I mean by that, turn to Chapter Ten.) For people with central nervous system diseases such as stroke, spinal cord injury, traumatic brain injury, and multiple sclerosis, fatigue and the effect of their conditions on muscle function sometimes prevents them from experiencing the health benefits of exercise. In these cases, if photobiomodulation can help these people manage their conditions and heal, it can mean they're able to return to exercise as it helps them build up the energy reserves that are required—and meanwhile, it provides some similar benefits even in the absence of the ability to exercise.[132] Aside from its benefits for wound healing, its effects of reducing pain and inflammation are well established.[133, 134, 135, 136, 137, 138] Because of its ability to reduce markers of inflammation, photobiomodulation has the potential to reduce joint pain and swelling for people with arthritis.[139]

Photobiomodulation has no real downside, and it's actually enjoyable. Although the "heating pad effect" is not the reason it works, the heat is pleasant and may help with pain separately from the effects of the light. (Australian brain scientist John Mitrofanis reported that in his research with photobiomodulation, the mice seemed to enjoy it, staying close to the lights even after they were turned off.) As mammals, we respond to warmth—we are programmed to seek it out. (Think of the way newborn puppies crowd close to their mother even when not nursing, and a human baby also prefers to sleep on its mother.) The light pad can, at least in some small sense, make up for the deficit of human touch most of us experience. As I'm writing this nearly two years into the COVID-19 pandemic and resulting social isolation, we're especially missing hugs and human contact, yet most of us don't get enough of it even in normal times. If humans benefit from the healing power of touch and the pleasant sensation of warmth, the light pad may not be a perfect substitute, but it still has some benefit in the comfort it provides. We need to let the light into our lives—sunlight for vitamin D and the lightness or levity that comes with social interaction—but in the absence of these, photobiomodulation can be at least a partial substitute.

INTRODUCING YOUR JOY SCORE

One of the most fascinating parts of scientific research—at least in my mind—is the way it is always revealing new and more precise ways to measure our well-being. One of the metrics that's recently emerged is *heart rate variability*, or HRV—a term it seems like nobody knew a few years ago, and yet suddenly it's everywhere.

If you ask people which they think is better—a steady, predictable heartbeat like a metronome, or a heartbeat that is more erratic and chaotic—most people will answer that they think the steady, regular heartbeat is better. But in fact, it's the opposite. We want more *variability* in the heart rate, meaning that the length of time between beats is less consistent. Remember how I said it's not about avoiding stress but about teaching your body how to adapt to stress? It's the same with your heart rate. A rigid, regular heart rhythm indicates a nervous system that's a little less flexible and adaptable to changing conditions.

HRV is measured by monitoring your heart rate for several minutes and measuring the intervals between beats; some intervals will be longer and some shorter. The variability measurement is obtained by calculating the difference between the longest and the shortest interval. Higher HRV is considered a sign of a more balanced nervous system, indicating an ability to speed up and slow down more nimbly. Greater adaptability to respond to conditions in your environment—ramping up quickly but also slowing down and relaxing easily—indicates a healthier nervous system, which affects our overall health on many levels. With practice, as you monitor your own measurements, you may start to recognize the feeling of high or rising HRV. Think of it as your "joy score"—a feeling of contentment and bliss, a feeling that all is right with the world.

When we monitor HRV, we are observing our sympathetic and parasympathetic nervous systems at work. You may recall that the peripheral nervous system (the system that covers the entire body outside of the brain and spinal cord) has two components: the *somatic nervous system*, which is under our conscious control, and the *autonomic nervous system*, which regulates all sorts of functions that take place beneath the surface of our consciousness. The autonomic nervous system regulates digestion, breathing, blood pressure, and, yes, heart rate—and it has two components that work in opposition to one another, the sympathetic and parasympathetic nervous systems.

The *sympathetic nervous system* is responsible for the fight-or-flight response we have all experienced. Stress hormones like adrenaline and cortisol pump through our systems, signaling our bodies to direct blood flow away from the digestive system into the muscles to literally prepare us to flee (or fight). Breathing and heart rate accelerate; thinking becomes quick and defensive rather than deep and nuanced. This state of sympathetic activation serves a very clear evolutionary purpose (priming us to flee from danger), but it's not good for us to have it chronically activated. We need the *parasympathetic nervous system* to turn down the volume on sympathetic activation and bring us out of fight-or-flight.

Parasympathetic activation leads to the exact opposite set of symptoms—and in fact, the term *activation* might be confusing since these telltale signs are things we more typically think of as *deactivation*. Muscle tension dissipates, heart rate and breathing slow down, and blood is directed back into the digestive system. (The nickname for parasympathetic activation is the "rest and digest" response.) Parasympathetic activation has its own set of markers, such as the neurotransmitter acetylcholine—but the important thing to know is that accessing this state is much more within our control than you might think.

We will explore many ways to activate your parasympathetic response later in the book. For now, I just want you to understand that HRV is like a tug-of-war between the sympathetic and parasympathetic nervous systems. High HRV indicates that both are functioning well and providing signals that influence your heart rate. Given the stresses of modern life, we all have plenty of sympathetic activation, but your HRV will be lower (i.e., your heart rate will be less variable) if you have *only* sympathetic activation. As the parasympathetic nervous system starts to tug in the other direction, prompting your biology to slow down and relax, this will show up as increasing HRV (i.e., your heart rate becomes *more* variable). A variety of everyday activities cause our HRV to decrease—including physical exercise[140] and even just speaking[141]—with sympathetic activation. It's not that we never want our HRV to drop; it's that when it does, we want it to have the capacity to recover quickly.

Interestingly, this balance of sympathetic and parasympathetic response seems to take some time after birth to develop. Babies seem to spend the first six months of life calibrating this response, showing a sympathetic (fearful/defensive) response to almost all stimuli at first, then gradually learning to relax in certain conditions (e.g., being fed and comforted). It seems that traumatic experiences in the earliest years may interfere with this process, leading to chronically low HRV.[142]

HRV varies quite a bit from person to person, but within each person, it typically declines dramatically with age. Athletes in their early twenties can log HRV scores as high as 180 milliseconds (ms), while athletes in their fifties max out at around one-third of that value. Note that this pattern persists even in older athletes with uncharacteristically low resting heart rates.

Low HRV has been shown to be a strong predictor of cardiovascular events[143] and mortality.[144] It predicts the risk of death for cancer patients[145, 146, 147] and terminally ill patients in hospice care[148, 149]—and indeed, low HRV is correlated with lower life expectancy overall.[150] Recent research highlighted abnormally high sympathetic nervous system activity (i.e., low HRV) during sleep as a risk factor for stroke.[151] In people with chronic fatigue syndrome, higher HRV is associated with reduced symptom severity,[152] reflecting that the nervous system is involved in that condition. HRV can be used to help predict a person's risk of sudden cardiac death,[153] and critical care medicine has recently identified ways to use it to predict the onset of sepsis.[154] Lower HRV is associated with a higher risk of death after myocardial infarction, a correlation the researchers interpret to mean that our nervous systems are healthier when they are more adaptable and can cool down just as efficiently as they ramp up in the face of danger.[155] Low HRV during sleep may be a biomarker that can serve as an early warning sign for dementia risk.[156]

Recall the concept of allostatic load from the previous chapter—the manifestation of stress in the body with multiple indicators that your body has recovered well (low allostatic load) or hasn't (high allostatic load). You probably won't be surprised to learn that a higher allostatic load is correlated with lower HRV.[157] People with major depression tend to have lower HRV[158]—a fact that might seem counterintuitive in that it indicates depression is an indicator of a chronically overactive (and stressed) sympathetic nervous system. High HRV, on the other hand, is associated with positive mood,[159] and higher resting HRV is associated with greater cerebral blood flow[160]—a fact whose importance will become clear as you read further in this book.

Extensive research has documented the association between HRV and emotions[161]—and has even associated low HRV with certain mental health conditions. The association between low HRV and depression is well documented.[162] Low HRV is also correlated with subjects' self-reported difficulty in regulating their emotions.[163] In addition, heart rate variability is considered to be an indicator of a person's resilience level in the wake of traumatic experiences like military combat,[164] deadly explosions,[165] and natural disasters.[166] One recent study found that the higher someone's HRV at the beginning of the COVID-19 pandemic, the more likely they were to report feeling safe and the less likely they were to report feeling worried or depressed as a result of these extraordinarily stressful circumstances.[167] You know the feel-good hormone oxytocin that bonds mothers with their newborn babies and which is also released after sex? One study found that giving subjects a nasal spray containing oxytocin had an instant boosting effect on their HRV.[168] This is an area research is still exploring and elucidating. Still, it's quite exciting because it hints that whatever influences HRV may help us feel better—and may even help treat chronic and debilitating mental health conditions. One study with members of the U.S. Army National Guard Special Forces found that subjects with higher HRV at the beginning of the study were more resilient (i.e., recovered faster) after experiencing stressful events of different types (whether emotionally charged or not).[169] This study also observed that flexibility, emotional control, and spirituality were predictors of high HRV at the beginning of the study, offering some clues for areas to focus on if we want to raise our HRV.

Lower HRV is associated with more severe disease in schizophrenia and bipolar disorder[170] and, more broadly, is associated with greater likelihood of developing a psychiatric disorder after experiencing stress.[171] Low HRV is believed to be a risk factor for developing PTSD, and monitoring this metric among those at risk of PTSD can serve as a way to identify people in need of greater support and more intensive intervention.[172] Stroke patients with lower HRV upon admission to the hospital for treatment are more likely to experience post-stroke depression.[173] People with major depressive disorder have lower HRV, on average, and their HRV does not increase to normal levels even with successful treatment of depression through established methods such as cognitive behavioral therapy.[174]

Interestingly, although the medical world has struggled to understand the underlying basis of chronic fatigue syndrome, HRV may be a missing link. At least one study found that people with symptoms of chronic fatigue syndrome had lower HRV than a healthy control group and took longer on a cognitive test (although they were just as accurate). Their HRV also took longer to recover than the control group's did following a cognitive challenge.[175]

HRV is gaining popularity as a measurement of the success of mental health treatments. One study noted its value as a tool for measuring the success of thought field therapy (a method in which the therapist guides the client to tap on meridian points in the body while focusing attention on the emotions the client is seeking to resolve and which is used to treat phobias, anxiety, trauma, obsessions, compulsions, addiction, and more).[176] Another study found that the effectiveness of expressive group therapy for cancer patients could be observed in changes in their HRV.[177] Some researchers have suggested that HRV can be used as part of a "precision medicine" approach to determine what combination of medicines, talk therapy methods, and other treatments would be best for a given patient.[178] This line of thinking is supported by the fact that low HRV is correlated with some depressive symptoms (suicidal ideation, lack of will for work and activities of daily life) but not others (difficulty concentrating, pessimistic thoughts, a sense of emotional numbness)[179]—indicating that HRV might help us better understand the nuances of these complex conditions and how to treat them.

As fitness trackers and wearables become more sophisticated and can reliably and accurately measure HRV,[180] I believe this will give rise to a whole new dimension for monitoring our health from moment to moment—and doing something about it. The sooner we can catch ourselves heading into a worried or distressed state, the sooner we can do something about it and return ourselves emotionally and physiologically to a state of balance.[181]

BREATHE YOUR WAY TO BETTER HEALTH

HRV depends, to some extent, on factors beyond our control—including the conditions of early life and even (some evidence indicates) geomagnetic activity.[182] However, despite the fairly reliable pattern of declining with age, there are actions you can take to raise your HRV—at any age. You will find many of them in the "recipe" chapters of this book—and one of the key practices is photobiomodulation, which is why I've included the HRV concept in this chapter of the book. A growing body of research is illustrating photobiomodulation's potential to activate the parasympathetic nervous system and move us toward relaxation and healing;[183, 184, 185, 186, 187, 188, 189] indeed, this is what I have seen with my own clients and in myself as well.

Other shortcuts encompass just about anything that will elicit a positive emotion in you;[190] many studies have documented the rise in people's HRV when they watch videos meant to evoke laughter or joy.[191] This has become a common way researchers manipulate people's feelings for the purpose of an experiment, and there's no reason you can't "engineer" your own feelings for a similar effect. (It sounds a little misleading or deceptive when phrased this way—but when it comes down to it, if you can manipulate your own emotions to get yourself out of a funk, then why wouldn't you?) A growing body of research also suggests that exposure to nature is a sure bet for boosting HRV.[192, 193, 194, 195]

We are beginning to see evidence that photobiomodulation helps HRV. Interestingly, laser acupuncture (another modality that uses light and, at this point, is more well-studied when it comes to this metric) has been shown to boost HRV in animals[196, 197] as well as humans—including night shift workers struggling to get their nervous systems to adjust to their new schedules.[198]

But there's one practice that influences HRV that is even simpler. In fact, you can do it right from where you're sitting without going outside or even getting up to put on your light pad or opening YouTube to find a funny video. You can start by using one simple, basic tool: your breath.

With a technique called resonance frequency breathing, you can learn to synchronize your breathing and heart rate and thus use your breath to *influence* your heart rate—and your HRV—in what's known as HRV biofeedback. With the help of a chest strap heart rate monitor and one of the many biofeedback breathing apps that are available, you can breathe in time with the expanding (inhalation) and contracting (exhalation) circles displayed on your phone screen and watch in real time as your HRV rises.

This type of breathing has shown efficacy for a variety of clinical outcomes.[199] When you practice resonance breathing, you are training your nervous system to let go and let you recover. You will experience a feeling of safety and well-being, along with the physiological "signature" of parasympathetic activation: lower cortisol, lower blood pressure, vasodilation.

A single session of HRV biofeedback has been shown to enhance HRV and decrease self-reported anxiety in musicians during a stressful performance.[200] One study found that a mindfulness-based stress reduction program including biofeedback breathing offered to subjects with traumatic brain injury and post-concussive syndrome (more on that in the next section of the book) resulted in improvements to their perceived self-efficacy and quality of life as well as memory and attention.[201] Another study found that a practice of biofeedback breathing, followed for six weeks, helped coronary artery disease patients get their hostility—a factor that carries a risk of worsening disease as well as implications for social and family life—under better control. This improvement in hostility was accompanied by an increase in HRV.[202]

Numerous studies have noted the promise of HRV biofeedback in treating depression,[203, 204, 205] and it has also shown promise for the treatment of PTSD[206] and attention deficit hyperactivity disorder (ADHD) in children.[207] In one particularly intriguing study, when HRV biofeedback was combined with psychotherapy, it led to not only increased HRV but also a larger decrease in depressive symptoms than with psychotherapy on its own.[208] Another one found that psychotherapy patients' higher HRV during therapy sessions was correlated with higher therapeutic alliance ratings—a measurement of the quality of the relationship between therapist and patient[209]—and yet another concluded the practice held promise for reducing stress and improving sleep for mothers in the early postpartum period.[210] One of the most important effects of biofeedback resonance breathing is its ability to influence blood pressure[211]—which, as you'll learn later in the book, has major implications for brain health. A study involving correctional officers found that HRV biofeedback training led to improvements in blood pressure, blood sugar and cholesterol levels, and optimism, as well as reducing psychological distress.[212]

Observing what happens to the human body during devotional practices such as meditation and prayer tells us that HRV and biofeedback may help to explain these practices' benefits for mental and physical health. Interestingly, prayer and chanting practices commonly slow the breathing rate down to around the rate typically used for HRV biofeedback breathing and achieve similar coordination of high-amplitude heart rate oscillations[213] (the technical term for how biofeedback breathing works its magic).

Improving our HRV may have downstream effects on some of the other biomarkers that contribute to allostatic load and influence our overall health. Several lines of research have found a link between autonomic dysfunction and chronic inflammation, which may help to explain why major depression is linked to cardiovascular disease independent of other risk factors.[214] In addition to low HRV, people who report experiencing loneliness also tend to have higher cortisol and dysregulated immune function.[215] People with low socioeconomic status (a designation that increases allostatic load and, consequently, risk of many chronic health conditions) also tend to have low HRV.

PROMOTING DESIRABLE OUTCOMES OR INHIBITING UNDESIRABLE ONES?

As we move toward the end of our first "recipe" chapter for better brain health, let me connect the dots for why I've included photobiomodulation, HRV, and biofeedback breathing all in the same chapter. Yes, photobiomodulation and biofeedback have both been shown to improve HRV, but that's not the only connection. The concept of balance—like the balance between sympathetic and parasympathetic activation that ensures our survival with an efficient response to threats but also allows our bodies to recover and regenerate when the threat is gone—is absolutely core to my message in this book.

The interplay between the two branches of the autonomic nervous system is an example of an essential category of relationships and interactions in the body: promotion and inhibition. Aside from sympathetic and parasympathetic, you already know about one more example of this type of relationship: pro-inflammatory and anti-inflammatory. What is crucial to know about this category of relationships is that none of the players are inherently good or bad. It's all about how they balance each other.

Many of the lifestyle recommendations given in this book are aimed at creating or restoring balance, the ones you've read about so far—photobiomodulation and biofeedback breathing—among them. By giving a boost to HRV, you are bringing your autonomic nervous system into balance, but this can also be framed as inhibiting the sympathetic nervous system, which, for most of us, is overactive.

Cutting-edge research (again, no pun intended) on the topic of pain applies a similar model. People who don't feel pain literally do not survive—they take risks that most of us long ago learned not to. People with numb patches of skin from a burn or a surgical scar need to take extra care to make sure the area without feeling does not get cut or burned since they won't feel it right away and pull back the way they would if the injury happened on an area with sensation. Pain is not inherently bad—in fact, it's vital to our survival. And yet, for people burdened with chronic pain, it drains the enjoyment from life. This new vein of research views the problem not as "too much pain" but rather as "not enough inhibition." The solution, then, becomes not finding and eliminating the source of the pain but rather figuring out how to activate the body's innate mechanisms that inhibit pain. Proponents of this approach believe we all encounter innumerable potentially painful stimuli as we go about our days. The pressure of sitting on a chair, the feeling of clothing brushing against our skin, the sensation of food with high fiber content traveling through our intestines—all of these are stimuli our bodies learn to tune out because they're no big deal. They don't signify danger. But for people with certain chronic pain conditions, those suppression mechanisms seem to go haywire, and their bodies overreact to these everyday, non-threatening stimuli.

In one such disorder—glossodynia, or "burning mouth syndrome"—patients report a burning sensation in the mouth and tongue without any obvious physical cause. After it was hypothesized to be a disorder of the autonomic nervous system, researchers tested photobiomodulation of the stellate ganglion (a bundle of nerves located at the sixth and seventh cervical vertebrae at the bottom of the neck) as a treatment and found that seventy-five percent of the study subjects achieved symptom relief. Following up on this finding, the same researchers found that abnormalities in the autonomic nervous system can be observed in the glossodynia patients' HRV and that photobiomodulation restores normal autonomic function as measured by HRV.[216]

Some kinds of neuropathic pain have been attributed to a similar type of sympathetic overactivity, and photobiomodulation applied to the stellate ganglion region has been successfully used as an alternative to a conventional sympathetic blockade (which involves the injection of local anesthesia). Researchers found that HRV can be used as a measure of how well this pain relief method is working and use that information to determine dosing.[217]

Within the beneficial effects of photobiomodulation, this ability to influence the parasympathetic nervous system—and to help the body inhibit pain and danger signals that are higher than they need to be—is one of the most intriguing. This benefit seems to come about through photobiomodulation's influence on HRV, which can be observed to drop (sympathetic activation) when someone experiences pain and then rise again (parasympathetic activation) as the person recovers and the perception of pain fades.[218]

Anxiety disorders, too, can be characterized as a failure of inhibition, as hypervigilance, worries, and panic take on an outsized role, becoming a threat of their own rather than warning us about threats in our environment.[219] Diminished HRV has been observed for many mental health conditions,[220, 221] indicating that a disturbance of autonomic balance (tipped in favor of sympathetic activation) may be a causative factor or at least a common symptom and a target for treatments and therapies.

Raising HRV is one potential mechanism by which photobiomodulation has positive effects for mental health issues. In a study of patients with anxiety disorder and major depression, symptoms improved for virtually all the subjects at the two-week and four-week marks after a single photobiomodulation session.[222] Another study showed that a six-session course of photobiomodulation treatment significantly improved patients' self-reported symptoms of depression.[223] The more studies establish the efficacy of this treatment—and the absence of any negative side effects of any kind—the more likely it is to become part of the standard of care.

Of course, the benefits of inhibiting sympathetic overdrive extend beyond mental health. One study found that adding photobiomodulation made acupuncture (considered by the World Health Organization to be an evidence-based treatment for hypertension) more effective at reducing blood pressure as it increased HRV (which may have helped to reduce the blood pressure).[224]

The parasympathetic response is often referred to with the shorthand "rest and digest," and the example of digestion shows just how important a role this autonomic balance plays throughout our bodies. In patients with chronic constipation, a single session of sacral photobiomodulation markedly affected autonomic nervous activity, reflected in changes in HRV.[225] Another study involving cognitive behavioral therapy (CBT) provides strong evidence of the mind-body connection and the role HRV plays as a marker. If our minds can't relax, our bodies can't relax—and it will show up as low HRV. The study found that CBT was an effective tool for managing constipation-predominant irritable bowel syndrome (IBS-C), with patients' symptoms coming under control with an eight-week course of CBT and staying under control sixteen weeks later. Subjects showed a significant increase in high-frequency power (a sub-measurement within a heart rate variability reading), and the greater the increase, the greater the subject's reduction in symptoms, indicating that HRV can act as a measurement of whether therapy is working and that restoring balance to the nervous system with parasympathetic activation can make a difference for digestive disorders such as IBS-C.[226] We all know that awful feeling of not being able to "go" as well as that nervous feeling of having to "go" too much—and tools including photobiomodulation can help bring the nervous system into balance and eliminate the issue (pun intended this time).

This concept of balancing promotion and inhibition also applies to inflammation. As you'll recall from Chapter Two, we want inflammation in the body to be not too much and not too little, but *juuuust* right. Impressively, photobiomodulation seems to work exactly this way, producing reactive oxygen species in normal cells but reducing reactive oxygen species levels in stressed cells.[227] "One of the most reproducible effects of photobiomodulation is an overall reduction in inflammation," this paper from Dr. Hamblin notes.

You'll recall from Chapter Two that inflammation in the brain is believed to be at least part of the cause of depression—and it turns out that photobiomodulation helps with this as well, providing another mechanism by which this therapy can yield mental health benefits. Interestingly, one study documenting this benefit identified an interesting potential pathway: the endocannabinoid system.[228] You might have heard of this system in the context of marijuana or, more recently, the cannabidiol (CBD) products that are seemingly everywhere and offer some of the same benefits without getting you high. Scientists' working theory about the endocannabinoid system is that it's what returns our bodies to homeostasis—an overall feeling of well-being. This system of molecules (either produced by the body or introduced from external sources) and receptors acts as a signaling system throughout the body, affecting appetite, digestion, metabolism, pain, inflammation, sleep, and the functioning of the liver and the reproductive system, among other bodily processes. This may help to explain how photobiomodulation impacts inflammation—and if cannabinoids have helped you with an issue such as pain, photobiomodulation may just have a similar effect for you (or provide an inexpensive substitute).

Chronic inflammation can lead to all sorts of problems for the brain—including lasting repercussions from supposedly mild head injuries (a topic you'll learn a lot more about in Section Two of this book) and the worsening of symptom severity in dementia and Alzheimer's disease patients (a topic we'll dig into in Section Three). That's why photobiomodulation is such an important ingredient in my brain health recipe. It not only enhances the function of mitochondria in the brain—and therefore literally enhances your brain power—but also promotes hormesis, helping the brain become equipped to handle stress better and adapt rather than becoming overwhelmed.[229] Recent research has shown how photobiomodulation—specifically, with a so-called intranasal device that shines the light through the thin skin inside your nostrils—improves circulation within the brain and also increases oxygen levels of the blood that's circulating within the brain.[230] This is one more way that with photobiomodulation, your brain gets more of the good stuff—all the nutrients from the nutritious diet you'll learn about in Chapter Six and all the oxygen you're taking in with your biofeedback breathing.

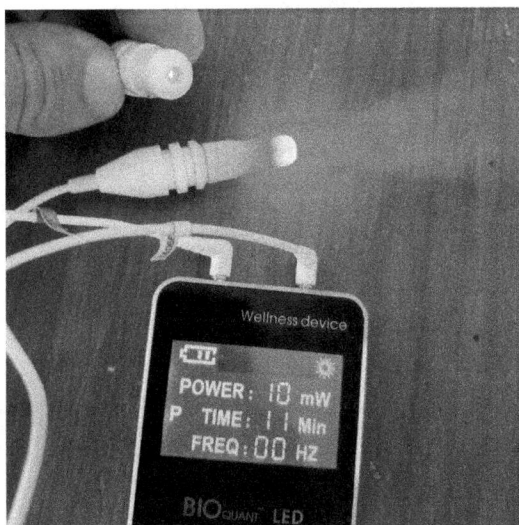

An intranasal photobiomodulation device of the type sold by ProNeuroLight

My personal practice of photobiomodulation is to incorporate it into my daily routine, morning and night. In each session, I do transcranial, intranasal, and body pad for twenty-four minutes. I do this in bed upon waking (before I check email, eat breakfast, or do anything else) and again in bed as the last thing I do before going to sleep.

Photobiomodulation is something I recommend for everyone because it helps our bodies recover from the stresses of daily life and helps reduce our risk of many different illnesses and disorders. But it becomes even more important in cases of brain injury—which is actually much more common than most people realize, as you'll see in the next section of the book.

Throughout the remainder of the book, as we explore the topics of traumatic brain injury and neurodegenerative disease in more detail, we'll also look at some of the clinical studies that have demonstrated the benefits of photobiomodulation in humans with those conditions. Many of these, to date, have been observational rather than a randomized controlled trial design, in which one group of subjects gets a placebo. However, some researchers have devised a "sham photobiomodulation" method in which subjects don't know whether light is coming from the device. This is a new and rapidly developing field, and as we have ever more and larger studies, we will learn more about the benefits of photobiomodulation—but the evidence so far is extremely promising.

It's possible our ancestors sensed the healing power of light. Some scientists have hypothesized that the traditional Japanese practice of worshiping the sun during sunrise and sunset may have been driven by intuitive or subconscious knowledge of the biological effects of red and near-infrared light.[231] Chalk it up to one more way modern science is validating ancient wisdom!

In summary, photobiomodulation has proven benefits in various areas—neurodegenerative, traumatic, psychiatric—and these benefits are almost too good to be true. Research in mice indicates a single exposure to light can have effects lasting up to a month. It's safe, gentle, simple, and pain-free—and universally well tolerated without any known side effects. This makes it a desirable alternative to medication, and it's much easier to implement than other lifestyle changes people may struggle to stick with.

Although I may give specific recommendations to some clients for when, where, and how to apply the light, in general, you can't go wrong—just put it wherever your body hurts or needs healing or anywhere on your body that's accessible and convenient. I usually recommend that my clients start out by applying it for twenty minutes a couple of times a day, but there's no harm in going longer. (People with darker skin or lots of body hair will generally need longer treatment times to see the benefits.)

You can even sleep with the light pad or just place it on your low back while watching a movie or reading a book.

By starting with this easy first step to enhance your brain power, you are empowering yourself to take better care of your health overall. This approach to healing—and the research that led me there—have been deeply transformative for me, as they've taught me that my issues with mood and memory weren't just in my imagination and I didn't need to just think my way out of them with the sheer force of willpower. As you'll see in the next section of the book, mood and memory issues have a physiological cause—and as you've already seen in this chapter, these issues have clear, concrete solutions that are eminently doable.

SECTION TWO

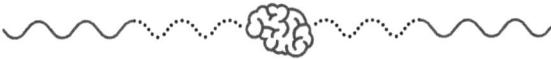

Heart of Darkness

CHAPTER FOUR

Brain Damage and Brain Healing

"Trauma is a fact of life. It does not, however, have to be a life sentence."

—Peter A. Levine

I now realize that my brain damage started at birth.

I don't know all the details—it wasn't something my mother spoke about—but I do know that I had a forceps birth and that it was a traumatic experience for her (and, by definition, for me, too). The human body's capacity for healing is at its best at the beginning of life; this is probably why doctors don't make a big deal about using forceps and simply say the child will heal, if they even mention the consequences at all. But make no mistake—having forceps applied to your head, and the consequent force transmitted to the base of the spinal cord as the doctor pulls, is a type of brain injury.

I know from my training as a chiropractor that pulling the child from the mother's womb can create traction injuries to the neural tracts that run from the brain out through the neck. This long-axis traction is similar to what happens when you are in a car accident. Your shoulders are held in place, in this case, via a seatbelt and shoulder harness, and when the car stops short, your head continues to move forward and pull away from your secured body. At this point, everything above your chest—muscles, ligaments, tendons, joints, bone, and the much more delicate nerve tracts—is placed under extreme tension, so much that they may even rupture. Likewise, a forceps birth is not harmless, as the head is pulled out, but the body drags behind—yet so little attention is paid to the consequences of this relatively common procedure. Can an infant heal from this trauma? Absolutely. But it's an injury nonetheless.

As I learned more about the effects of trauma and stress on the brain, I realized that not just my birth but many other incidents throughout my life created a need for healing. As I share more examples, it's likely you'll see some of yourself in them and begin to call to mind your own experiences that compromised your brain health. You might even want to have a journal handy so you can jot down notes. It's fine if you don't know all the details—just jot down what you do remember. (There's also a questionnaire at the back of the book if you want to take a comprehensive inventory.)

As you read my story and make notes about your own experiences, you may find yourself wondering, "Do I have brain damage, too?" The answer is probably yes—but don't worry. It's not as catastrophic as it might sound. (However, I do want to warn you to proceed with caution—you'll never see *America's Funniest Home Videos* in the same way again. I can't even watch that show anymore because all I see is brain injury after brain injury as people slip and fall, hit their heads, and walk into glass doors. Who will fix all these people and help them heal?)

Note that when I say many people have brain damage, I'm not saying we're all "damaged goods"—but rather, we can all heal from the trauma we've experienced. To create the conditions necessary for healing, it is helpful to first acknowledge the impact (no pun intended) of the trauma and the fact that healing is needed.

It might seem melodramatic to describe what happened to me as *brain damage* and *brain injury*—but part of my goal with this book is to broaden the definition of those terms and bring awareness to just how widespread this damage and these injuries really are. Many activities we view as perfectly healthy actually have a significant impact on our cognitive function.

We are already seeing attitudes start to change as our understanding of this topic grows. You don't often see kids skateboarding or riding bikes without helmets anymore. Many schools and youth sports leagues are adopting changes to the sports offered and the rules of play to protect

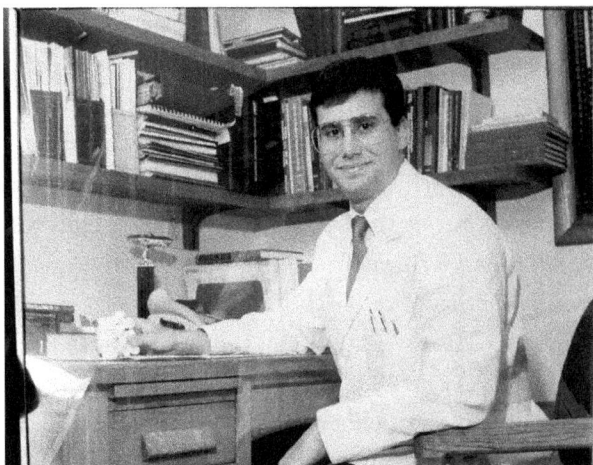

In the office at my first chiropractic practice in Geneva, New York (picture taken for the opening in 1987)

brain health. Attitudes are also changing with regard to adults, with increasing recognition of the long-term effects of brain health for American football players and also of the personality changes that can result from frequent head trauma. (You may recall the 2015 movie *Concussion*, starring Will Smith as Dr. Bennet Omalu, whose research played a key role in bringing attention to the issue of chronic traumatic encephalopathy, or CTE, among retired NFL players. An excellent series of articles by journalist Matt Chaney detailed how the NFL has been skirting the issue of traumatic brain injury-induced cognitive issues and emotional regulation problems in its players for more than a hundred years.[232]) It's my fervent hope that this book can help drive even greater awareness of the issue and, ultimately, get more people engaged in creating and maintaining healthy brains.

Knowing what I know now, I wouldn't want my kids to play tackle football, participate in boxing, or even execute the "header" move in soccer. Everyday lifestyle habits can also deal a blow (metaphorically speaking) to our brain health—but the most important takeaway here is not the need for prevention but rather the fact that we can heal, especially if we understand the conditions that best enable healing.

Back when I was in chiropractic college, we were taught that you couldn't grow new neurons as an adult. Indeed, there are "critical periods" for certain functions—for example, it's much harder to learn a new language or learn to read music as an adult than it is as a child, and full development of the visual system is impossible for children who were deprived of visual stimulation during the first year of life. But scientists understand today, based on plenty of evidence accumulated during the second half of the twentieth century, that the brain can regenerate and rewire well beyond childhood. (The work continues today—it was only in 2016 that the University of California's Michael Merzenich received the Kavli Prize in Neuroscience for his work demonstrating the potential of the brain and the entire nervous system to recover after injury.[233])

So, as you read through this chapter and reflect on your own experiences, don't allow yourself to become too alarmed. The act of letting your worries spiral into worst-case scenarios produces stress hormones that can stand in the way of healing! Later in the book, we'll get into more detail about how to create the optimal conditions for regeneration and recovery. For now, just rest assured that healing is possible—and it is within your control.

A NEW LENS ON LIFE

I first realized I had brain damage while assisting Dr. Gregory Hipskind, one of the leading scientists who studies the consequences of traumatic brain injury (TBI) and how photobiomodulation can help. I was helping him prepare a conference talk about his work with TBI. This was a talk I had reviewed multiple times, but this time, standing in front of the screen and clicking through the slides, something clicked in me. As I reviewed the presentation about the prevalence of chronic TBI and the list of symptoms, I understood that this presentation was describing my personal experience.

One of Dr. Hipskind's studies involved military veterans with traumatic brain injury who had developed PTSD. Their lives were going down the drain; they couldn't concentrate, they couldn't work, they were irritable. Their spouses didn't want them around anymore; they said it was like living with a monster.

I stood there in front of the slide show that described what happens to the lives of people who do not completely recover from a mild TBI and then go on to suffer the additional misfortune of an accidental fall or a car crash, and suddenly it dawned on me: "That's me." I realized that my personality—my irritability, my crankiness, my sleep difficulties—was really not *who I was* at my essence and core, but that those traits were the result of brain damage. My whole perspective shifted in that moment. It was the first time I was able to show myself compassion for those tendencies—and for the first time, I saw that I had the power to change them. That was the moment I said, "These things aren't my fault. They were accidents. But it's my responsibility to fix them."

Once that clicked for me, I started finding more and more examples of brain damage in my life history. My mother always said one of her earliest memories of me involved me getting knocked out. I was an adventurous kid and not particularly cautious. One time my cousin came over and hit me in the head with a tennis racquet. There was another time when I was climbing up a ladder to our treehouse, and I got startled and fell all the way down, banged my head against the riding lawnmower, and was knocked out cold.

I remember, at age six, being taught by my father in our driveway how to ride my bike without training wheels. He and a neighbor friend were so excited and were cheering as I headed out of the driveway and made my first turn left. Unfortunately, as I rode off down the street and gained speed, a car was coming up the street, and I panicked. I couldn't quite manage the left turn, so I crashed into a fire hydrant, flipped my bike end over end, and knocked myself out on the concrete curb. If you're sensing a theme here, you're not wrong—but it's also probably not all that different from the experience of most active kids.

Another of my childhood memories involves competing with my friends to see how many "stingers" we could give each other during football practice. This feeling of tingling and numbness (an electric shock, lightning bolt type feeling) happens when the brachial plexus—the bundle of nerves that runs from the neck and shoulder down the arm—gets stretched away from the neck. Sensations such as this and seeing stars (in which the receptors in your eye that usually respond to light are instead responding to pressure) are evidence of the nervous system discharging. It might seem like harmless child's play—but, actually, it's brain damage. It's an injury, however minor, that your nervous system will need to heal from.

As a collegiate lacrosse player (a sport that, by the way, was developed by the Iroquois to prepare their men for battle), I weathered *many* head injuries. There were also car accidents, which almost by definition create concussions—they say a fifteen-mile-per-hour impact has the same effect as having an eighty-pound bag of cement dropped on your head.

One of my most serious brain injuries was in December 2005. While living in Davenport, Iowa, working on my master's degree, I was out running along the Mississippi River. It was a bright, sunny day—but very cold. As I was running, I saw a puddle, and the childlike impulse to splash my foot in the puddle took hold. I timed my stride to hit the puddle directly in the center—but when I hit it, it wasn't water. It was sheer ice that had looked blue because of the sky's reflection. My feet went straight out from under me, and I landed directly on the back of my head. I don't know how long I lay there unconscious on the ground. When I finally did wake up, the back of my head hurt, and I thought to myself, "Brrrrr... Why am I cold? Why am I lying on the sidewalk? What happened to me?" I got up and just continued running because I had no sense of anything serious having happened. It was only when I got home and my wife asked in a panicked voice, "Where have you been?" that I realized I must have gotten knocked out. I had gone out for a forty-minute run, and I'd been gone for two hours.

That incident had a big effect on me. It changed my personality. I remember sitting in class and the professor asking me, "Joe, are you all right?" because I looked so sullen. It was nearly impossible to concentrate for a while afterward. Statistics class felt impossible. I enjoy a challenge, but trying to perform statistical computation with a recent brain injury was a little much even for me.

That day reviewing the presentation in Dr. Hipskind's office, I felt a renewed sense of hope from my newfound realizations. Once again, life had placed me exactly where I needed to be to solve a problem and take the next step in work that was not only meaningful to me personally but had the potential for widespread impact.

WHAT WE CAN LEARN FROM WOODPECKERS

When a boxer gets hit in the face, the brain sloshes forward, and then when he hits the ground, it bounces to the other side. This is the classic understanding of traumatic brain injury.

But what's also happening, before the moment of impact, is that the nervous system is being stretched—similar to the way the brachial plexus was stretched in those "stingers" my friends and I used to give each other or the way the neural tracts stretch during a forceps birth. This, too, is part of the injury and is part of the reason you don't need to hit your head to have brain damage.

The extent of the brain damage, either with or without impact, depends on the strength of the protective factors in place—and when it comes to protective factors, woodpeckers have a lot to teach us.

As it turns out, these birds are the ultimate experts in traumatic brain injury. They bang their heads against hard surfaces tens of thousands of times a day. How do they do it without suffering debilitating consequences?

Once high-speed cameras allowed for observing birds' movements in finer detail, this technology enabled scientists to make a fascinating discovery: While woodpeckers are pecking, they wrap their exceptionally long tongues around their own necks, constricting the jugular vein and thus increasing the blood volume within the bird's skull. The extra fluid cushions the bird's brain (such as it is) from the constant, jarring impact of pecking.

Taking a cue from nature, researchers are investigating whether a device that constricts blood flow out of the brain might be useful for preventing injuries in athletes—but short of that, there's a very low-tech way to reduce risk: Stay hydrated.

When you see athletes chugging electrolyte drinks on the sidelines, this is not just because they're sweating a lot. Staying well hydrated quite literally reduces the impact on their brains of hitting their heads or running full speed and then coming to a quick stop.

Think of it like shipping your grandmother's tea set. You wouldn't just place this treasured family heirloom into a box and close the box, would you? No—you'd wrap each piece carefully in bubble wrap, so if some clumsy delivery worker happens to drop the box, the tea set would be well protected. We have to do the same thing with our brains, and letting ourselves get dehydrated is like shipping the tea set without bubble wrap.

This points to an important fact. What determines the severity of the brain damage is not just the injury itself—it's the conditions in your body that help determine the severity of the injury as well as the speed and success of the healing. And one of the simplest protective factors—hydration—is also one of the most powerful. As we continue to unfold the **PRONEURO** recipe for healing, you'll learn more about hydration (how much and how?) as well as additional protective factors that will leave you well situated for healing when injury occurs, as it inevitably will for all of us.

Remember that at one time in my chiropractic career, I was the guy teaching everyone else about injury prevention. I was educating my colleagues on how to prevent chiropractic stroke and how to identify the patients who were most at risk. But as I learned more about photobiomodulation and that became more of a focus for me, my approach shifted from avoiding injury to promoting healing.

Yes, prevention is important—and it took me until the age of fifty to make an informed decision to no longer participate in any sports that require a helmet. But complete avoidance of risk is not the goal. The analogy of wrapping ourselves in bubble wrap only gets us so far. We are going to have the beer and get dehydrated. We are going to get in car accidents and slip on ice. Kids are going to give each other stingers and hit each other with tennis racquets. My message in this book is not to avoid all of those experiences. My message is that we can have those experiences and heal from them.

Now, of course, I'm not recommending you go out and take risks recklessly. But when your brain and your nervous system do sustain some type of injury, my goal in this book is to set out—step by step—a plan for you to create the optimal conditions for healing and to remove the factors that interfere with healing.

As it turns out, the factors that set us up for optimal healing generally set us up for optimal functioning—because the body is constantly healing damage within itself every single day of our lives. My new, broader definition of brain damage actually includes damage caused by chronic lifestyle factors that prevent our bodies from healing the way they should—and this, too, is a type of brain damage I myself have suffered.

As a chiropractic student, as a young parent, as a master's student—even though I understood the value of a healthy lifestyle, I had trouble practicing it. The lifestyle interventions chiropractors were focused on a century ago evolved into today's functional medicine, fitness and lifestyle coaching, and personal training industries as well as nutritional supplement companies. They were part of the functional, integrated approach I was using to help my patients—but I didn't yet understand, for the sake of my own life and health, why it was so important to manage stress, to get enough sleep, to pace my exercise routines, to pay attention to what I was eating. These are all things I realized as I started to learn more about mitochondrial function and how much better the body works when it is "operating on all cylinders," so to speak, with mitochondria working at their full capacity. As I learned more about brain injury and how the nervous system heals, I realized I was not creating the optimal conditions in my own life for my body to heal from past trauma and chronic insults.

Watching my mother grapple with dementia also brought my own lifestyle and habits into sharper focus, as you will learn more about in Section Three of this book. In the chapters that present the **PRONEURO** recipe for healing, I'll share with you everything I've learned over the years—but please recognize that your own personal recipe for optimal health may not be the same as mine.

For instance, I've heard it said that a man is as old as his flexibility. That's true to some extent, as a loss of flexibility and mobility can lead to a loss of function that, in turn, leads someone to become less active, lose strength, and suffer an injury. But other people are hypermobile. They have *too much* flexibility. In their case, what would be more useful is to learn to practice and preserve their flexibility in healthy ways while also building strength and stability to keep them from getting injured. This example illustrates why I like to work with people one on one in my coaching practice. Still, in this book, I'm offering guidelines that are useful for all—a basic recipe, if you will, that could be adapted to individual tastes and circumstances.

Once I recognized the damage that had been done to my brain over the years—and once I realized I had the power to set myself up for healing and optimize my own brain health—I took responsibility for creating the lifestyle I personally needed to support a healthy nervous system going forward. This is the kind of ownership I want to encourage you to take as well, and it's never too late in life to start.

I want you to understand that *you* are in charge of your brain, and the choices you make have an effect one way or another—positive or negative. If you skimp on sleep, you're damaging your brain. If you subject your body to chronic stress and inflammation, you're damaging your brain. This is the harsh reality. Although sleep deprivation and chronic stress may not be your fault per se, it's up to you to do what you can to manage them and facilitate recovery.

I think this empowerment piece is what can be missing from support groups for chronic conditions. One of my clients was part of an Alzheimer's support group to help him deal with the strain of caring for his ailing wife; he asked me whether it was supposed to feel comforting to hear that drugs were being developed to slow Alzheimer's patients' decline. "Why would we want that?" he asked me, explaining that, to him, this just meant drawing out his wife's suffering for a longer period of time. In an effort to express compassion, these groups can accept the condition—and the fact that it will progressively worsen—as a given. Having a listening and sympathetic ear is a powerful source of comfort, no doubt. But sometimes the group functions to support you as your condition gets worse to the exclusion of offering a sense of agency or hope for healing and recovery.

There is a concept called the Hero's Journey—a framework developed by Joseph Campbell, the American scholar of literature and mythology—that describes the narrative arc followed by most books and movies. As the story takes you through the development and eventual resolution of a conflict, you, the reader, identify with and root for the main character. Perhaps you are doing that in this book—rooting for me to overcome my brain damage and help my mother grapple with hers. But I want to propose that *you* are the real hero in this saga.

Each of us is facing challenges to our brain health—posed by environmental factors, stressors, injuries, and other hazards. By reducing the harm and healing the damage, we can fulfill our full cognitive potential. This not only leads to breakthroughs in science, technology, and other realms of learning and discovery. It also leads to better relationships, as our brains—no longer clouded by the consequences of injury—can provide a more balanced foundation for our emotional life. And if we can accomplish this as individuals, we can "level up" as a society.

Life is not about (literally or figuratively) wrapping yourself in bubble wrap and staying away from all risk (although I still don't recommend shipping your grandma's tea set without some padding). Things are going to happen; your mission, should you choose to accept it, is to recover. Your brain matters.

Remember, that's not the same thing as saying your mission is to cope. The **PRONEURO** method is not part of the support group that comforts you while your condition gets worse. Why cope when you can heal?

CHAPTER FIVE

Brain Damage: The View from Inside

"The trouble with the rat race is that even if you win,
you're still a rat."

—Lily Tomlin

According to the U.S. Centers for Disease Control and Prevention (CDC), approximately 1.7 million incidents of TBI are documented in the U.S. each year, with an approximately equal number believed to go undiagnosed (making the total number of injuries more than three million a year). Of the cases that are reported, about one-fifth fall into the severe category and the remaining four-fifths are classified as mild. Since we can assume the ones that go unreported are probably *not* severe—and if the total number of cases is double the number actually reported—then the severe cases that make up twenty percent of *reported* cases would make up about ten percent of *total* cases (both reported and unreported). These numbers add up over time, as these injuries do not always resolve within a year, and the CDC estimated in 2013 that 5.3 million Americans were living with TBI-related disabilities.

Of course, this is just one country, and per capita rates may be even higher elsewhere (for example, in places that have a much higher incidence of road accidents). But the point is that on a societal level, the fallout from brain injury is massive—especially when we consider that it's not just the severe injuries that have lasting consequences.

Of the people who have so-called mild TBI, an estimated fifteen percent go on to develop (also so-called) permanent brain damage. Not only is this latter group walking around with lasting consequences but, if they suffer subsequent brain damage, they are even less prepared to heal from it because the healing is not complete from the prior injury—and therefore they are at risk for more severe consequences the next time.

According to the definitions commonly used by the scientific establishment, up to half a million people each year in the U.S. suffer a mild TBI that leads to permanent brain damage. I would argue that a more accurate term for this is *chronic traumatic brain injury*. It is not permanent damage, but rather an opportunity for healing. It may be lasting, but it is not permanent—because the brain can heal.

As discussed in the previous chapter, awareness is growing with regard to the consequences of head trauma, but we still have a long way to go. All the way back in 2003, the CDC recognized TBI as a "silent epidemic," and in 2014, the World Health Organization declared mild TBI a "prominent public health problem." A 2017 review article that examined forty-five previous studies found that "in contrast to the prevailing view that most symptoms of concussion are resolved within three months post-injury, approximately half of individuals with a single [mild TBI] demonstrate long-term cognitive impairment."[234] Yet, the American Medical Association (as of this writing) still maintains that mild TBI symptoms "generally resolve in days to weeks, and leave the patient with no impairment."

When even the world's leading health authorities can't get their story straight about TBI, you know it's an issue that merits deeper examination so we can understand the true impact and the best methods of treatment. In this chapter, I'll pull together insights from research about how TBI affects the brain and what helps it heal. It's my hope that this book might even influence health policy at the national and international levels to recognize and respond to brain injury's toll on human health, happiness, and productivity.

AN INJURY THAT ROBS YOU OF YOURSELF

According to the American Congress of Rehabilitation Medicine, diagnostic criteria for a mild traumatic brain injury include:

+ Loss of consciousness for up to thirty minutes
+ Loss of memory for events immediately before or after the accident for as much as twenty-four hours
+ Alteration of mental state at the time of the accident (e.g., feeling dazed, disoriented, or confused)
+ "Focal neurologic deficits that may or may not be transient, but where the severity of the injury does not exceed loss of consciousness exceeding thirty minutes, post-traumatic amnesia lasting longer than twenty-four hours, or a Glasgow Coma Scale score falling below 13 after thirty minutes." To help you unpack that a bit, focal neurologic deficits are problems that can be traced to a specific brain region (such as problems with speech, hearing, or vision). Someone with a score of 13 or higher on the Glasgow Coma Scale is very close to fully responsive (the maximum score is 15) in terms of visual, verbal, and motor responses to what's happening around them.

I think it's worth giving this definition so you can understand that the way the medical community defines the term *mild* includes head injuries that most of us would not necessarily consider mild. If you hit your head so hard that you lost consciousness for half an hour or you experienced memory loss (even for just one day), would you consider that minor? I think, to most people, that would feel pretty major (or at least moderate). I honestly think the terminology is part of the problem. In the parlance of the doctors who treat the injuries, there's only mild or severe—nothing in between. But when a layperson hears "mild," it doesn't sound like a big deal at all. So, the field would benefit from recasting its terms and definitions. But setting that aside, it's important to understand that some of these so-called "mild" brain injuries are really pretty serious—and in addition, even a head injury that doesn't knock you unconscious or knock out your memory (or doesn't even consist of impact at all) can have serious repercussions.

By the way, are you noticing how many metaphors in the English language use imagery of collision and impact? It's actually been quite difficult to write this book without making bad puns and double entendres—which I think speaks to the importance of these experiences in our lives and how we all implicitly understand that these can be life-changing events, even if science has been slow to recognize that fact.

Interestingly, another native of Geneva, New York, has been instrumental in bringing this issue to light. Ray Ciancaglini, a former professional boxer whom I had the privilege of interviewing for my own research, founded a nonprofit called Second Impact to bring attention to the lasting impact of TBI after he developed Parkinson's disease and dementia. Ray's story has been published as a book,[235] and he also speaks at conferences and other events; his efforts helped to get some safety protections for boxers passed into federal law with the Professional Boxing Safety Act of 1996. Although lots of people are talking about TBI now, Ray brings a unique perspective in that he talks about the importance of treating concussions promptly rather than about avoiding them altogether—an approach very much in line with what I present in this book. Although Ray suffered numerous concussions throughout the course of his boxing career, he traces the beginning of the cognitive changes to a "second impact" that took place when he was sixteen years old. After suffering one concussion, Ray assumed everything was fine since he hadn't been knocked out (which was conventional wisdom back then) and got back in the boxing ring the next week—and immediately sustained another concussion. His story highlights the way the damage can escalate if we don't give our brains a chance to heal.

The term "punch drunk syndrome" was coined and first described by Harrison Martland in a 1928 paper in the *Journal of the American Medical Association* that noted the way boxers sometimes seemed drunk after receiving blows to the head. The paper described how the boxers would become disoriented and have trouble speaking and walking.

Since Martland first described this phenomenon in a medical context, treating it as a neurological condition rather than a punchline, scientists have learned a lot about what happens inside the brain to produce these symptoms. The symptoms that appear immediately after a TBI incident give way to another set of symptoms that unfolds over the weeks and months after the injury—and for the people who develop these secondary symptoms, they are often more severe than the immediate aftermath of the injury.

Early symptoms include headache, dizziness or vertigo, memory problems, lack of awareness of surroundings, nausea, and vomiting. The symptoms that develop later include persistent low-grade headache, light-headedness, poor attention and concentration, excessive or easy fatigue, intolerance of bright light or difficulty focusing vision, intolerance of loud noises, tinnitus, anxiety and depressed mood, irritability, and low frustration tolerance.

The late-developing symptoms can be doubly frustrating because they appear at a time when the initial symptoms are resolving, and those around the injured person might assume they are recovering and becoming better able to return to normal functioning—when at the same time, the injured person is feeling worse and suffering more emotional and cognitive disturbances. Although issues with memory and cognition are well-known consequences of TBI, neuroscientists are becoming increasingly aware that what might seem like emotional issues—impulsivity and violent behavior—actually often result from TBI, so much so that some in the field believe these behavior patterns are a more reliable way to diagnose TBI than brain imaging.[236] (Separate from the research on "mild" concussions—but very related—is the research on the effects of "subconcussive" impact to the head, such as the "header" move soccer players may execute multiple times in a single game or practice, adding up to a rough estimate of two thousand headers throughout the career of a professional soccer player.[237])

Concussions are typically considered to be a functional rather than structural injury in that it doesn't show up on structural brain scans such as a CT or MRI but, rather, are diagnosed based on symptoms such as headaches, dizziness, blurred vision, sensitivity to noise and light, and diminished strength and motor abilities. Because of how they are diagnosed, it's tempting to consider them resolved once those symptoms fade—but researchers are learning that another measurement holds clues to concussions' lasting impact. That measurement is something you learned about in Chapter Three: HRV.

In a nutshell, HRV provides a way to observe the effects of a brain injury after the initial symptoms have resolved—and it also helps us understand why other symptoms persist (or even emerge for the first time) after the initial symptoms' resolution. Something is going on with the nervous system. The body is having trouble bringing the sympathetic and parasympathetic branches of the autonomic nervous system back into balance. Ultimately, HRV may prove to be a more reliable indicator of whether full recovery has been achieved than simply relying on self-reported symptoms.[238] The world of sports would do well to keep this in mind. Once the initial effects of TBI have healed, secondary effects may persist; cognitive tests as well as measuring HRV can provide insight into which athletes are still suffering from lingering effects and should be given more time to heal before returning to play.[239]

Discussions of TBI often make reference to *primary injury* and *secondary injury*. There may be physical injury from the impact of the brain sloshing around in the skull—this is the primary injury. But the impact also sets off a chain reaction of cellular processes inside the brain: "free radical generation, calcium-mediated damage, hypoxia, and increased intracranial pressure."[240] Disruption of the neurovascular unit—i.e., disruption to the blood-brain barrier—initiates something called a *neurovascular cascade*, resulting in alterations of the sodium/potassium pump functioning, calcium influx into the mitochondria, an increase in neuro-excitatory amino acids such as glutamate and aspartate, neuroinflammation, decreased cerebral blood flow, and brain edema (also known as swelling).[241] Essentially, the body maintains a finely calibrated balance of minerals such as sodium, potassium, and calcium that support vital processes throughout the body. This delicate balance is just as important for brain function as it is for bodily functions like heartbeat and maintaining the proper fluid balance—but TBI can upset that delicate balance in the brain, with consequences such as a buildup of calcium that leads to cell death or, on the other end of the spectrum, the survival of cells that aren't working correctly and therefore *should* be killed off and recycled by the body for optimal functioning.[242] In other words, when you upset this balance, it can either result in too many cells dying or too many cells surviving—and neither is good.

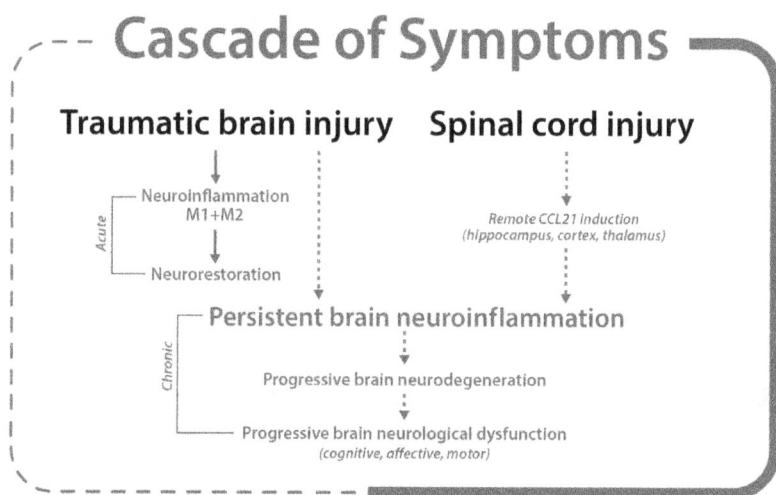

Cascade of Symptoms

Traumatic brain injury   Spinal cord injury

Acute
- Neuroinflammation M1+M2
- Neurorestoration

Remote CCL21 induction
(hippocampus, cortex, thalamus)

Chronic
- Persistent brain neuroinflammation
- Progressive brain neurodegeneration
- Progressive brain neurological dysfunction *(cognitive, affective, motor)*

In both TBI and spinal cord injury, neuroinflammation leads to neurodegeneration and neurological dysfunction, with effects on movement, cognition, and emotion. If the body successfully reduces inflammation after the acute phase of TBI, neurorestoration and recovery are possible; if inflammation persists, the subject will continue into a chronic phase of secondary injury.

Since evidence of a secondary injury does not show up on an MRI, patients are sometimes told they've healed and there is nothing wrong with them. This can be a blow to their self-esteem. People may even feel crazy when they're told everything is normal—and meanwhile their inability to focus is affecting them at work, and at home they are having trouble with their relationships, experiencing problems with emotional regulation, acting out of character, feeling like they are just not themselves. (It probably goes without saying that being told nothing is wrong when everything feels off only compounds the emotional challenges that can accompany TBI.) Depression and other mental health conditions affect a large percentage of TBI survivors in the first year post-injury.[243, 244] In fact, one 2020 research paper characterized TBI as "the single most common biological cause of psychiatric symptoms" amid a discussion of how injuries, infections, inflammation, gut-brain dysregulation, and other physiological causes can be identified for psychiatric illnesses much more commonly than we typically believe.[245] This can have wide-ranging consequences in people's lives: Disproportionately high rates of TBI are seen in homeless shelters and prisons.[246]

Recent developments in imaging have allowed for the identification of four separate ways TBI causes long-lasting effects in the brain:

+ Lesions of the gray matter and white matter
+ Disconnection of the networks that enable high-order cognitive, emotional, and social functioning
+ Disruption of the activity of essential neurotransmitters such as serotonin, dopamine, acetylcholine, and norepinephrine
+ Lesions that affect the HPA axis (a system you will learn more about in the next section of the book; for now, just know that it influences the parasympathetic nervous system's ability to respond to changing conditions in an agile fashion)[247]

One fascinating finding is that the aftermath of a brain injury shares certain features with age-related neurodegeneration. Half a century after Martland's groundbreaking "punch drunk" research paper, a different team of researchers examined the brains of fifteen boxers posthumously. They found "neurofibrillary tangles"—the aggregates of hyperphosphorylated tau protein that are considered a primary marker for Alzheimer's disease.[248] A 2014 survey of the literature on CTE (a phenomenon defined in reference to repetitive sports-induced head injuries) characterized the tangles of tau protein as resulting from a "pathological cascade" involving "a series of metabolic, ionic, membrane, and cytoskeletal disturbances" that can play out years after the primary injury or injuries.[249] Other studies have noted "diffuse axonal injury"—damage to the part of the neuron responsible for transmitting electrical signals—as a consequence of TBI that predisposes a person to neurodegenerative conditions in an epigenetic process.[250] This diffuse axonal injury has implications for the Krebs cycle, mitochondrial function, and ATP production in the brain.[251] We will go into this more in the third section of the book, but mitochondrial damage is a key feature of the aftermath of brain injury,[252] and we can look at it as an issue of the brain not having enough energy to function on all cylinders. Here again, brain injury upsets the delicate balance, causing a condition called *excitotoxicity* in which an overload of a common neurotransmitter causes injury to the neurons, which, in turn, upsets the calcium balance and, through effects on the mitochondria, eventually leads to cell death.[253]

In a healthy brain, tau proteins play a role in regulating and stabilizing the microtubules that are key to mitochondrial movement—but after a brain injury or in a neurodegenerative condition, they detach from the microtubules and adhere together to form tangles, which are toxic to the surrounding neurons and glial cells (that is, the other types of cells that are part of the nervous system aside from neurons). But recent research is showing that photobiomodulation can facilitate the clearance of these tau proteins as well as the amyloid beta associated with Alzheimer's disease and is more effective the sooner the therapy is begun.[254, 255]

The physiological basis for these symptoms has been further substantiated by research with mice. Like humans, mice display increased risk-taking, sleep disturbances, cognitive issues, and depression after being subjected to TBI.[256] This chain reaction is the secondary injury that causes a drop in HRV, indicating the nervous system still has healing to do before it is fully recovered. Some more sophisticated imaging methods can pick up on changes in blood flow to capture the symptoms of secondary injury, but the average person with mild TBI doesn't have access to this and doesn't need it. You can use HRV instead to measure whether you've created the conditions for healing or have more work to do to get there.

It's been well documented that a drop in HRV typically follows TBI, and one study connected these lower HRV scores to the impaired social and emotional functioning that is often seen in the wake of TBI. The same study showed that HRV biofeedback improved HRV scores for both the TBI patients and the control group, thus providing a promising avenue for treatment of TBI—and for improving social and emotional functioning for all of us.[257] (That's right—don't forget the breathing techniques you learned about in the last chapter!) Researchers have found that among TBI sufferers, reductions in HRV are proportional to the severity of the injury and are also associated with worse outcomes.[258] This may seem obvious—more serious injuries lead to more serious symptoms and worse outcomes—but I would like to propose that if we can achieve improvement on the mediating factor, HRV, we can interrupt this vicious cycle and pave the way for healing.

An estimated one-third of sports-related concussions and ten percent of non-sports concussions result in what's called *postconcussive syndrome*, defined as having three or more of the following symptoms that do not resolve within three to six weeks of the injury: headache, dizziness, fatigue, irritability, insomnia, concentration difficulties, or memory difficulties. A case study of a competitive athlete who was coached in a ten-week course of biofeedback breathing after she suffered a concussion documented the improvement in both her postconcussive syndrome symptoms and overall physiological indicators of her readiness to return to training. Although a case study involves just one subject and does not have a control group for comparison, the authors noted that they considered it unlikely that this subject's symptoms would have resolved on their own "since the patient was symptomatic for many months prior to the HRV biofeedback program and did not improve after ... three months of standard treatment."[259] Other papers have documented similar case studies showing improvement of low HRV following TBI with the help of biofeedback breathing.[260]

Studies have shown that persistent low HRV can continue to affect athletes returning to training after their concussion symptoms have faded,[261] reminding us of the importance of gradually building up training intensity after an injury and monitoring the nervous system's recovery— and of practices like biofeedback breathing to help support this recovery.

The aftereffects of TBI can be seen even more clearly by digging into the components of HRV[262]—for example, the low-frequency and high-frequency values—and although we won't get into that level of detail in this book, I expect that the scientific understanding of HRV will continue to develop, and that within a few years, we will understand much more about it and be able to monitor and analyze it with much greater specificity. Certain types of cognitive tasks can help reengage the prefrontal cortex—an area of the brain you'll learn much more about in Section Three—and bring about an accompanying rise in HRV[263] (a finding that can help inform therapeutic approaches).

Recall the relationship between HRV and emotions—HRV can be thought of as your "joy score," and low HRV is correlated with depression. It turns out that HRV can help predict when the fallout from a head injury may be leading into depression. For example, one study found that diminished HRV following mild TBI predicted the onset of depression eighteen months later.[264] If we can help the nervous system shift into parasympathetic activation, it seems we may be able to interrupt this chain reaction or at least reduce its severity and duration.

In general, the impact of TBI on the autonomic nervous system seems to play a role in how primary injury compounds into secondary injury, as the sympathetic nervous system becomes hyperactive and the body is not able to shift into parasympathetic rest-and-digest (and heal) mode.[265] Inflammation also plays a role, as the chronic inflammation that persists after the primary injury heals is a hallmark of secondary injury and seems to provide the conditions for progressive neurodegeneration—that is, for things to get worse instead of better.[266]

Although I have divided brain injury and age-related neurodegeneration into separate sections of this book, keep in mind that they are not completely separate. They share some symptoms and pathways in common, and in fact, one of the main points of this book is that injuries and brain damage can add up over time to contribute to the changes we commonly attribute to aging. Those changes are not inevitable. *We do not need to accept cognitive decline as part of aging. We are not doomed to become* absent-minded or emotionally volatile, either with aging or in the wake of a brain injury. This book provides a reason for hope and a path to healing.

A BRAIN WITHOUT SLEEP IS A BRAIN THAT DOESN'T HEAL

In your recipe for creating the conditions for healing brain damage, sleep is one of the key ingredients, and you can find plenty of information about how to get better quality sleep in Chapter Ten. For the purposes of this chapter, I want to take a moment to focus in on how sleep is involved in the vicious cycle of secondary injury following TBI.

Research shows that after suffering a TBI, people typically get less REM sleep (the sleep phase during which we are dreaming with rapid eye movement—and the phase that's essential to consolidating learning and memory).[267] Insomnia and sleep apnea are also prevalent among TBI sufferers[268]—and the causality can go both ways. People with chronic insomnia are at higher risk for TBI because they are more likely to get into a car accident or take a fall. Insomnia can amplify TBI's cognitive effects, such as interfering with memory, attention, and executive function. Research has even found structural changes in the brain associated with poor sleep.[269] That's right, the awful feeling of being chronically sleep-deprived is not just a matter of perception—the size and shape of certain brain regions are altered when we don't get enough high-quality sleep. See what I mean about a vicious cycle?

Disrupted or low-quality sleep seems to be one way head injuries lead to mood and personality disorders. It's shocking, actually: Every major psychiatric illness is associated with a high prevalence of sleep disturbances. Not just a few. Not most of them. *All* of them. Quite simply, if you aren't sleeping well, you are at a higher risk for mental as well as physical illness.

One research study examined how sleep helps us consolidate memories and process the emotions associated with them by comparing subjects who had experienced concussions but had healed from the primary injury (it had been at least one year since the incident that caused the concussion) with another group of subjects who had never experienced a concussion. Study subjects were shown negative stimuli (pictures with disturbing or upsetting content) twice; some remained awake for twelve hours between the viewings, and others slept between the viewings. Electrodes were used to measure the subjects' brains' responses to the images. Subjects who had never had a concussion showed evidence of their brains habituating to the pictures while they slept—the magnitude of their response to the same image was less after sleeping. But for the subjects with a history of concussion, this consolidation did not occur. In fact, in the concussion sufferers, the response magnitude was slightly *less* for the group that stayed awake than for the group that slept between the two viewings. In other words, the subjects with a history of concussion did not habituate to seeing the negative images while they were sleeping the way the subjects who never suffered a concussion did—indicating the injury may have interfered with their brains' ability to help them cope with disturbing experiences in everyday life. This study shows how sleep plays a role in emotional and mental health—and how this process goes haywire after a head injury, with consequences for emotional well-being.[270]

Photobiomodulation helps you sleep better (turn to Chapter Ten for more on that). We also know from animal studies that photobiomodulation can help reduce the effects of sleep deprivation on our bodies and brains. One study found that sleep-deprived mice that received photobiomodulation once a day for three days showed less evidence of cognitive impairment than sleep-deprived mice that did not receive the treatment. This study also identified mitochondrial damage and oxidative stress as the mechanisms by which sleep deprivation causes memory impairment; photobiomodulation was able to temper this effect, activating the antioxidant defense system and maintaining mitochondrial survival.[271]

One of the ways acute TBI becomes a chronic issue is when the injury slows down or prevents the healing process by interfering with one of the very things that would make the biggest difference for healing: high-quality sleep. It does appear likely that photobiomodulation helps with sleep quality, although more research is needed to solidify the link.

What is clear, even setting aside the effect on sleep, is that photobiomodulation can help break the vicious cycle of secondary injury after TBI.

PHOTOBIOMODULATION CAN HELP THE BRAIN HEAL

There is currently no drug that can interrupt the chain reaction and stop the progression of primary injury into secondary injury—but there are plenty of steps you can take to activate your body's innate healing power. It starts with a practice that will be familiar to you at this point. At least in mice, studies have shown that photobiomodulation can prevent primary from progressing into secondary injury. (It's pretty fascinating how they arrived at this specific finding. They identified a specific gene that, when missing, predisposes mice to develop secondary injury, rather than healing completely, after a TBI—and then they showed that photobiomodulation helps even the mice that are missing that gene heal, probably due to its effects on the mitochondria and inflammation.[272]) Across numerous studies in humans, photobiomodulation has been shown to have beneficial effects in treating TBI—improving memory, learning, and overall cognitive function by stimulating neurogenesis, reducing inflammation, and protecting the affected neurons from dying.[273]

I can't emphasize enough the quality-of-life improvements that correlate with these changes. This isn't just about abstract concepts used as variables in a research study. People see enormous improvements on a practical level because of photobiomodulation. In a study from a research team including my friend Dr. Hamblin, whom you met earlier, eleven subjects received photobiomodulation three times a week for six weeks. All had a history of concussion—some as long as eight years before the study started—and all saw improvements to their memory, verbal skills, and executive function.[274] In one case, the improvements were pronounced enough that they enabled a subject to return to work when that had not been possible before. Another subject went from nonverbal to verbal. Another case study involved a woman who had been greatly hindered in her ability to work and apply herself to cognitive tasks after suffering a TBI in a car accident seven years earlier; after receiving photobio-modulation weekly for two months, she was able to increase her time on the computer to three hours per work session from her previous limit of twenty minutes.[275] In yet another case study, just five photobiomodulation treatments over the course of a week resolved a TBI sufferer's migraine headaches to the point that he could actually get a good night's sleep for the first time in two years.[276] Imagine the difference these improvements could make for the quality of life of TBI sufferers everywhere if more people had access to photobiomodulation.

Some studies have documented changes to brain structure as well as function with photobiomodulation. For example, an MRI of a hockey player who tried photobiomodulation to help with the lasting effects of a concussion found changes including increased volume in the hippocam-pus, a crucial brain area for memory, after eight weeks of treatment.[277] Photobiomodulation has also been tested for the emotional repercus-sions of TBI, with encouraging results: Depression after TBI went into remission for thirty-six out of thirty-nine subjects in one study.[278] Chronic TBI patients who received ten photobiomodulation treatments over the course of two months showed improvement in symptoms, including sleep disturbance, cognition, mood dysregulation, anxiety, and irritability.[279] Upon completion of a twelve-week photobiomodulation program, the cohort of thirty patients with mild to moderate TBI (with symptoms per-sisting for six months or more) all saw significant improvement in symp-toms for at least two of the four domains evaluated (cognitive, mood, daily functioning, and sleep problems).[280] And in a study of patients with moderate and severe traumatic brain injury, their memory, attention, and mood improved significantly when they received photobiomodulation treatments three times a week for six weeks, compared to a control group that received placebo treatments with a device that delivered a different type of light.[281]

In most human studies of photobiomodulation, there is no control group for comparison, so there's always the chance that subjects would have improved on their own even without the treatment. That's why I'm thankful animal research allows us to have more certainty that the healing we're witnessing is actually due to photobiomodulation. Ethical concerns prevent us from inducing brain injuries in humans as part of a research study, and it's sad even to think about inducing them in lab animals, but I'm grateful for the contribution these animals are making to human health. Photobiomodulation has been shown to improve neurological performance in studies with mice that suffered traumatic brain injuries.[282] Mice with moderate to severe TBI had a significant improvement in Neurological Severity Score compared to controls four weeks after a single treatment.[283] Four weeks post-TBI, mice that received photobiomodulation treatments showed better healing of their brain lesions and less depression (measured by whether they actively swim or give up when dropped into a tank full of water) than their counterparts that did not receive the treatment.[284] In a study of rats, photobiomodulation after surgery or TBI was associated with improvement at the behavioral, cellular, and chemical levels relative to the control group that did not receive the treatment.[285] And because the hippocampus—a crucial brain region for memory—is one of the brain regions most affected by TBI, researchers tested injured rats with a cognitive test that specifically requires the involvement of the hippocampus and found that the rats that had received photobiomodulation performed significantly better on the test than did their counterparts that did not receive the treatment.[286]

Incidentally, there is also evidence that starting photobiomodulation soon after the injury occurs can help stem the resulting damage.[287] In a study of mice that suffered TBI, the mice that received photobiomodulation within the first eight hours after their injuries had better recovery scores than the mice that did not receive the treatment. Various timing and formats were tested for the photobiomodulation treatments; in one treatment group, sixty-three percent of the mice achieved full recovery by two months after their injuries.[288] This knowledge probably won't apply to you as you're reading this book, but keep it in mind for future reference. Knowing how common head injuries are, we're all bound to know somebody who hits their head in a car accident or a hard fall before long.

In a study of sixty-eight men and women with moderate TBI, photobiomodulation treatment (applied through the skull with a helmet) was begun within three days of the injury. After three treatment sessions, MRIs of the patients who had received the treatment showed statistically significant differences in the brain's white matter from scans of patients in the placebo group (who sat for sessions of equal length but wore a helmet that did not actually deliver near-infrared light). The paper notes that not enough is known about what healing and improvement look like in the brain to conclusively interpret the MRI results on their own, but the differences, in this case, correlated with improvement in symptoms for the group that received photobiomodulation (that is, relative to the control group, the treatment group's symptoms improved more).[289]

So, how exactly does photobiomodulation help the brain heal? For starters, it has the same effect on mitochondria in the brain as it does on mitochondria everywhere in the body, helping them produce more ATP—thus improving the bioenergetic capacity of cells in the brain, or in simpler words, helping the brain cells have more energy.

Daniel Bourassa—like me, a scientific researcher who studies photobiomodulation and also started out as a chiropractor—describes photobiomodulation as "mitochondrial resuscitation." One of the most amazing things about it is that the mitochondria seem to use light to bring them back into optimal balance—whether the initial problem was an overactive or an underactive inflammatory process. Remember how inflammation needs to be not too little and not too much—but like Goldilocks and her porridge, *juuuust* right. Photobiomodulation seems to help the body recalibrate to reach that "just right" level of inflammation to deal with an acute threat but not overdo it with a response that is too broad or stays active too long. As Michael Hamblin puts it: "Over-irradiance of injured tissue does not result in a worse outcome than if photobiostimulation was not performed at all. Therefore, photobiostimulation is a very safe modality and can be employed early in acute phase treatment, even before the full extent of the injury is known."

Most importantly for the purpose of brain injury, photobiomodulation has this effect on the mitochondria of neurons. Inflammation has been shown to be an important marker that may help to predict when TBI will develop into CTE.[290] This is why it is critical to start using photobiomodulation as soon as possible after brain injury—or to use it as a preventive measure throughout life to optimize the body's innate healing abilities and help us recover from daily stressors and minor damage we may not even be aware of. Light applied to the tibia has been shown to have beneficial effects for both the brain and the heart (most likely through a phenomenon involving stem cells that I'll explain later in this chapter), and light applied to the low back has been shown to have benefits for depression sufferers.[291]

What's more, this mitochondrial resuscitation takes place without an increase in reactive oxygen species when it comes from photobiomodulation.[292] Here are Bourassa's words so you can marvel along with me at just how powerful photobiomodulation actually is: "From a neurobiological perspective, the cascade of beneficial cellular activity includes increased mitochondrial membrane potential, nitric oxide release, and modulation of intracellular calcium. Signaling pathways and transcription factors are activated, leading to the production of anti-apoptotic, pro-proliferation, antioxidant, anti-inflammatory, and pro-angiogenic factors. Regeneration of neurons through neurogenesis and synaptogenesis aids in restoration and maintenance of cognitive function and supports neuroplasticity during the recovery process. Brain repair is directly affected by the expression of genes related to cell proliferation and indirectly through regulation of the expression of genes related to cell migration and remodeling, DNA synthesis and repair, ion channel and membrane potential, cell metabolism, and suppression of apoptosis. Cognitive function benefits by stimulation of these brain repair pathways and reduction of neurofibrillary tangles. Neuroplasticity is supported by an increase in brain-derived neurotrophic factor (BDNF) and synapsin-1 that encourages synaptogenesis and is significantly upregulated by photobiostimulation."[293] With results like that, how could anyone concerned about brain health *not* want to use photobiomodulation?

In a study conducted in Brazil, ten patients with severe TBI received photobiomodulation treatments three times a week for six weeks and experienced improved cerebral blood flow and, consequently, improved cerebral oxygenation.[294] (This particular effect is going to become even more important when we get to the third section of this book.) Photobiomodulation can also help people improve sleep quality and quantity for people recovering from TBI,[295, 296] setting their brains up for more efficient healing.

TBI causes both a continual release of excitatory neurotransmitters and an impairment of uptake mechanisms for those neurotransmitters—leading to excessive levels that can result in excitotoxicity.[297] Notice how, as with so many aspects of our health, this is a case of dose-dependent response. Vital as these neurotransmitters are to our brains' functioning, they become poisonous to neurons when they build up to a certain level of concentration—and this is a key factor in how primary injury cascades into secondary injury in TBI. Our observations of photobiomodulation show us that it does not contribute to excitotoxicity. In fact, where this condition exists, photobiomodulation can help alleviate it. I like to say that photobiomodulation is acceleratory, not excitatory. It speeds the engine up to as fast as it can go but not so fast a speed that it overheats and burns out.

Noting that "repeated LED application of red and near-infra-red light can improve cellular activity of the damaged brain tissue and promote synaptic plasticity, which can enhance therapeutic outcomes" after TBI, one Boston-based expert on TBI rehabilitation recommends including photobiomodulation in treatment plans along with transcra-nial magnetic stimulation and computer-based "brain training" programs designed for rehabilitation.[298] While I certainly recommend making use of all the available tools, the advantage of photobiomodulation is that it can be done at home and does not rely on a level of precision that requires an expert's oversight.

Photobiomodulation has similar pro-survival effects for neurons as it does for cells elsewhere in the body: "Mitochondria are thought to be the principal photoreceptors, and increased ATP, reactive oxygen species, intracellular calcium, and release of nitric oxide are the initial events. Activation of transcription factors then leads to expression of many protective, anti-apoptotic, anti-oxidant, and pro-proliferation gene products."[299] To maximize the effects for the brain, I recommend using a light helmet and an intranasal photobiomodulation device. (In case you're wondering, yes, there is scientific proof that the light penetrates the skull to reach the brain tissue underneath.[300, 301]) Remember that no matter where you apply the light, it will have effects throughout your body, but it makes sense that the effects would be the most concentrated for the area closest to the light.

Nevertheless, if you don't have a light helmet or intranasal device, using a body pad will still have beneficial effects for your brain. As you'll recall from Chapter Three, this is because of the abscopal effect—the indirect effects of photobiomodulation applied somewhere on the body to areas beyond that specific area. Part of this is due to the effects of photobiomodulation on fluids that travel around the body. This encompasses multiple mechanisms—some of which may not have even been discovered yet—but an important one is the mitokine (signaling) function. When the body senses damage, it shifts into energy conservation mode. The bioenergetic enhancement that occurs where photobiomodulation is applied results in signals that travel throughout the body. When inflammation is out of control, it actually impedes healing rather than enhancing it—but thanks to photobiomodulation, the signals that travel to the brain via the mitokine effect convey the message that it's safe to let healing processes get underway instead of staying in the stalled-out protective state represented by all the symptoms of secondary injury after TBI.

Key to this process is something called the *cell danger response*, which happens when a cell encounters a chemical, physical, or microbial threat that could injure or kill it. This happens because of infections or ingested toxins that enter our bloodstream—and it's probably part of the explanation for how stress and trauma contribute to ill health via allostatic load. Many components of the cell danger response—e.g., the mitochondrial unfolded protein response, the oxidative stress response, and inflammation—have been studied in isolation, but viewing these components as part of a coordinated danger signal has allowed scientists to see the role the cell danger response plays in the development of a widely varied list of diseases: from asthma and emphysema to Tourette's syndrome; from diabetes to schizophrenia; from lupus and multiple sclerosis to ADHD and autism spectrum disorders. And, yes, the list also includes neurode-generative conditions such as Alzheimer's and Parkinson's diseases.[302]

In the cell danger response, the body mounts such defenses as stiffer cell membranes and releasing antiviral and antimicrobial substances to kill invaders. The cell danger response also includes epigenetic features—that's right, your gene expression is literally altered when your body is under threat. And metabolism is lowered so you'll feel tired and have the urge to rest.

When this goes on for too long and the cell danger response fails to resolve, chronic disease can result. Our systems were never meant to stay in this state indefinitely. And through its effects on the mitochondria, inflammation, and autonomic nervous system balance via HRV, photo-biomodulation can help quiet the response down and signal that the body can turn down its defenses and enter healing mode. (Remember, you can't heal when you're in fight-or-flight mode; the body and brain must sense safety in order to move into healing and regeneration mode.)

Photobiomodulation also has the potential to help people with more serious brain injuries than concussions. For example, hypoxic-ischemic injury is one of the most common serious birth complications, affecting four in every thousand newborns in the U.S.—with twenty percent of these not surviving and another thirty percent dealing with long-term neurological impacts. Research in rats (since it is not ethical to induce this type of injury in humans) has shown that photobiomodulation mitigates the effects of such injuries on the brain—effects that include cognitive impairment, brain volume shrinkage, neuron loss, and dendritic and synaptic injury. The researchers also found that photobiomodulation restores healthy mitochondrial dynamics and prevents neuronal apoptosis.[303]

About half of the people who survive cardiac arrest experience impaired memory, attention, and executive function afterward. This is believed to be due to *global cerebral ischemia*—that is, temporary low oxygen conditions in the brain due to the heart stopping. Induced hypother-mia is currently the only approved therapy for global cerebral ischemia after cardiac arrest. This treatment has adverse effects—such as electrolyte imbalances, heart arrhythmia, and blood sugar dysregulation—and the evidence isn't even conclusive on whether it actually has any benefit.

There is some evidence that mitochondrial function plays a role in determining which cardiac arrest survivors will go on to develop cognitive issues. (Surprise, surprise! Are you starting to see how nearly everything comes back to the mitochondria?) For this reason, photobiomodulation is a promising treatment for helping cardiac arrest survivors avoid these cognitive consequences, and at least in animal studies, photobiomodulation has been shown to protect neurons from dying after they are deprived of oxygen.[304, 305] This makes sense since mitochondrial dysfunction is known to play a pivotal role in the chain of events that leads some neurons to die off in the wake of global cerebral ischemia.[306] In one study, the control group of rats that did not receive photobiomodulation after experiencing global cerebral ischemia lost eighty-six percent of the neurons in a key region of the hippocampus to cell death; the rats that were treated with photobiomodulation lost between eleven and thirty-five percent of the neurons in that region.[307] That's a significant difference!

Similar effects were seen in rats that suffered hypoxic-ischemic injury as newborns. With seven days of photobiomodulation treatment after the injury, the baby rats had significantly reduced damage and cell death in key brain regions compared to the control group. The researchers also observed reduced oxidative damage and improved mitochondrial dynamics in the rats that received photobiomodulation.[308]

Doctors still learn in medical school that brain damage from a stroke is irreversible, and you saw at the beginning of this chapter that the medical field still considers brain damage resulting from a severe TBI to be "permanent." But the way we understand these types of brain damage is changing rapidly as science shows us that much more of the damage is reversible than we once thought. As scientists come to understand more about stem cells, their discoveries are revealing more about the role stem cells can play in healing—and how photobiomodulation can help.

STEM CELLS AND HEALING:
PAVING THE PATH FOR NEUROREGENERATION

Across multiple realms of scientific inquiry, from space exploration to inward exploration on a subatomic scale, "the ultimate frontier extending across all these vast scales happens to be light." Just as light has transformed diagnostics and surgery, it can now transform regenerative medicine. This was the theme of a 2016 special issue of the journal *Photomedicine and Laser Surgery* that focused on stem cells and photobiomodulation.

Although the term *stem cells* might call to mind the ethical controversies that have dominated popular news stories about the topic, the research about stem cells and photobiomodulation has nothing to do with the embryonic stem cells that elicit religious objections. Rather, this research has focused on *mesenchymal stem cells*. These are cells each of us has within our own bodies—so when I discuss photobiomodulation's effect on stem cells, know that I am not talking about injecting another person's stem cells.

Mesenchymal stem cells are present in the bone marrow, among other locations, and they are able to differentiate into multiple different tissue types, including bone, cartilage, muscle, fat, and connective tissue. (Whether this mechanism exists for neurons is a topic of scientific debate,[309] but either way, we know that photobiomodulation promotes neurogenesis and synaptogenesis via other mechanisms.) In addition to stem cells, as adults, we also still have *progenitor cells* that are more limited than stem cells in the kind of cells they can become but which can nevertheless divide into new, healthy cells to replace damaged ones. (Recall the discussion of epigenetics in Chapter Two and remember that the new cells will be developing in your body's present-day environment—so they have the potential for developing in a healthier way than the cells they're replacing if you have recently made some lifestyle improvements such as changing your diet, sleeping more, or sitting for a daily session with your light pad.)

When you sustain a physical injury, mesenchymal stem cells come out of the bone marrow and into our circulation to help replace the cells that were damaged. This process works best when we are young, and its effectiveness declines with age. But photobiomodulation can turn back the clock on aging, in a sense, by helping that process work better—especially when applied to the long bones of the leg and arm or to thin bones where the bone marrow is closer to the surface, such as the sternum. Studies in the *Photomedicine and Laser Surgery* special issue showed that applying photobiomodulation enhanced mesenchymal stem cell activity after injuries to the kidney, heart, and knee. Other research in the same issue identified some of the mechanisms by which photobiomodulation promotes wound healing, decreases scar tissue, and reduces pain and inflammation.[310]

To understand more about how this works, let's look at the typical model of tissue damage and death. When a tissue loses its blood supply, this is known as *ischemia*; if ischemia goes on for too long, it results in tissue death, or *infarction*. With ischemia, the tissue recovers when blood flow returns. With infarction, the neurons (or whatever type of cells we are speaking about) cease to work. It is harder to recover from infarction than ischemia—but if we can keep ischemia from proceeding into infarction, we boost the odds of recovery. Putting this in a brain injury context: If we build the resiliency of our neurons, we can actually reduce our likelihood of sustaining a more severe injury that will be harder to recover from. The concept of hormesis, introduced in Chapter Two, applies throughout the body—including in the brain, where cells grow stronger and more resilient in response to stress as long as the stress does not overwhelm them. So, there are two ways photobiomodulation can aid neuroregeneration: by improving mitochondrial function so cell death never occurs in the first place and through its effect on stem cells, which allow for the replacement of cells that weren't able to survive.

The first section of the book focused on mitochondrial function because the average reader has much to learn about that—but photobiomodulation's effect on stem cells is equally important. Remember that before the 1960s, when the concept of neuroplasticity became widely accepted and understood, medical students learned that neural networks were fixed in early adulthood and no new brain cells developed after that. Until then, it was widely believed that any brain cells that die once someone becomes an adult could never be replaced! We know now that neural networks can rewire and brain cells can regenerate throughout the life course—and mesenchymal stem cells are the reason this is possible. (By the way, it's not *only* the effect on stem cells that is important for the brain;[311] there is also evidence that mitochondrial dysfunction plays a role in neurodegeneration, and thus the effect on the mitochondria is important for the brain, too.)

Let's pause to review the mechanisms and benefits of photobiomodulation. I'll quote one particular journal article that lists them all out in a compelling way, ending with the most recent benefits discussed in this chapter. Photobiomodulation, the article states, "has been scientifically proven as a beneficial therapeutic modality for numerous diseases and diseased conditions. Using very specific laser and light-emitting diode irradiation parameters, specific cellular activities can be induced, namely, cellular proliferation and viability while stimulating mitochondrial activity, thereby increasing [ATP] production, synthesis of DNA and RNA, and activating cell-signaling cascades including the production of reactive oxygen species, nitric oxide release, activating cytochrome c oxidase, and modifying intracellular organelle membrane activity, calcium flux, and expression of stress proteins. ... Low-intensity laser irradiation has been shown to induce stem cell activity by increasing migration, proliferation, and viability; activating protein expression, and inducing differentiation in progenitor cells."[312]

Across many journals, studies in rodents and humans have documented both of the ways photobiomodulation helps damaged cells heal and regenerate. Studies have shown photobiomodulation's ability, via its effect on mesenchymal stem cells, to reverse ischemic damage to both the heart and the kidneys in rats and pigs.[313, 314, 315]

In a study that used diabetic rats, photobiomodulation and mesenchymal stem cell therapy both aided the healing of wounds infected with methicillin-resistant *Staphylococcus aureus* (MRSA), a common kind of antibiotic-resistant bacteria that can be life-threatening if not properly treated.[316] In rats with osteoporosis, photobiomodulation was able to activate bone marrow stem cells, indicating the treatment could be helpful in reversing bone loss from the condition.[317] In a task called the Morris water maze test—commonly used in experiments with mice, it tests how quickly they can swim through a maze to find a platform that allows them to climb out of the pool and usually also tests how well they learn by measuring the improvement in the time it takes to get to the platform in subsequent rounds—brain-injured mice that received photobiomodulation treatment got faster at swimming to the exit compared to their peers that suffered similar brain injuries and did not receive photobiomodulation.[318] Pivotally, another study of mice that suffered brain injuries found that photobiomodulation increased the mice's levels of brain-derived neurotrophic factor (BDNF), an essential molecule for neuroplasticity.[319]

Hamblin's own research with mice showed that photobiomodulation stimulates neurogenesis in the hippocampus (the part of the brain that encodes memories) and the subventricular zone (a key brain area for neurogenesis, and thus neuroregeneration, throughout the brain).[320] Describing the significance, Hamblin and colleagues wrote: "The likelihood that [photobiomodulation] can induce the brain to repair itself after injury suggests that laser therapy may have much wider applications than previously considered. ... [Photobiomodulation] appears to be a viable and efficient stimulus for enhancing neurogenesis and to exert a survivability-enhancing effect on the neuroprogenitor cells, thus increasing their chance to get functionally integrated into the preexisting neuronal circuitry."

Photobiomodulation can also be used to enhance the growth rates of cell lines outside the body, with applications such as increasing the rate of production for certain vaccines.[321] Cells such as fibroblasts (the most common cell type in our connective tissue), keratinocytes (the cells that make up the outer layers of our skin), lymphocytes (white blood cells that produce antibodies), and two types of cells essential to forming new bone (osteoblasts and bone marrow stromal cells) have all shown increased proliferation when photobiomodulation is applied to cell cultures of these types in a lab.[322, 323, 324] Also based on results from animal studies, treating mesenchymal stem cells with photobiomodulation seems to supercharge those cells' healing capabilities.[325, 326] What's more, applying photobiomodulation to astrocytes enhances the proliferation of these cells, which have the ability to act as a kind of neural stem cell and differentiate into new neurons.[327] This gives some sense of the various cell types that may be affected when we apply photobiomodulation to our bodies. Intriguingly, this line of research might offer the potential to bridge from lab to life, as cell cultures enhanced by photobiomodulation might then be used in procedures such as skin grafting and reconstructive surgery.[328] Photobiomodulation has also shown potential for helping skin cells heal the damage caused by exposure to ultraviolet light.[329] Photobiomodulation may even be able to help restore hearing by enhancing the differentiation of the specific type of stem cell that replaces lost hair cells in the cochlea, a complex and delicate cell type that has thus far not been possible to restore once lost.[330]

Photobiomodulation stimulates transcription factors in stem cells, activating their power to regenerate.[331] Through its effect on stem cells, photobiomodulation has the potential to promote the healing process for a wide range of injury types, including recovery from dental work and dental injuries (through its effects on human periodontal ligament stem cells and dental pulp stem cells).[332] Patients who've received bone grafts heal faster and are less likely to develop infections when they receive photobiomodulation.[333] In addition, a new treatment option for heart transplant candidates combines photobiomodulation with stem cell therapy to help the heart heal and regenerate—and, in some cases, to eliminate the need for a transplant.[334]

It also holds promise in the treatment of post-operative cognitive dysfunction, a condition in which memory and overall cognitive function are compromised for a period of time following surgery. As one team of scientists that researched the connection noted, it makes sense that photobiomodulation would help since postoperative cognitive function is believed to result at least in part from neuroinflammation. The researchers also noted that photobiomodulation affects the microtubules of neurons (hence affecting the neurons' mitochondrial function) and brings about other changes in the brain that alleviate pain; they recommend using photobiomodulation before surgeries to decrease the likelihood a patient develops postoperative cognitive dysfunction afterward.[335]

After someone suffers a stroke—in which a blood vessel blockage leads to ischemia and infarction—we see a suite of symptoms that you'll recognize as components of the cell danger response: an increase in reactive oxygen species, inflammation, mitochondrial dysfunction, and neuronal cell death. Neurogenesis (the formation and growth of new neurons) can turn this around, but the conditions in the brain after a stroke—including inflammation and impaired mitochondrial function—make this difficult. Because of its ability to convert microglia from the pro-inflammatory M1 type to the anti-inflammatory M2 type and to activate stem cells, photobiomodulation provides a promising avenue for enabling the brain to better recover from stroke.[336]

A study of rabbits recovering from strokes also documented the benefits of photobiomodulation; if the rabbits received photobiomodulation six hours after the stroke, they showed improved recovery compared to the rabbits that didn't receive photobiomodulation until twenty-four hours after their strokes.[337] Photobiomodulation was shown to have beneficial effects for rats following an acute stroke,[338] leading to "a marked and significant improvement in neurological deficits" for the rats that received photobiomodulation.[339] What's more, applying the treatment to rodent cells in the lab resulted in changes to the cells suggesting that, if these results hold true for humans, photobiomodulation could interrupt the inflammatory processes that lead to a cascade of damage after a brain aneurysm.[340]

A study of acute stroke survivors who were in an unresponsive or minimally responsive state found that photobiomodulation for ten minutes a day for six weeks significantly improved subjects' scores on the Coma Recovery Scale.[341] Several studies have found that transcranial photobiomodulation significantly improved outcomes in acute stroke.[342, 343, 344] One study specifically found that photobiomodulation improved cognitive function in people with chronic aphasia (difficulty with spoken and written communication) after a left hemisphere stroke.[345] A study of more than eight hundred subjects in Russia with a history of cerebral ischemic stroke found that one hundred percent of the subjects who received photobiomodulation treatments showed improvement in their motor and mental functions, whereas, in the control group (which received other treatments but not photobiomodulation), the likelihood of improvement varied according to the severity of the stroke. These results continued in the year after the treatments ended: Again, one hundred percent of the study subjects who had received photobiomodulation exhibited "the maximum positive clinical results" possible under the study's measurement parameters.[346]

SHOCK TO THE SYSTEM: MILITARY BLAST INJURIES

Although this book focuses primarily on so-called mild TBI—attempting to bring more attention to this topic since it is much more common than most people realize and causes longer-lasting and more debilitating symptoms than the medical field admits—it's worth taking a brief detour to discuss military blast injuries. Perhaps because this matches our mental concept of the "typical" TBI—a head injury sustained due to an explosion or impact during combat—this type of injury has been relatively well studied compared to the effects of repeated mild TBI like the fall I took when running or the head impacts kids experience while playing sports.

A military blast injury is a very specific type of injury in which the shock wave causes a vascular surge from the chest through the neck vessels, creating an air embolism (a bubble that pushes fluids up into the brain) and even generating electrical currents due to the intense mechanical energy and heat. This type of injury delivers a kind of shock to the brain tissue; the effect happens on a time scale of nanoseconds, and the damage it delivers to affected cells can lead to apoptosis—and, consequently, neuroinflammation, systemic inflammation, and all their downstream effects. This type of injury also increases soldiers' risk of PTSD, with physical (neurological) damage compounding the emotional risk factors of combat service. This helps to explain why PTSD often accompanies TBI—and not just because the TBI resulted from involvement in emotionally disturbing events.

This combination is especially common for military veterans, where their injuries are more likely to be accompanied by violent and emotionally traumatic memories. The proportion of military veterans who experience TBI and who also experience PTSD is estimated to be one-quarter to one-half.[347] Incidentally, recent research proposes that HRV can be measured to help identify which veterans are suffering from PTSD and help

Overlapping Symptoms of PTSD and TBI

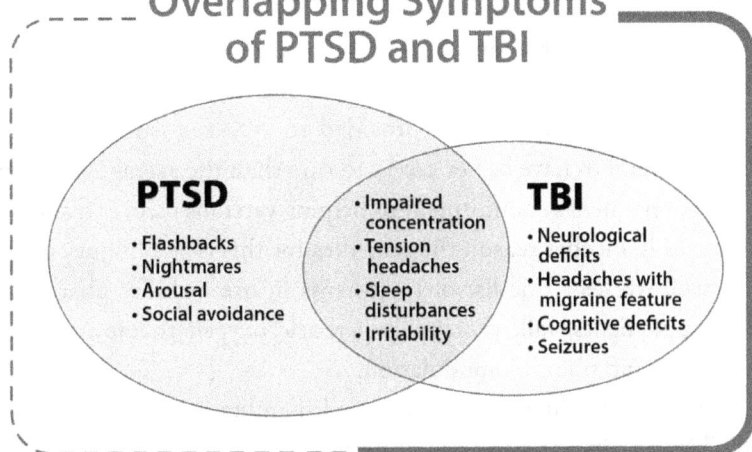

PTSD

- Flashbacks
- Nightmares
- Arousal
- Social avoidance

- Impaired concentration
- Tension headaches
- Sleep disturbances
- Irritability

TBI

- Neurological deficits
- Headaches with migraine feature
- Cognitive deficits
- Seizures

Post-traumatic stress disorder and traumatic brain injury have overlapping symptoms that sometimes mean one of the conditions goes undiagnosed in a person suffering from both concurrently or even that the person is misdiagnosed when one condition is mistaken for the other. These common symptoms include impaired concentration, tension headaches, sleep disturbances, and irritability. PTSD's distinctive symptoms include flashbacks, nightmares, physiological arousal and hypervigilance, and social avoidance; TBI's include neurological deficits, migraine headaches, cognitive deficits, and seizures.

professionals know which subjects need treatment for PTSD separately from other consequences of TBI.[348] In addition, making HRV part of the physical exam upon enlistment or before deployment may help to predict which members of the military are at the greatest risk of developing PTSD in the course of their service.[349] Interestingly, an animal study found that photobiomodulation could help to protect against a specific type of memory deficit that contributes to PTSD;[350] if that finding holds true for humans, this treatment has the potential to reduce suffering on a vast scale.

Taking one recent conflict that is far enough in the past to have solid numbers, an estimated fifteen to forty percent of soldiers returning from Iraq or Afghanistan as part of Operation Enduring Freedom and Operation Iraqi Freedom reported at least one TBI.[351] (By the way, combat injuries are not actually "typical" per se, even for military veterans: The U.S. Department of Defense estimates that service members suffered 255,852 TBI incidents between 2000 and 2012 and that more than eighty percent of these occurred in non-deployed status. These incidents include injuries suffered during training, sports, and accidental falls as well as the blast injuries we more typically associate with military service.)

Although the health care provided to veterans isn't perfect, this group does tend to have better access to care than the average American, and the government's commitment to helping veterans recover from combat injuries is another reason the remedies for this type of injury are relatively well studied. The list of treatments in use includes pharmaceuticals, supplements, talk therapy, hyperbaric oxygen therapy, cognitive training[352]—and photobiomodulation.

Research conducted specifically with military veterans who suffered TBI has documented the improvement of symptoms they experience with photobiomodulation. One study found that even long after the injury (the average time since injury for the study was 9.3 years), subjects who undertook photobiomodulation treatment experienced improvement in lingering symptoms including headaches, sleep disturbance, cognitive issues, mood issues, anxiety, and irritability.[353] One case study by Hamblin and colleagues delivered nightly photobiomodulation treatments to a fifty-two-year-old female military officer with a history of repeated head trauma; after four months of treatment, she was able to return to work (after having been out of work for five months prior to the start of treatment) and also reported improvements in her PTSD symptoms and overall cognition.[354]

In a case series by Hipskind and colleagues, twelve veterans with a history of TBI received photobiomodulation treatments for twenty minutes, three times a week, for six weeks. These subjects were medically disabled due to their symptoms, but they didn't qualify for benefits because their CT scans were normal. After six weeks of photobiomodulation, all the participants reported significant improvement in their symptoms, and before-and-after SPECT imaging revealed increases in blood flow in many areas of the brain.[355] This line of research has helped to establish Dr. Hipskind as the nation's leading forensic expert in functional brain SPECT imaging evaluation of TBI, a technique that makes visible the abnormalities that do not show up in a CT scan or an MRI. Although we want to take the symptoms of TBI sufferers seriously regardless of what their scans show, it can be helpful for both the patient and the practitioner to see with their own eyes the functional changes in the brain and know that the symptoms have a clear underlying cause. As Dr. Hipskind notes, a picture is worth a thousand words!

One new syndrome that has been identified relatively recently is Gulf War Illness, a condition that affects more than one-quarter of veterans of that war (and would be presumed to affect, at similar levels, veterans who served in other conflicts under similar conditions). Gulf War Illness, believed to be the result of exposure to neurotoxins such as sarin gas and the smoke from oil well fires, is not just a cognitive disorder but rather a systemic mitochondrial disorder—with symptoms including fatigue, headaches, chronic pain, and digestive and skin complaints. Given the role of the mitochondria, it makes sense that photobiomodulation would be an effective treatment—and indeed, this is what research has shown.[356]

In a study of forty-eight subjects with Gulf War Illness—half of whom received transcranial photobiomodulation twice a week for a total of fifteen treatments while the other half received a placebo treatment—those who received photobiomodulation showed more improvement on a variety of cognitive tests (specifically, a subgroup that had the lowest scores on the tests at the beginning of the study). The subjects who received photobiomodulation also reported fewer physical complaints at the end of the study than the placebo group. Of the subjects who had the highest PTSD scores at the beginning of the study, receiving photobiomodulation was associated with reduction (that is, improvement) in their PTSD scores one month after the end of treatment, whereas the placebo group's scores regressed toward the scores they'd had upon entering the study.[357]

The truth is that military blast injuries are not as common as the movies would lead us to believe—or perhaps more to the point, even among service members, this is not the most common type of TBI. But at the end of the day, this type of injury reflects features of the cell danger response we see with other types of TBI, and it benefits from the same approach as the other types, too: doing what we can to interrupt the chain reaction of brain damage and set the body up for healing.

Pre-Treatment   Post-Treatment

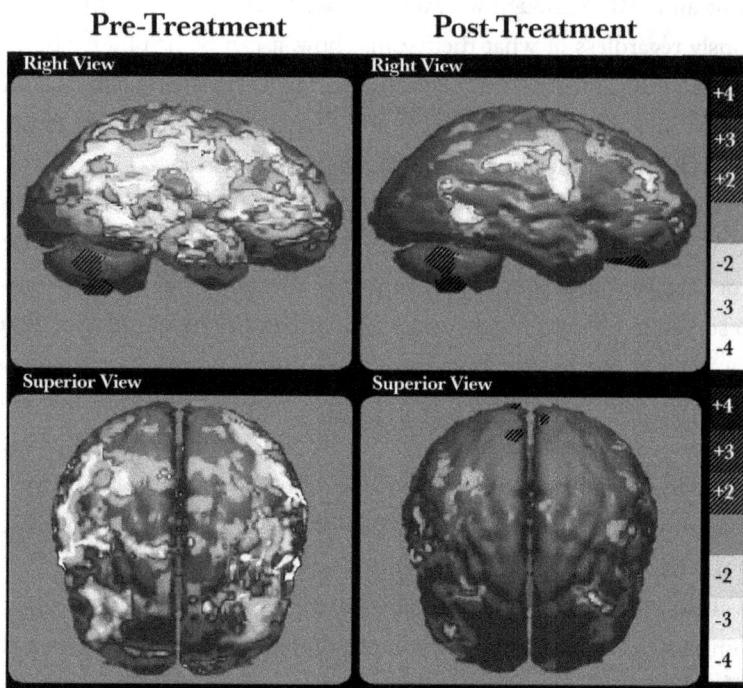

These images from Dr. Hipskind's study of military veterans with a history of TBI make visible functional abnormalities that would not show up on a CT scan or an MRI—and also show the impact of photobiomodulation. As far as we are aware, this is the only study to date that demonstrates objective improvement in cellular metabolism via brain SPECT images pre- and post-treatment with transcranial LED photobiomodulation. Unlike structural imaging such as CT and MRI, metabolic imaging with SPECT shows the disruptions in cellular metabolism that are causing a patient's symptoms. (Image courtesy of Dr. Gregory Hipskind)

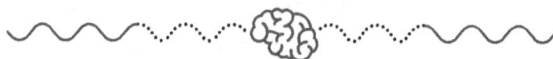

When it comes to healing brain damage, you can't go wrong with photobiomodulation and its ability to help bring our nervous systems back into balance. As Michael Hamblin writes: "The brain suffers from many different disorders that can be classified into three broad groupings: traumatic events (stroke, traumatic brain injury, and global ischemia), degenerative diseases (dementia, Alzheimer's, and Parkinson's), and psychiatric disorders (depression, anxiety, post-traumatic stress disorder). There is some evidence that all these seemingly diverse conditions can be beneficially affected by applying light to the head. There is even the possibility that [photobiomodulation] could be used for cognitive enhancement in normal, healthy people."[358]

Conditions that can be treated with photobiomodulation:[359]

Acute stroke	Lou Gehrig's disease (ALS)
Chronic stroke	Huntington's disease
Acute TBI	Primary progressive aphasia
Chronic TBI	Prion diseases (Creutzfeldt-Jakob)
Global ischemia	Depression (major, bipolar, suicidal ideation)
Coma (vegetative state)	Psychosis (schizophrenia)
Birth trauma (neonatal stroke)	PTSD
"Chemo brain"	Addiction
Alzheimer's disease	Insomnia
Parkinson's disease	Autism
Other types of dementia	ADHD

Remember that you don't necessarily need to apply the light to your head in order for your brain to benefit. Wearing a light helmet or an intranasal device will have the most direct effects for the brain, but even a body pad can create some benefit for the brain through abscopal effects. Due to the effect on stem cells explained in this chapter, photobiomodulation has the potential to help people not just with wound healing and pain relief but also with healing from conditions such as stroke, heart attack, spinal cord injury, brain injury, and neurodegeneration. What's more, as you'll see in the next section of the book, photobiomodulation helps to improve circulation—which is yet another mechanism that contributes to its beneficial effects for the brain and the whole body.

Some of the other healing practices we've already touched on in our discussion of HRV—such as mindfulness-based stress reduction[360]—have demonstrated benefits for people dealing with TBI's aftermath. Biofeedback resonance breathing is also a promising modality for treating chronic TBI symptoms due to the effect it has on HRV. It works by increasing parasympathetic (and, conversely, decreasing sympathetic) activation. A study of subjects suffering chronic post-concussion symptoms found that, in combination with low-resolution electromagnetic tomography neurofeedback (a treatment delivered by placing electrodes on the scalp to help subjects visualize and self-regulate the electrical activity of their brains), HRV biofeedback improved the subjects' symptoms of post-concussive syndrome and also reduced their response time in a driving simulation (a measurement of how well different brain regions are working together).[361] A study of athletes who had suffered concussions found that subjects who practiced HRV biofeedback breathing showed significant improvements in mood, headache severity, and other postconcussion symptoms.[362]

Remember that low HRV is a marker of poor cardiovascular health and increased risk of death and high HRV is associated with heart health, a well-calibrated autonomic nervous system, and a high level of cognitive function and emotional regulation. When we take action to increase our HRV, we can move ourselves out of the constellation of symptoms associated with low HRV into the constellation of benefits that accompany the increase. This is why scientists are increasingly pointing to biofeedback breathing for inclusion in treating concussions from sports and military service. As one paper on the subject notes, "Diet, endurance/cardiovascular exercise, and biofeedback are effective interventions. Of these three, HRV biofeedback breathing can be accomplished with minimal hardware, software, time, cost, and effort constraints upon an individual over a period of a few days. Additionally, biofeedback provides real-time feedback ... allowing the athlete or soldier to exercise cognitive control over their physiology."[363]

You've seen in this chapter that brain damage is much more common than most people realize. In fact, I'd venture to say that it's nearly universal—in that almost all of us experience it at one time or another, even if we never have a head trauma that knocks us unconscious. Photobiomodulation and biofeedback breathing are familiar tools that can aid in healing; the next chapter will take a look at some others.

CHAPTER SIX

The Recipe: Repair, Optimize, Nourish

"Shame corrodes the very part of us that believes we
are capable of change."

—Brené Brown

B ased on my own story and the statistics given in the last chapter, you
might be feeling paranoid about your own chances of having had a
traumatic brain injury that is causing lasting effects for your health. You're
not wrong to be concerned—but I want to encourage you to focus on the
positive side of the message. Your body has the ability to heal, and this
chapter will show you exactly what to do to activate and optimize that
healing process. For starters, turn to the back of the book, where you will
find questionnaires you can use to evaluate your own TBI history as well
as your ACEs score. The higher your scores, the more seriously I encourage you to take the recommendations in this chapter.

There is a concept called the "three T's" that's commonly used by
chiropractors (and was originally developed by the field's founder, Dr.
Palmer). It stands for *trauma, toxins,* and *thoughts*—but I like to rewrite
that last one as *auto-suggestion* to emphasize the control we have over our
thoughts.

This triangle of disease represents an equation in which both inputs
and outputs matter. Your past traumas are not your destiny; your body
has natural detoxification mechanisms built in to help you clear out the
biological markers of injuries and stressful experiences. Your body's complex and powerful detoxifying equipment includes your lungs, liver, kidneys, skin, intestines, and more. The better your innate detoxification

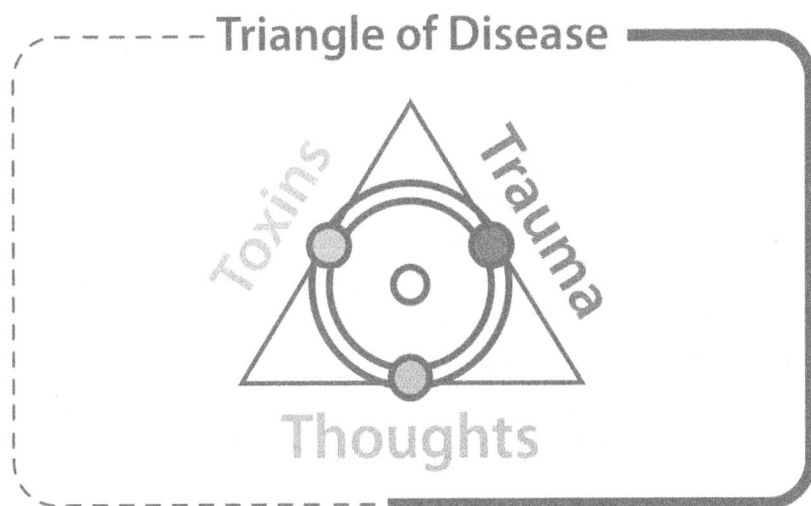

Triangle of Disease

Toxins

Trauma

Thoughts

mechanisms are working, the better you'll be able to recover from any of the three T's. Efficient detoxification processes maximize the output side of the equation.

But the magnitude of the input side also matters. If you're eating fish that's high in mercury or vegetables that were treated with lots of pesticides, you're giving your body a big detoxification job to carry out. When you put lotion on your skin or fabric softener on your clothing, compounds are absorbed through your skin that your body then needs to work to clear (again, through those innate detox mechanisms). The more polluted the air we breathe or the water we drink, the bigger the job of detoxification we are asking of our bodies.

So, we need to look at both sides. We want to simultaneously minimize the *input* side and maximize the *output* side of the equation to give our bodies the best chance of achieving balance or even coming out ahead.

We minimize the inputs by reducing the load of toxins we take in but also by being smart about not exposing ourselves to head trauma and conditions that stress the brain, such as sleep deprivation. Lastly, for the third side of the triangle—auto-suggestion—we can work to break the habits of worrying and negative self-talk. On the flip side, we can work to choose positive, optimistic thoughts that won't tip us into sympathetic activation and trigger the release of stress hormones that add to our allostatic load and, thus, our bodies' detox burden.

Throughout this book, I've been referring to the **PRONEURO** approach as a neurometabolic solution, and the detox concept also ties back to energy and metabolism. Since mitochondrial function affects every process in the body, using photobiomodulation to help your mitochondria work better will also help your body detox better. This effect has also been shown specifically for the brain: The power of photobiomodulation to help neuron cells not only continue to function in the presence of neurotoxins but to process those toxins for removal was demonstrated in an *in vitro* study (conducted with cell cultures in a lab rather than live subjects) by researchers in Wisconsin. The study noted that photobiomodulation "was able to completely reverse the detrimental effect" of the toxic substance that was applied to the neurons and that the study results provide further evidence for photobiomodulation's effect of upregulating cytochrome c oxidase and, thus, increasing energy metabolism in neurons.[364]

As our discussion of the recipe for healing continues, you'll also notice that rest is a common thread. Healing requires energy. That's why sick people lie down (and perhaps you've noticed by observing your pets that animals are better than we are at honoring the need to heal by resting while dealing with an illness or injury). Conserving energy lets your body redirect that energy into recovery. The fast pace of modern life, with a focus on productivity no matter the cost, makes it all too easy to forget this principle. To relate it back to another concept we've covered, HRV can be viewed as a measure of your energy reserve. If your HRV is very low, your body is already stressed, and you need to help it move into parasympathetic activation so healing can occur. Burning up a lot of energy in sympathetic drive will not aid in your healing process.

One more factor can hinder the healing process: inflammation. (In fact, this is part of how toxins can make it harder to heal: In some cases, they promote inflammation.) Once the acute injury phase has passed (if applicable), reducing inflammation will help create the conditions your body needs for healing. You've already seen how photobiomodulation can help with chronic or systemic inflammation, and many of the other ingredients in the **PRONEURO** formula also work to calm down inflammation.

In Chapter Three, you discovered all the beneficial effects of photobiomodulation—the ice cream for our sundae. Now it's time to start layering on the toppings with the next three letters of **PRONEURO**: Repair, Optimize, and Nourish.

R: REPAIR, REGROW, REGAIN

To help illustrate how stress can lead to disease, let's take a look at how the stress response starts in the brain—with certain brain regions becoming more active and certain regions less active under stressful conditions.

The human brain is distinctive in its size and complexity. Still, it's important not to lose sight of the fact that our cerebral cortex sits like a cap atop the brain structures we share with other mammals, which, in turn, have another layer of brain structures beneath them that we share in common with all vertebrates. From the bottom up, you have your "lizard brain" (with the cerebellum and brainstem, which control basic bodily functions such as balance, breathing, blood pressure, and coordinating movement), then the limbic system (which includes the hippocampus and amygdala as well as the hypothalamus—and, broadly speaking, represents the hardwiring of emotion and memory into our brains), and lastly, the neocortex (the front portion of the cerebral cortex, which adds such capabilities as language, music, abstract thought, planning, and logic).

The thing is that when our sympathetic nervous system is highly activated, the lizard brain is the *only* part of the brain we have access to. The body redirects energy from the neocortex and the limbic system to give us a better chance of surviving danger by getting away from the (literal or figurative) predator.

Have you ever noticed that you can't think clearly when you're under stress? And have you noticed that the response is the same whether the stressor is emotional or physical? This is beautiful evidence

Brain Regions and Functions

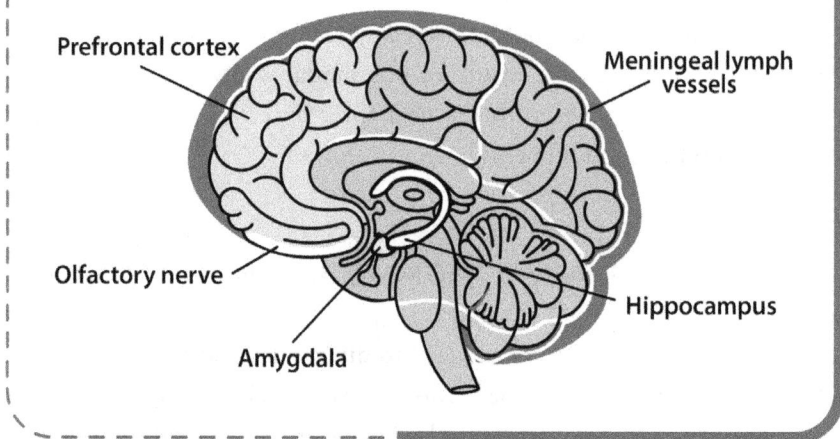

Prefrontal cortex

Meningeal lymph vessels

Olfactory nerve

Hippocampus

Amygdala

Rather than an exhaustive depiction of all brain structures and regions, this image is meant to show the general location of several structures and areas that are significant in this book. The **prefrontal cortex** plays a crucial role in executive function, planning, working toward goals, and moderating emotional responses and impulse control. The **meningeal lymph vessels**, located along the outer lining of the brain, provide an elimination route for the brain to clear waste products while we sleep. The **hippocampus** plays a key role in learning and memory and is one of the regions that becomes impaired in dementia. The **amygdalae** (you actually have two, one in each brain hemisphere) are almond-shaped structures (the name actually means *almond*) that drive emotional responses such as fear, anxiety, and aggression and influence decision-making when these emotions factor in. The **olfactory nerve** is responsible for our sense of smell—a sense that is commonly affected by conditions that cause neuroinflammation, such as Alzheimer's disease and COVID-19 infection. The nerve's close proximity to the amygdalae and the hippocampus may explain why scents can have such a strong influence on emotion and memory.

of how our physiology evolved to keep us alive. The problem is that it wreaks havoc with our health when this response is activated too frequently or for too long.

Anyone who's driven a car has probably come close to rear-ending another vehicle at some point. If you mentally transport yourself into that situation right now, I bet you can feel the physiological response. Your whole body tenses up. Your heart races. Your breath becomes shallow. Your eyes are fixed straight ahead, unblinking, with singular focus on the scene playing out in front of you. You feel a jolt of adrenaline pumping out to your fingers and toes to improve your response time and your strength when you hit the brake pedal or steer to avoid impact. And whatever you were thinking about a moment ago is completely gone.

What you feel in the moment of realizing the risk of a car accident and trying to avoid the collision is pure sympathetic activation, brought to you by the more primitive parts of your brain that are concerned with keeping you alive. The moment your brain sensed the imminent threat, energy was redirected from the big, fluffy, beautiful cortex into the limbic system and the hypothalamic-pituitary-adrenal (HPA) axis it controls.

The HPA axis concept represents a chain reaction that explains how the stress response that starts in the brain has a widespread effect on your physiology. In fact, this may be the "missing link" that connects allostatic load (high burden of stress) to disease. In the first step of the chain reaction, a stress signal in the environment makes its way to the *hypothalamus*, which initiates a fight-or-flight response in your body. The *pituitary gland*, taking its cues from the hypothalamus, secretes hormones that further contribute to your readiness to fight or flee. Then the *adrenal glands*, which sit atop your kidneys, get into the act too, secreting stress hormones. This threefold response is what produces the hyper-focused feeling you get when your survival is threatened.

Notice that emotional triggers can activate this same survival instinct—and this, too, is an evolutionary adaptation. Social and familial rejection triggers this response because there was a time when being cast out of the herd was literally a death sentence since it would make us vulnerable to predators. As frustrating as the fight-or-flight response can be sometimes, do you see why I say we should be grateful for it? It allowed our ancestors to survive in a world that was much more dangerous than the one we live in today with all our modern comforts.

Once you've sufficiently calmed down from visualizing the impending car crash, mentally transport yourself to another experience we've all

HPA Axis

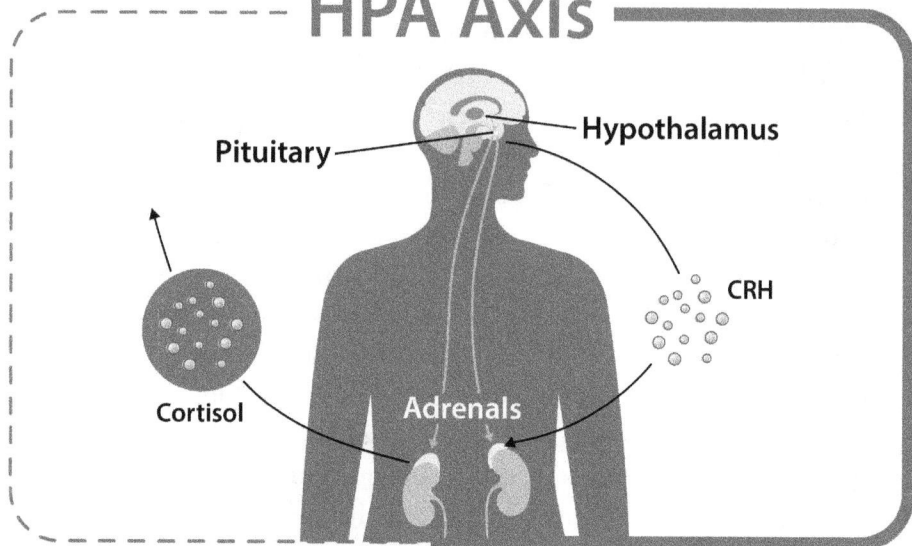

In the hypothalamic-pituitary-adrenal (HPA) axis, the hypothalamus and pituitary gland respond to stress signals in the environment, initiating a fight-or-flight response that travels from the brain to the body via corticotropin-releasing hormone, or CRH—which, in turn, cues the adrenal glands to release the stress hormone cortisol and send it out throughout the body.

had: having someone you care about "push your buttons" and say something so hurtful you feel like you can't breathe. There's an emotional response—perhaps feeling defensive and being tempted to "hit back" with a cruel comment. There's also a physiological response that has a lot in common with the car crash scenario: sweaty palms, rapid heartbeat, shallow breathing. Perhaps you even have the impulse to turn and leave. Notice that this, too, is a fight-or-flight response, despite the fact that there is no actual threat to your physical safety and survival.

This is an example of how the sympathetic nervous system (via the limbic system and HPA axis) gets activated much more often than it needs to in today's world. Deadlines at work, "keyboard warriors" making nasty comments on social media, scary or violent movies and TV shows—these and many more common features of modern life alert the brain that we're in danger, and it responds accordingly. The end result is that we spend much more time in the stress response than is necessary for our survival and far more time than is healthy.

Integrating the input from various other parts of the brain is the role of the prefrontal cortex, a brain region that is crucial for executive function, planning, working toward goals, and moderating emotional responses and impulse control. Section Three of the book goes into more detail about the prefrontal cortex, but for now, just know that this brain region has been shown to be key to the emotional changes that accompany TBI and neurodegenerative conditions. This relationship has been observed in fascinating ways, such as studying the HRV and facial expressions of patients watching film clips designed to elicit specific emotions—and noting a significant difference in responses of patients who've recently undergone neurosurgery involving the prefrontal cortex.[365]

When things start to go wrong in the brain, changes in the prefrontal cortex seem to be driving many of the symptoms that make these conditions hard to live with. The damage of mitochondrial dysfunction, inflammation, and neurodegeneration compromises prefrontal cortex activity. But when we set our bodies up to detoxify and heal, we can shift from sympathetic to parasympathetic activation, thus redirecting energy into the prefrontal cortex and parts of the brain and body that need healing.

HRV plays a key role in mediating this redirection of resources—which makes sense since HRV is a measurement that captures the shift from sympathetic to parasympathetic. For example, among PTSD patients, low HRV predicts which patients suffer from intrusive thoughts, involuntarily being reminded of or reexperiencing disturbing memories; decreased HRV and intrusive thoughts are markers of reduced ability to control one's thoughts and stay focused in the present moment instead of ruminating and fixating on worries.[366] Compared to healthy controls, subjects with PTSD show suppressed prefrontal cortex activity during memory retrieval (based on brain scans).[367] This may be an indicator of the prefrontal cortex falling down on its functions of inhibition and suppression—a finding that would help to explain why people with PTSD have trouble suppressing unwanted memories. Although this is surely a frustrating combination for someone who is experiencing it, the interrelationship among HRV, prefrontal cortex activity, and intrusive thoughts also offers us hope because it suggests that by impacting one, we can also influence the others.

The high-frequency domain of HRV, specifically, has been found to be correlated with working memory, sustained attention, mental flexibility, and inhibition (in a study of naval cadets,[368] among others). We see that people with higher HRV are better at resisting temptation, and this capacity seems to operate via the prefrontal cortex.[369] We know some ways to influence HRV—such as biofeedback breathing—and you're about to learn more ways in this chapter. As HRV increases, it tells us healing is occurring, but we can also influence healing with practices that raise HRV.

Do you see how the triangle of trauma, toxins, and auto-suggestion can be self-reinforcing? If we're stuck in "survival brain," we are more likely to choose instant gratification—but when thinking with our rational brain, we can make choices that serve our long-term health. Trauma can lead to toxic stress and toxic thoughts, compounding the body's need to detoxify. If we can build habits that interrupt the cycle and short-circuit the stress response, we can choose healing thoughts and behaviors—but you can only choose better thoughts if you first turn down your stress response enough to see that you have a choice.

In a sense, the entire **PRONEURO** approach supports the Repair (Regrow, Regain) part of the formula, and this is why it comes right after photobiomodulation as the next most important item in the recipe. (Maybe it's the chocolate sauce on top of the ice cream? The sundae is good without nuts and sprinkles, but if you have to pick one topping, I'd go with hot fudge sauce.) Photobiomodulation enhances mitochondrial function to allow everything in your body to work better—including all the processes of repair and recovery. Many of the recipe ingredients we'll be covering later in the book—supplements, nutrition, hydration, stress alleviation, and especially sleep—achieve their beneficial effects at least in part by helping your body come out of the stress response and get into repair mode. So, the first R in **PRONEURO** is, in some respects, an "umbrella" that covers other elements of the formula. But let's take a moment to look at a couple of specific habits that can help your body and brain Repair-Regrow-Regain.

One of these is cold exposure. Cultures with a tradition of heating up in a sauna and then plunging into a cold pool or lake were onto something! And as unpleasant as it might sound, the polar plunge into icy water to celebrate the new year is actually a great idea for your health. Humans intuitively sensed these benefits long before science substantiated them.

Regular cold exposure has been linked to an increase in brown fat—the health-promoting type of fat that boosts metabolism. (Side note: What gives brown fat its color is that it's packed with mitochondria—so everything you've learned about the mitochondria applies even more to this type of tissue.) Immersing yourself in cold water increases your metabolic rate and also drastically increases serum levels of dopamine (a neurotransmitter that mediates our experience of pleasure) and norepinephrine (a hormone that boosts energy, mood, and focus and also improves sleep).[370] This practice also triggers neurogenesis. Plunging into cold water does put the body under stress—but as long as you don't stay too long, it's the good kind of stress that leads to hormesis, not toxic overload.[371]

You don't have to do a polar plunge to activate these benefits. Just turn on the cold water for a few minutes at the end of your shower. Even just splashing cold water on your face produces physiological changes by stimulating the parasympathetic nervous system—and leads to observable changes in heart rate variability.[372] The area behind the eyeballs is actually an easy and powerful locus of stimulation for the vagus nerve—a powerful activator of the parasympathetic nervous system, as you'll learn in the next section of the book—so this adds to the calming effect.

Heat exposure may have almost as many beneficial effects as cold exposure. (Even better, follow the Eastern European tradition of heating up in a sauna, then jumping in a cold lake afterward!) A 2016 study of Finnish men found that the more often the study subjects used a sauna (up to seven days a week), the lower their dementia risk.[373] In 2018, the same research team published findings that sauna usage reduces the risk of stroke[374] and also demonstrated that sauna usage may achieve its health-promoting benefits by lowering systemic inflammation.[375] Sauna usage also has favorable effects on the autonomic nervous system and HRV.[376, 377]

The concept of hormesis might help us understand why these practices work. By exposing the body to mild stress, we help it get better at adapting to stress. We are not exposing ourselves to such cold conditions that we get hypothermia or frostbite, nor are we exposing ourselves to such extreme heat that we develop heatstroke. By subjecting our bodies to conditions that are near the edge (or just beyond the edge) of our usual comfort zone, we force our bodies to adapt—and in the process, to operate more efficiently under the "normal" conditions of a comfortable room temperature.

Another condition that seems to affect the body in a similar way is hypoxia—mild deprivation of oxygen. (Not so much, of course, that it leads to tissue death—just enough to force the body to work a little harder to oxygenate the blood.) This is why training at high altitude makes athletes feel like superheroes when they return to lower altitude—their bodies have adapted. This may also be why slowing down the breath has so many health benefits—it forces the body to work more efficiently with the oxygen that's coming in and develops excess capacity in the breathing muscles so they don't have to work as hard during normal breathing. There is also some evidence that temporary hypoxia stimulates mitochondrial biogenesis in the brain![378]

Practices like cold exposure, sauna usage, and biofeedback breathing are, in a sense, exposing the body to a mild stressor to help it learn to respond to stress without breaking out of its equilibrium. They are ways of keeping us out of HPA axis activation and out of the fight-or-flight response driven by the limbic system. Learning to get out of your stress response quickly and spend as much time as possible in repair-regrow-regain mode is the goal of the remainder of the **PRONEURO** recipe.

O: OPTIMIZE

Do you *need* to take supplements? Not necessarily. Think of this as an optional ingredient on our sundae. But I think of them like choosing to pay a toll to take the road that gets you to your destination faster. If your organs are overburdened in carrying out their detox processes, supplements can help support them. If certain nutrients are depleted in your body after years of chronic stress, supplements can help rebuild those stores. If you have genetic factors that make your body less efficient at these detox processes than some of your fellow humans, supplements can help close that gap.

These are just a few reasons you might want to take supplements. If you end up working with me as a client, you'll receive personalized recommendations for specific supplements, forms, and dosages. But for the purpose of this book, here are a few individual supplements and categories that I believe are most important for brain health. Before adding any new supplements, it's always a good idea to consult a physician you trust about possible prescription medication interactions and any other concerns.

Vitamin D is a supplement that just about everyone can benefit from, especially if you live someplace far from the Equator that doesn't get much sunlight for a good chunk of the year. You may be familiar with the role it plays in bone health and immune function—but a lesser-known function of vitamin D is the role it plays in brain health. It plays a key role in the function of neurons and glial cells (the nervous system cells that do not produce electrical impulses, i.e., the cells other than neurons). Vitamin D deficiency has been implicated in the development of dementia as well as diabetes—which itself has a cascade of effects that impact the brain, as you'll learn more about in the next section of the book. Vitamin D deficiency appears to put diabetic patients at higher risk of developing neuropathy.[379] It is also linked to higher levels of inflammation in the brain and elsewhere—and to higher depression risk due to the impact of vitamin D on calcium levels in the brain.[380] You can see why it's concerning that up to half of seemingly healthy adults are deficient in vitamin D! In addition, the higher someone's allostatic load, the lower their level of vitamin D—and although it's not clear which one is causing the other, this relationship tells us that most people experiencing chronic stress would probably benefit from taking vitamin D for the host of beneficial effects even if it does not directly influence allostatic load indicators.[381] (Make sure you are also getting enough vitamin K—and especially the form found in grass-fed meat and dairy as well as fermented foods like natto—since this vitamin works in tandem with vitamin D to regulate the balance of calcium in your bones.)

Given research linking magnesium deficiency with anxiety, I also recommend **magnesium** as a supplement most people could benefit from. This mineral is essential for proper muscle and nerve function. It is what allows the muscles to relax. If you don't have enough of it, the result is tense muscles and even spasms. Magnesium regulates the activity of several enzymes involved in mitochondrial function; magnesium deficiency has been linked with worse outcomes after TBI.[382] You don't necessarily need to supplement with oral magnesium—you can actually absorb it through your skin in an Epsom salt bath. Thus, a warm bath at the end of the night can serve a double function of delivering magnesium to enable muscle relaxation and helping your body temperature to drop once you get out of that warm tub. When that parasympathetic activation kicks in, you can sleep soundly and wake up with a brain that's repaired and ready to go for the next day.

Zinc is another mineral that most people may benefit from supplementing. In addition to being vital for brain function—it is needed for axonal and synaptic transmission—it also plays a key role in immune function, and emerging research is highlighting the role it plays in mitochondrial function.[383, 384, 385]

B vitamins are a class of vitamins that may have preventive value. A review article noted that several studies found an association between supplementation with vitamins B_6 and B_{12} and reduced atrophy of the gray matter and of the whole brain for subjects with mild cognitive impairment or dementia.[386] Since we know that B vitamins are important for a wide range of cellular functions, including transporting nutrients throughout the body and keeping our brains running properly, it makes sense that they would be helpful for people already beginning to experience neurometabolic problems.

Another category of supplements to consider is **mitochondrial nutrients**. These include coenzyme Q10 (CoQ10), acetyl-L-carnitine, and pyrroloquinoline quinone (PQQ). CoQ10 plays a crucial role in the electron transport chain by which the mitochondria produce ATP; the declining levels associated with aging may play a role in the fatigue that comes with growing older.[387] Carnitine, the generic term for a number of compounds, plays a crucial role in energy metabolism by transporting long-chain fatty acids into the mitochondria for beta-oxidation and aiding with the removal of waste products for excretion. Supplementing with acetyl-L-carnitine has been found to reduce the mitochondrial decay that can accompany aging.[388] Studies of PQQ supplementation in both rodents and humans have shown it activates PGC-1α, the main regulator for gene transcription and replication in creating new mitochondria.[389, 390, 391, 392]

One last mitochondrial nutrient to consider is **pomegranate extract**. A recent study from Swiss scientists identified a compound called urolithin A, a compound generated by our gut bacteria after we eat pomegranates or drink pomegranate juice, which has the effect of enhancing mitochondrial function.[393] This may help to explain earlier research that found adding pomegranate extract to the diet of mice with Alzheimer's disease improved their synaptic function.[394]

As I'll go into more detail about in the next section of the book, vasodilation is an important part of how photobiomodulation produces its beneficial effects, and improvements to circulation are also part of the reason exercise holds such healing power. Photobiomodulation prompts the discharge of nitric oxide, which, in turn, causes nearby blood vessels to dilate—but you can supplement with **nitric oxide** for the same (or a more pronounced) effect. Another option is to supplement with arginine, a precursor to nitric oxide in the body. (Note that this is different from the *nitrous* oxide you sometimes get at the dentist's office—we're not talking about laughing gas!)

Another category of supplements to take a close look at is **adapto-gens**. These are herbs that support your body in handling stress in vari-ous ways—that is to say, they support hormesis. With the help of these herbs, you can increase your capacity to handle more stress without breaking a sweat, so to speak. Ginkgo biloba has a reputation for improv-ing brain function, but the research findings when it comes to that are mixed; we do, however, know that it is a powerful antioxidant that helps fight inflammation—and also protects mitochondria[395, 396] and improves circulation and heart health by increasing nitric oxide levels![397]

Another herb in this category is rhodiola, which has been shown to reduce fatigue in people who work night shifts and to reduce perceived fatigue during exercise—and, at least in a petri dish, to inhibit the growth of cancer cells.[398, 399, 400, 401, 402, 403, 404, 405, 406, 407]

Astragalus is an herb from traditional Chinese medicine with reputed anti-aging properties; modern-day scientists have discovered that its active compounds act to increase telomerase activity—and thus, have the potential to reverse aging on the cellular level since shortened telomeres on the ends of your chromosomes are a marker of aging.[408, 409]

One final herb on the adaptogen list, ashwagandha, has mul-tiple desirable benefits. To name a few, it acts to reduce inflamma-tion; induce apoptosis in cancer cells; increase the activity of natural killer cells, a key immune system component; and reduce cortisol lev-els, helping your body downregulate the HPA axis and exit the stress response.[410, 411, 412, 413, 414, 415, 416, 417]

I recommend that my clients with sleep problems (which, honestly, is most people) use **melatonin**. This is a hormone your body naturally produces to make you feel nice and sleepy at bedtime. It can help you fall asleep faster or get your circadian rhythm back on target if you've become too much of a night owl. Our ability to produce melatonin declines as we age, so I especially recommend this for my older clients.

Branched-chain amino acids are especially important for my older clients since research has shown that this category of supplements can support mitochondrial biogenesis, prevent oxidative damage, and enhance physical endurance later in life.[418]

Nicotinamide adenine dinucleotide, or **NAD+**, is a molecule found in every cell of the body and is essential to cellular energy and mitochondrial health. When scientists discovered in the early twentieth century that niacin (vitamin B₃) deficiency caused pellagra—an illness characterized by the "three Ds" of dermatitis, diarrhea, and dementia and which was once widespread in the American South—this was because niacin is a precursor to NAD+. In other words, if you consume enough niacin through food or supplements, your body will have what it needs to create this essential molecule—but you can also supplement with NAD+ directly.

Alpha-lipoic acid is a substance the body makes on its own; it's naturally present in the mitochondria and essential for producing ATP—but when present in the body in larger amounts, it acts as an antioxidant, scavenging free radicals.[419]

Quercetin is a flavonoid—a class of substances that gives fruits and vegetables their vibrant colors. (Yes, its neon yellow color is completely natural, not artificial!) In the brain, it acts to protect neurons from inflammation and oxidative damage—and, importantly, does the same for endothelial cells, which play an important role in the brain's vascular system.[420] It also affects several aspects of mitochondrial metabolism in beneficial ways,[421] which may help to explain how it brings about these positive effects in the brain.

In addition, taking an amino acid called **N-acetylcysteine** (NAC) may enable your body to produce more of the powerful antioxidant glutathione and can help support your body's detoxification functions during times when they become overburdened and the molecules involved may become depleted. Glutathione depletion is believed to contribute to bipolar disorder, schizophrenia, obsessive-compulsive disorder, and addictive behavior through its effects on the brain.[422, 423]

Research suggests that **guaraná**, a plant native to Brazil whose seeds are used in a similar way to coffee beans, has similar cognitive benefits to caffeine without caffeine's effect of stimulating sympathetic drive.[424]

In general, I recommend a diet high in **anti-inflammatory** substances, and many of these could be considered foods rather than supplements. What I'm saying is that when you see turmeric, ginger, garlic,[425] and cayenne on my supplement list, you can simply season your meals with them instead of purchasing supplement capsules. Many of the substances that give fruits and vegetables their vivid colors—like fisetin[426, 427] in strawberries and resveratrol in grapes and berries—have documented health benefits. While you may get a more potent dose in a pill than you do in eating a handful of fruit, there is also something to be said for the process of savoring your food, chewing it slowly, tasting it, and taking in the nutrients that way.

N: NOURISH

When it comes to nutrition, popping a pill or blending some powder into your smoothie is the easy part—but the food you eat also makes an enormous difference to the health of your brain and nervous system, and in this section, I'll try to sum up the most important nutritional habits to add in.

1. Invest in a good probiotic.

The balance of bacteria in your gut affects your immune function. It affects your body's ability to absorb and use the nutrients you take in with your food. There is also evidence that the gut microbiome affects inflammation and mood and that it can influence metabolism and weight gain or loss—and even more serious conditions such as diabetes, colon cancer, and schizophrenia. Did you know that nearly all of the feel-good neurotransmitter serotonin is produced in the gut, not the brain? Recent research even indicates that the gut microbiome influences blood pressure and cholesterol levels.[428, 429, 430, 431, 432]

We are learning more and more about the wide-ranging influence of the gut microbiome. Hippocrates claimed that all disease begins in the gut; modern scientists are demonstrating that statement's proof points. Researchers recently found a connection between compromised gut health and damage to the hippocampus[433]—which, of course, is a key region of the brain for learning and memory. Indeed, research has shown that probiotic supplementation can improve Alzheimer's symptoms as well.[434] Other studies have found associations between gut bacteria imbalances and the development of Alzheimer's disease,[435, 436] and a recent study found that the greater the diversity of one's gut bacteria, the higher one's scores across all areas of cognitive function are at midlife.[437] If that's not an argument for paying attention to gut health, I don't know what is!

As it turns out, gut microorganisms can actually activate the vagus nerve.[438] Stay tuned for more information in Chapter Eight about why that's important—but know that this is the express route to get your body out of fight-or-flight mode and into rest-and-repair mode. Ongoing research is exploring whether enhancing the gut microbiome with probiotics may be able to interrupt the negative feedback loop and prevent secondary damage after TBI.[439, 440] Early research is also pointing to a role for probiotics in healing the gut, tempering inflammation, and protecting the health of the mitochondria in the aftermath of COVID-19 infection.[441] For all these reasons and more, it is vitally important that you maintain a healthy gut microbiome. By taking a probiotic, you populate your intestines with beneficial bacteria.

There are many different kinds of probiotics on the market, and the offerings are always changing. I have certain specific strains and brands that I recommend to my clients. Many of the probiotic supplements and food products on the market are not formulated in a way that enables the beneficial bacteria to survive the environment of the stomach and get to their intended destination (the intestines). The most important thing is to do some research before you spend a lot of money on these products or to get a recommendation from a trusted health professional like a doctor, nutritionist, or coach.

Instead of (or in addition to) a probiotic supplement, consuming fermented foods can improve the health of your gut microbiome. This list of foods includes fermented dairy, such as yogurt and kefir; fermented soy products such as tempeh, natto, and miso; fermented vegetables like sauerkraut and kimchi; and fermented drinks like kombucha. Like with any food or drink you consume, pay attention to production methods when selecting your fermented foods; for example, some sauerkraut is pasteurized, which kills all live cultures, thus destroying the probiotic benefit. (I feel strongly enough about the benefits of fermented foods and drinks that I actually started my own kombucha business, Pura Bucha. That's a story for another time, but if you ever come to Costa Rica, you can try it for yourself at many hotels and restaurants.)

Incidentally, this seems to be another area where photobiomodulation can help. In mice, it has been shown to increase health-promoting gut bacteria.[442] One study retrospectively analyzed stool samples from Parkinson's disease patients who had taken part in a previous study that showed a twelve-week regimen of photobiomodulation improved their symptoms. The new analysis showed positive changes in the subjects' gut microbiomes,[443] indicating this may be part of how photobiomodulation wields its positive effects—or at the very least, another benefit to add to the list.

In terms of factors that can affect your gut microbiome negatively, one category of food additives stands out: artificial sweeteners such as saccharin, aspartame, and sucralose. One headline-grabbing recent study found that consuming these sugar substitutes enabled gut bacteria to cross the intestinal wall and enter the bloodstream, a condition known as "leaky gut" that, in severe cases, can lead to an infection or even sepsis.[444] What's more, scientists have long since concluded that these sugar substitutes do not really help people lose weight and may actually increase risk of metabolic syndrome and type 2 diabetes, possibly due to how they affect the gut microbiome.[445, 446, 447, 448]

2. **Consider a new (to you) dietary approach such as the ketogenic diet, intermittent fasting, or intuitive eating.**

When it comes to the food we put in our bodies, the "how" is just as important as the "what." If we simply eat the way we always have and never try anything new, we are acting on force of habit. The way you eat may feel good because it's familiar, and change might feel scary.

Instead, I'd encourage you to treat your dietary habits as a science experiment. When you take a more flexible approach and try new things, you get used to changing up what you eat. You increase your tolerance for change, and your body starts to realize that even when the familiar foods are not available, or show up in different patterns and combinations, you are still receiving the nourishment you need. Think of it as a form of hormesis. If you're trying to give up processed sugar, on the first day it might feel impossible—you might literally feel like you're going to die— but with practice, you develop a tolerance. Your body gets used to it and realizes it's still getting plenty of nutrients.

You can choose from many different dietary approaches to help you gain this experiential learning. Here are a few of my favorites. If you decide to try approaches not listed here in your science experiment, keep in mind that it's always best to get a wide variety of nutrients in the food you eat and to avoid anything overly restrictive (such as the "grapefruit diet" that was popular in the 1980s, which consisted of eating only grapefruit and nothing else). In general, malnutrition seems to contribute to neurodegeneration, so eating a nutrient-dense diet that includes a variety of whole foods is a good baseline for reducing your risk. There is also some evidence that a Mediterranean diet (think olive oil, seafood, lots of vegetables, and sparing use of processed foods) reduces one's risk of neurodegenerative diseases.[449, 450, 451, 452, 453]

Each of the approaches described below has specific benefits, and you might wish to try each of them for a period of time. (Remember: It's a science experiment!) You can track the changes in how you feel, your energy levels, and even biomarkers such as HRV, sleep quality, blood sugar, and blood lipids, depending on what you have the ability to track.

Some of the approaches (such as a ketogenic diet) are not meant to be permanent, but when you try them out temporarily, you will gain insights you can incorporate into a longer-term approach to nutrition. The overall goal is to learn through experience how much agency and choice you have in what you eat and to no longer let cravings and well-worn habits run the show.

A **ketogenic diet** depletes your body of carbohydrates, forcing it to burn fat as fuel. Carb depletion puts your body in a state called *ketosis* in which fatty acids are released from your body's fat stores, oxidized by the liver, and turned into molecules called *ketones* that can provide energy for the body in the absence of glucose. Think back to the different methods of producing ATP in the mitochondria. (You can refer back to Chapter Two if your memory needs refreshing.) When fatty acids instead of carbohydrates are the energy source, ATP output is about twenty-five percent greater. Fatty acids also provide cleaner fuel in the Krebs cycle, whereas the free radicals produced when glucose is the fuel source promote inflammation and oxidative stress.[454] When in a state of ketosis, the brain can use ketones for energy and can also convert ketones into glucose in a process called *gluconeogenesis*.

You will need to keep your carb intake quite low to achieve ketosis and will need urine test strips to verify that your body is in ketosis. The amount of carbs you can take in without kicking your body out of ketosis varies from person to person but is generally less than fifty grams per day and, for some people, as low as twenty grams (less than the amount in a single serving of most fruits). Also, keep in mind that all carbohydrates count—not just processed carbohydrates—so natural carb sources like chickpeas, quinoa, and sweet potatoes will be off-limits along with candy and cookies. Because carb intake is pushed so low, a ketogenic diet consists primarily of protein and fat.

The reasons that a ketogenic diet works well for people with epilepsy also explain why people without epilepsy would want to eat this way. One study found that epileptic rats suffered less mitochondrial damage from their seizures when they were fed a ketogenic diet. Upregulation of cytochrome c, along with other signals, indicated a decrease in mitochondrial apoptosis—meaning that, apparently, something about the changes in the brain due to following a ketogenic diet had a protective effect and kept cells from dying.[455] Activation of the maternal immune system due to a viral or bacterial infection during the first trimester is a risk factor for autism; in mice with autism symptoms (such as repetitive behaviors and disinterest in social interaction) due to maternal infection during pregnancy, a ketogenic diet reduces these symptoms—at least for the male off-spring. This effect is believed to result from the ketogenic diet's impact on inflammation.[456] In general, a ketogenic diet has anti-inflammatory effects, and research has shown that this diet works well in supporting the brain's recovery from injury, so it can be useful if you are recovering from TBI or chronic effects of stress on the brain.[457, 458, 459] Ketogenic diets have also shown promise for slowing, stopping, and even reversing the progression of Alzheimer's disease,[460, 461] very likely because of the mechanisms that TBI and dementia have in common (stay tuned for more on that in the next section of the book). From animal studies, we know that a ketogenic diet preserves vascular function as the animals enter old age. It also reduces oxidative stress, preserves mitochondrial function, restores neuronal structure, and enhances cognitive function.[462] It also improves the efficiency of the electron transport chain.[463] Although a strict ketogenic diet can be a hassle to follow, it may be worth the trouble at least for those most at risk of Alzheimer's disease and, in particular, may be worth considering for people who aren't able to engage in vigorous exercise.

Developed in Japan with roots in Zen Buddhism, the **macrobiotic diet** consists mainly of vegetables and whole grains with smaller amounts of legumes, soybeans, fruits, seeds, and nuts. The only animal product included is fish (recommended to eat two to three times a week). It also includes superfoods such as seaweed (rich in essential minerals) and miso (a fermented soybean paste that enhances the gut microbiome). In a certain sense, this is the opposite of a ketogenic diet; it's hard to eat an extremely low-carb diet when not consuming animal products since plant-based sources of protein tend to contain carbohydrates, too. But what the two diets have in common is that they'll get you to eliminate heavily processed carbohydrates such as cake, chips, and soda from your diet—and that's ultimately one of the best things you can do for your metabolism and brain health.

Many books about the macrobiotic diet ask you to buy fruits, vegetables, grains, and herbs that are native to Japan but can be hard to find in other parts of the world. I think it's important to keep in mind that one of the most important principles of the macrobiotic diet, as originally designed, was to emphasize plant foods that are locally grown and in season—so in my opinion, you can make some adjustments to this meal plan instead of paying top dollar for exotic foods in specialty stores.

Intermittent fasting is an approach that's recently gained popularity because of its longevity benefits. Studies of bacteria, yeast, worms, and mice have found that depriving them of nutrients increases their lifespan (through increasing the reactive oxygen species stress signal and inducing a mitohormetic response[464]) and has benefits for mitochondrial function,[465] neurogenesis,[466] and cognition.[467] There is some debate over just how much humans would need to reduce our caloric intake to get the same benefit, and it's hard to answer that question for certain without the kind of randomized controlled trial we conduct with non-human animals (assigning subjects to the experimental or the control group without giving them a choice). But we do know that fasting provides benefits for humans, with those benefits probably becoming more pronounced with longer fasting times, and that for people who aren't able to exercise, fasting can provide some of the same benefits (such as reducing circulating levels of inflammatory molecules[468]) as it forces your body to switch fuel sources once the liver's glycogen stores run out.[469]

In general, intermittent fasting is defined as fasting at least twelve hours per day—something that's easy to achieve without changing how you eat too much. If you finish dinner by seven p.m. and you don't eat breakfast until seven a.m. the next day, you're golden. Even better if you can fast for a little longer—say, by pushing your breakfast back to become brunch at eleven a.m. Then you eat what you want during your "feeding window." (I still recommend choosing real, whole, nutrient-dense foods and keeping highly processed foods to a minimum, but technically there are no rules about *what* you eat with intermittent fasting—it's all about *when* you eat it.) The hard-core intermittent fasters confine their feeding window to four hours per day (say, between noon and four p.m.), but a twenty-hour fast really starts to restrict your options socially—say, if you enjoy eating breakfast with your family or getting dinner with friends. You may also find that you're so hungry when your fast ends that you make less-than-optimal food choices, and you might decide to do a shorter fast (and give up some of the benefits) to improve your overall food quality (and get different benefits). It's all just part of the science experiment.

Intermittent fasting has demonstrated benefits for neurodegenerative conditions[470] and age-related memory loss[471] (reducing the symptoms of Alzheimer's disease, Parkinson's disease, and Huntington's disease in mice) and for promoting recovery after TBI, spinal cord injury, and stroke. Also in rodents, it has been shown to increase lifespan,[472, 473] to increase neurogenesis in the hippocampus,[474] and to prevent and even reverse metabolic syndrome (a condition that involves weight gain and insulin resistance and usually indicates type 2 diabetes is coming next)—and to mitigate damage to the heart after a heart attack. In mice, fasting is believed to slow tumor growth and protect cells against metabolic ailments because of the ways it affects antioxidant defense and oxidative stress via proteins called sirtuins.[475] Intermittent fasting increases levels of human growth hormone, with the effect of increasing lean muscle mass and reducing body fat to shift body composition. (In fact, declining levels of human growth hormone are thought to be part of the reason people tend to lose muscle mass and gain fat as they get older.[476]) In rats, caloric restriction and intermittent fasting both lead to a reduction in blood pressure and an increase in HRV;[477] in rats that are deficient in estrogen and thus at higher risk of cognitive decline, intermittent fasting has a protective effect.[478] Studies in humans have shown promising indications for hypertension,[479] high cholesterol,[480] metabolic disorders,[481] and multiple sclerosis,[482] among other conditions. A review article concluded that intermittent fasting is effective at inducing the all-important process of autophagy[483] (the body's equivalent of reduce-reuse-recycle), and thus can potentially provide similar anti-aging benefits to a calorie-restricted diet.[484]

When you eat a meal, assuming that your pancreas is working properly, your insulin levels rise to help balance your blood sugar. Insulin acts as a signal to your fat cells to take in, rather than release, energy—so it's impossible for your body to access the energy stored in your body fat unless you are in a fasted state (with the corresponding low insulin levels). In addition, the body's "repair, regrow, regain" processes (such as the reduce-reuse-recycle process of autophagy) only begin once your body is in a fasted state. If you eat too close to bedtime, you'll see that your resting heart rate takes a long time to drop—indicating that your body was directing energy into digestion and couldn't drop into the deep parasympathetic state that's so important for recovering from stress, trauma, and injury.[485, 486, 487, 488, 489, 490, 491, 492, 493, 494, 495]

One last approach I recommend you consider, **intuitive eating,** focuses more on mindset than a specific dietary protocol. Intuitive eating involves learning to listen to your body's needs and desires. This approach can go hand in hand with tuning in to your body's circadian rhythms and learning to get better sleep. With the breakneck pace of modern life, most of us have gotten completely out of touch with our natural rhythms; tuning back in can be a beautiful practice.

Intuitive eating is not just "anything goes." It does not rule out eating according to the health-promoting attributes of certain foods—but it *does* require learning to honor our hunger and prioritize satisfaction. With practice, as we tune in mindfully to how food affects us, we can start to notice as we try out different foods how they affect our energy and satiety levels and use what we learn to inform our future choices. When we give ourselves unconditional permission to eat, it becomes easier to notice when we are using food to numb our emotions instead of responding to a physical need. When we unsubscribe from punishing ways of eating, it becomes normal to feel good—and this helps us tune in to the way different foods make us feel. Our bodies give us signals of what they need; it's just that many of us have gotten in the habit of tuning out those signals. When we start to listen, those signals get louder, and it becomes possible to pick up on what our bodies are asking for, whether that's the satisfaction of a high-protein meal, the refreshing crunch of a salad, or the quick energy of a sweet treat.

Intuitive eating is a combination of dietary approach and devotional practice. If you are just getting started with it, the book *Intuitive Eating* by Evelyn Tribole and Elyse Resch is a wonderful resource. Like the other approaches described in this chapter, intuitive eating might be something you choose to practice for a limited time before returning to something more structured, or it might become a long-term lifestyle—and like the other approaches, you will take what you learn with you into the rest of your life. Working with a coach can help you venture into a new dietary approach one step at a time, and it is part of what we offer if you choose to enroll in coaching with the **PRONEURO** approach.

3.   Don't forget that hydration is also part of nutrition.

The water you drink throughout your day supports your body's detoxification and elimination functions. Here's a quick calculation: Take your body weight in pounds and divide it by two. Now convert that number to ounces. If you're not drinking at least that much water in a day, it's time to make a change because that number is the bare minimum.

For example, a two hundred–pound person should be drinking at least one hundred ounces of water in a day. But I'll say it again: That's the minimum! I know plenty of smaller people who drink a whole gallon of water (128 ounces) each and every day. If you're still consuming significant amounts of soft drinks (even if they're non-caloric) or if all you drink is coffee all day long, switching to water is one of the very best things you can do to enable your body's healing powers.

Just drinking water—period—is the most important thing. But if you want to make this an even better habit, invest in a good filtration system. Bottled water that's stored in plastic absorbs compounds from the bottle that act as endocrine disruptors in your body, interfering with hormonal function and balance. It's better to drink tap water but use a filter that removes these compounds as well as other chemicals. (Did you know that your tap water likely includes molecules from other people's medications that they have either peed out or flushed down the toilet? It's pretty alarming to think we might be taking other people's medicine when we drink our water, isn't it? Most municipal water treatment systems ensure the water won't contain pathogens such as *E. coli*, but they make no such guarantees when it comes to antibiotics, antidepressants, and other pharmaceuticals.) Alternatively, you could run bottled water through the same kind of filter, but purchasing bottled water is an extra expense that probably isn't necessary. One more note on water filters: Exercise caution with reverse osmosis systems since they also remove beneficial minerals such as calcium and magnesium, so you may then need additional supplementation to compensate.

While we are on the topic of reducing exposures, let's take a quick look at some other ways you can reduce your toxic burden so your body doesn't have as much to do in terms of detoxification. (Because, remember, the more energy that goes into detox, the less energy is available for other functions such as healing.)

My instructions for bottled water apply to everything else, too: It's better to use glass, ceramic, or stainless steel containers than plastic, especially if the food or drink being placed in the container is hot or will be in the container for a significant length of time. If you must use plastic containers for food storage, take care not to run them through the dishwasher, as this can cause them to degrade faster and leach more chemicals into the food inside them. Also beware of nonstick cookware (stainless steel, ceramic, or cast iron is preferable), and especially be sure to discard nonstick items if they become scratched, as this makes the coating more likely to flake off into your food (and the chemicals to end up in your bloodstream).

Choose local, seasonal, and organic produce whenever possible. The less processed your food is, the fewer toxins you'll be taking in along with the nutrients you consume. Single-ingredient foods are best; anything that comes in a bottle, can, or box has the potential to contain additives or chemicals leached from the packaging material. Read ingredient labels and avoid anything that lists BHT, BHA, benzoate, sulfites, or artificial colorings. Look for BPA-free can linings. When possible, go for the glass bottle over the metal can or plastic bottle—especially when it comes to highly acidic foods like tomatoes.

Take special care when choosing meats and fish, paying attention to how and where the animal was raised and what it was fed. Remember that anything the animal consumed during its life is now coming into your body—so there *is* a difference between grain-fed and grass-fed beef or wild-caught and farmed salmon. If you eat animal products, higher-quality items are well worth the additional cost.

While food and water are the most important, once you've implemented the suggestions already given, the next level of removing toxins from your life is to pay attention to what you put on your body and in your home. Read the ingredient labels for bath and body products; the simpler and more natural, the better. You may want to consider a filter for your shower water. Switch to natural laundry and cleaning products, and avoid plastic or vinyl items anywhere in your home (swapping out your vinyl shower curtain for cloth is a quick fix and an important one since you apply hot water to it and breathe in the steam).

If you wear shoes in the house, it's time to start leaving them at the door so contaminants outside don't come in. (If you need the arch support, wear a pair of indoor shoes or supportive slippers.) Replace older items such as carpets, mattresses, and foam furniture, as they may contain chemicals that have been outlawed due to their effect on human health—and these types of items degrade as they age, creating more emissions. Use low- or no-VOC paints, and invest in a whole-house air filtration system or free-standing room filters. All of these chemicals in our food, water, air, and surroundings contribute to our toxic burden, creating more work for our bodies and diverting energy from other endeavors.

4. Find room for superfoods.

Overhauling your entire diet is a major lifestyle change. As worthwhile as it may be, it takes a lot of work and practice to change your habits that way. So, to close this nutrition section, I thought I'd give you a few "quick wins" in the form of foods you can add into your diet that pack a major health punch. These just might be the beginning of a delicious new healthy habit!

The first of these is **dark chocolate**. I'm not talking about the mass-produced grocery store brand that says "dark chocolate" but has more sugar than cocoa. To reap the health benefits, shoot for at least eighty-five percent cocoa or higher. Dark chocolate has one of the highest concentrations of magnesium in a food, with one square providing 327 milligrams, or eighty-two percent of the U.S. Food and Drug Administration's recommended daily value. The only other foods that are as concentrated are squash and pumpkin seeds. Dark chocolate also contains large amounts of tryptophan, an amino acid that works as a precursor to serotonin, and theobromine, another mood-elevating compound. A single dose of dark chocolate can increase your heart rate variability and give your parasympathetic nervous system a boost.

Second on my "quick win" list is **omega-3 fatty acids.** Think of the acronym SMASH: salmon, mackerel, anchovies, sardines, herring. If you enjoy any of these fish, know that they contain some of the most heart-healthy and brain-healthy fats that exist. A diet high in omega-3 fatty acids has been linked to vagus nerve activation (remember, the express route to exit your stress response) and higher HRV. When we see people eating a Mediterranean diet who seem to be enjoying the good life, it's not just because they live in a beautiful place—their diet is actually increasing their sense of joy and relaxation. Fish oil has been shown to have neuroprotective and neuroregenerative benefits such as modulating inflammation after TBI,[496, 497, 498] but if you are taking supplements rather than getting it from whole food sources, consult with a trusted practitioner for the appropriate dose for your specific situation.

A third "quick win" I recommend is getting in the habit of drinking some **bitters** before dinner. These botanical-infused spirits aren't just for cocktail snobs! Typically made by soaking fruit, herbs, spices, leaves, bark, or roots in clear alcohol, bitters are high-proof but are typically used in such small amounts (due to the potent flavor) that they are marketed as non-alcoholic (just like vanilla extract is alcohol-based but you can buy it without showing identification because nobody is doing shots of vanilla extract). Some varieties, known as potable bitters, are meant to be consumed on their own in slightly larger quantities. Whether you're having a small glass of potable bitters or using a few drops of cocktail bitters, stimulating the bitter taste receptors, in turn, stimulates the vagus nerve. This impacts digestion so nutrients are absorbed more quickly—and also activates the body's detoxification function, an evolutionary vestige from a time when eating something bitter meant there was a good chance it was poisonous.[499] Remember: It's all about the detox. Anything we can do to improve the efficiency of our body's detoxification processes will improve our brain health and overall health. Even better if it involves an *apéritif* that becomes an enjoyable ritual.

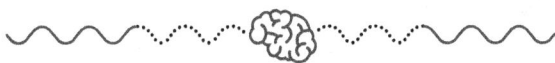

If you're starting to feel overwhelmed by all the information in this chapter, take a deep breath. (Literally—just take a single deep breath and notice how everything starts to feel more manageable. Do you feel the stress response start to wane as the HPA axis becomes less active, allowing your parasympathetic nervous system to come online?) Remember that you're building an ice cream sundae. Start with the foundation and build up from there.

Start by identifying one thing that stood out to you as you were reading—something that felt especially important, or simple, or easy. Don't try to do everything at once; start with one simple change. Once that change is solidified into a habit, you can take on one more change. You'll have a chance to assess how it's going and maybe even decide that particular change isn't working for you and you want to try something else. Even if you experience backsliding, which we all do sometimes, it won't be as tempting to throw in the towel and stop trying altogether. Lifestyle change is far more effective when taken one small step at a time than when we attempt a drastic, all-encompassing overhaul. I promise, you'll achieve *more* change in the long run by focusing on one area than if you try to address multiple areas all at once!

Also, remember that your thoughts and what you believe is possible for you are just as important as toxins and trauma. There are three sides to the triangle, all with equal length. If you find yourself feeling overwhelmed, it may be worth taking a look at the thoughts, assumptions, and beliefs behind your emotions. That feeling of overwhelm is usually a telltale sign of shame. The thought pattern might go something like, "Ugh! I'm not doing *any* of this yet. I'm such a failure at healthy living. I've gone all these years doing absolutely nothing for my health. There's no point in starting now."

Once you learn to notice your thoughts, you can start to reframe them to treat yourself with more compassion. For example, if you catch yourself thinking something like what I just wrote above, you might interrupt that thought pattern and instead say to yourself, "I've done the best I can so far. I didn't understand how important this was before. Now that I do understand, I can work on making some changes. Just the fact that I'm paying attention to this now and making an effort is meaningful." Do you see how this way of framing it produces a completely different feeling—you're doing great, you're being supported, you might make mistakes and mess up, but that just means you're human—compared to the first thought pattern?

Reprogramming your thoughts is one of the most powerful things you can do because it affects every aspect of your life. If behavior change feels impossible or if you routinely beat yourself up for failing, changing your thoughts can make life feel infinitely easier and more enjoyable. Accumulating quick wins by focusing first on small changes that feel easy to make is one way to build your confidence. Still, no matter how many quick wins you rack up, it will never be enough if you're constantly dwelling on where you're falling short instead of celebrating what you're doing right. If this feels like a significant factor that's inhibiting change for you or if it's something you've never really considered before, try keeping a journal to record your thoughts, how they make you feel, and the assumptions that underpin them. This could be a great habit to start with, perhaps while you're using your light device each evening.

Think of it as another form of hormesis. When things go wrong in life, you'll be able to bounce back faster and respond more effectively to a stressful situation if you've trained your thoughts and built up your capacity to treat yourself with compassion instead of compounding the stress of external events and circumstances by piling on and blaming yourself. By building your self-compassion "muscle," you are training your mind to respond in a more positive and productive way to the stressors that will inevitably come your way.

SECTION THREE

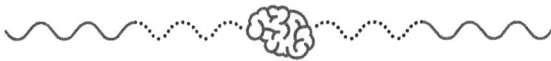

To Infinity and Beyond

CHAPTER SEVEN

Neurodegeneration: When the Professional Became Personal

"By the time you're eighty years old, you've learned everything. You only have to remember it."

—George Burns

You've seen how my own life has been touched by the concepts of brain damage and brain fitness, but it's my mother's story that explains the true depth of my passion for this topic. Watching her suffer from—and ultimately lose her life to—Alzheimer's disease added new urgency to my desire to share this message with the world and change lives with it.

In my thirty-plus years of clinical practice, I saw many, many people with brain diseases. Already, I felt like I had a front-row seat to see the havoc that was created in their lives and their loved ones', and I did my best to assist in each one's personal health recovery. But with the events of my mother's last few years of life, my vantage point changed to the front-row seat on a roller coaster, careening wildly over peaks and valleys with stomach-dropping speed—and it was definitely one of those roller coasters that's in the dark so you can't see what's coming next. I experienced for myself what I had been seeing in my patients' lives for so long: how being a caregiver for someone with Alzheimer's is its own diagnosis with its own effects on brain health. Caregiving is stressful, but we can take action to minimize the effects of this stress—and these actions rely on the same recipe for protecting our brains from disease and debility that you've already started to learn.

By the time my mom started to decline, I was already working with photobiomodulation and learning how it could be useful in treating neuropathy, which is a condition that tends to affect people later in life—often as a consequence of diabetes or a side effect of chemotherapy. But watching what she went through—feeling powerless and wanting to find some way, any way, to help—led me to delve deeper into researching light's power to heal. She was one of the first "clients" to try out what would later become known as the **PRONEURO** approach.

The approach described in this book did have some benefit for my mother, and the research has come along even further since she passed away. If she were alive today to benefit from these scientific advancements—or if she had started to follow the **PRONEURO** approach earlier in life before she declined so much—who knows what kind of difference it could have made for her?

In a sense, I wish I would have come out with my photobiomodulation devices and this book sooner because every new person who receives the message of this book represents a potential life saved—and, if they share what they learn with someone else, potentially more than one life and many additional years of a better *quality* of life. But I trust that events in life unfold at the pace they're meant to, with divine timing—and I know that personally experiencing the anguish of caring for someone with Alzheimer's gave me a perspective that is needed for this work. Caring for my mother was all-consuming, and only once that phase of life was over was I ready to write this book. Trying to get people to understand the urgency of changing their lifestyle habits to take care of their brains requires a level of passion and devotion that I'm not sure I would have had without that firsthand experience.

A SHARP AND CURIOUS MIND, REMEMBERED

My mother grew up in an Italian immigrant family in New York during the Great Depression. It would have been easy for her to just stay there and get married and start a family. That was what was expected of women at the time, but that wasn't in her nature. She did eventually get married and start a family, but first, she went to college—including a semester of study abroad in Denmark—and then she moved to California to complete her student teaching.

She was an independent woman back in 1949. I think she was an adventurer at heart (everywhere I lived, she came to visit me)—and she wanted her son to be independent, too. When I told her I'd decided to get out of New York and go to college in Montana, she simply said, "That's a good idea." There was never a thought in her mind to keep me close so she could see me all the time; she encouraged me to go out and explore the world.

Maybe I got my unorthodox and contrarian streak from her—because she definitely wasn't your typical housewife. She didn't even know how to cook when she got married. It's part of our family lore that because of her still-developing cooking skills, my father had to go to the emergency room twice to get his stomach pumped during the first year of their marriage!

During my childhood, she worked as a school librarian, and she used to say all the time, "I have a master's degree." She was very proud of that. (I would jokingly respond back to her, "Yeah, Mom. Me, too—and I'm a doctor!" These days, my own daughter, who is a naturopathic physician, tries the same thing on me.) Mom was very smart, and education was important to her; I definitely got that from her. It wasn't just her job to be a librarian; it was who she was. Her house was filled to the brim with books; we donated more than five hundred of them after she died.

Our first sign that something was wrong was in 2004. My mother had flown to California to visit my brother, and when the plane landed, she found that she couldn't get up from the plane seat. She couldn't figure out why—she just tried to get up and she couldn't. Her legs wouldn't work.

My mother was overweight and diabetic, and it turned out she had neuropathy. This was around the time they were discovering that statin medications—which she took to lower cholesterol—caused neuropathy. We got her off of the statins and using CoQ10 and photobiomodulation, and the next thing we knew, she was doing better. When she came to see me in Italy, we walked all over Venice together.

But neuropathy is progressive, especially if you don't make the necessary lifestyle changes and don't maintain your preventive care regimen. In 2008, my mom fell and hit her head. Nobody thought much of it, but eight weeks later she fell again, and this time it was worse. The second fall caused a subdural hematoma—like a bruise under the skull when blood pools because of damage to the blood vessels of the brain. For people with neuropathy, the risk of death greatly increases if they live in a house that has more than one story, and this is why.

There were no more major crises until 2017, when Mom was diagnosed with Alzheimer's, but that entire time, I could see she was slipping. My clinical work by that time had given me a certain perspective, such that I never really stopped looking for the subtle signs of brain damage and loss of function. So, I saw what was happening, but living far away, there was only so much I could do. I tried to warn my brothers, but for them, it seemed to be easier to wait and see—or, perhaps more accurately, *not* see.

By the time I moved back to New York to assist with caregiving responsibilities for my mom, she had full-blown Alzheimer's. In her surroundings, I could see the signs that her condition had been developing for a long time. Around the house, I would find notebooks with notes dating back as far as 2006 in her beautiful scrolling penmanship: "Paid $20 to Susan for birthday card," "Sent payment to AAA insurance." These notes were an early sign of dementia, the coping mechanism of someone who knows something is starting to go wrong with their memory and cognition.

WHEN THE CAREGIVER BECOMES THE PATIENT

Until I moved closer, Mom's primary caregiver was Howard, her companion of twenty-five years. They had known each other for longer than that—they were coworkers as schoolteachers in 1945 and developed a friendship that turned romantic almost fifty years later, once they both were widowed. They actually reconnected in the waiting room of my chiropractic office (and it may not have been a coincidence—I played matchmaker by arranging for them to be in the same place at the same time and mentioning that Mom needed some help putting up her storm windows for the winter).

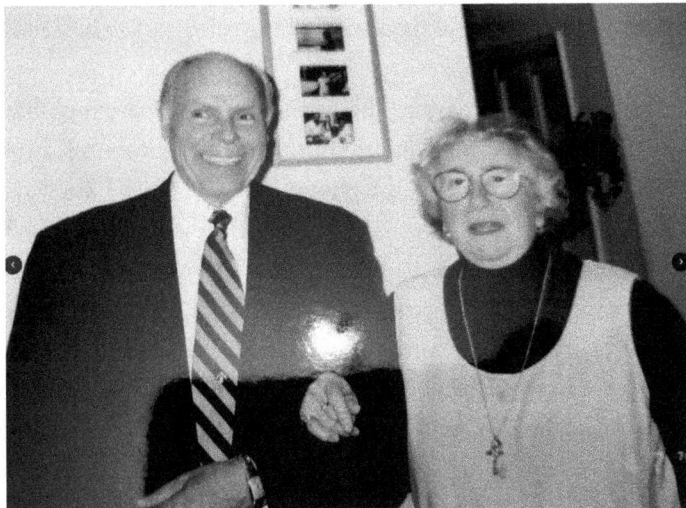

Mom with Howard

Howard was a wonderful man. That's pretty much the first thing everybody said about him. He took such good care of my mom, and he did it lovingly. We should all have that amount of tenacity.

At Mom's eighty-fifth birthday celebration in 2015, we had noticed that caregiving was taking its toll on Howard. He'd always been very athletic—he loved golfing with his children and swimming at the YMCA—but now he had a belly. He wasn't able to do his favorite activities anymore, and he'd become very socially isolated as Mom's needs escalated. I'm not sure he was fully aware of just how much he was declining. When you see yourself in the mirror each day, you don't notice the changes because they're so gradual. I first noticed the impact of caregiver stress on him, and I'd later experience it for myself.

Howard's catastrophe happened on Memorial Day in 2018. I'd walked over to my son's house to spend some time with my son watching *Cobra Kai* on Netflix. When I got home that evening, I opened the door and entered the house. I found Mom pacing around, looking distressed.

She was nonverbal by that time, so I couldn't ask her what had happened; a feeling of horror set in as my eyes scanned the scene and noted the open door leading down to the basement. Lying unconscious at the bottom of the stairs was Howard, his skin an ashen blue color and a trickle of blood coming from his mouth.

I called for help right away. The dispatcher didn't have me administer CPR due to a suspected head injury; in the forty-five minutes it took the ambulance to come, I stayed on the phone with them, but I knew it wasn't looking good for Howard.

I had cameras set up in the house where Mom and Howard lived—with their permission, of course—so I could see what was happening when I wasn't there. When I played back the video of what had happened before I'd come home, I could see that my mom had gone to the phone a couple of times. She knew she was supposed to do something, but she couldn't remember how to use the phone, much less what numbers to dial. The timestamp showed that he'd already been lying there for forty-five minutes by the time I saw him—so the first responders weren't treating him until an hour and a half after his fall. We got the call at three a.m. that Howard had sustained an "unsurvivable injury"—and just like that, Mom and I were on our own. She lived another year with me (and later, my brother) as her caregiver.

It is well documented that caregivers experience loneliness and social isolation due to the "double loss" they experience. They not only lose the person they loved, whose personality is receding as they require progressively more care. The caregiver also loses social connections outside the home, as they are no longer able to leave their loved one alone. In this domain, cognitive decline is just as harmful as physical decline: Even when the loved one can get out of the house for a social gathering, if they cannot participate fully in conversations, card games, and other interactions the way they once could, the social event is less fulfilling not just for them but perhaps even more so for the caregiver. Instead of feeling fun, it may just feel like a painful reminder of loss. It's no surprise that mental health conditions, including depression and anxiety, are significantly more common among caregivers.

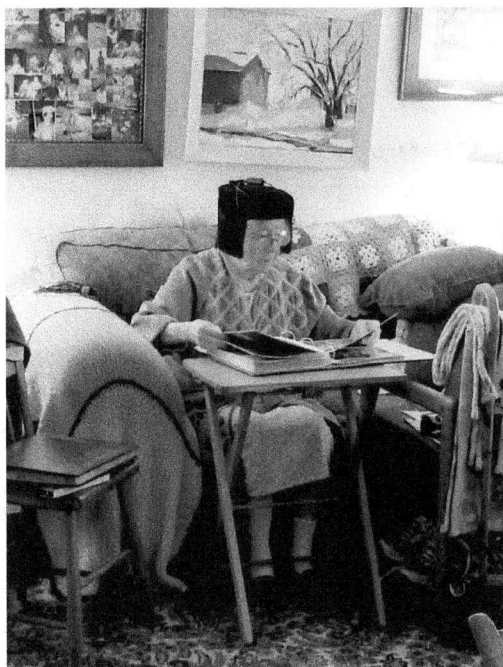

I got Mom using the transcranial photobiomodulation helmet to help improve her cognitive function. In this picture, she is also paging through photo albums to help trigger old memories.

Caregiving demands can also take an economic toll, as caregivers may be prevented from seeking employment outside the home if their loved one cannot be left alone—or they may be required to hire a paid caregiver, at significant expense, to ensure their loved one's safety. The AARP Public Policy Institute estimates that the value of unpaid caregiving provided to adults in the United States is nearly half a trillion dollars per year—a rough indicator of the lost wages of unpaid caregivers and a rough estimate of what it would cost to hire caregivers to provide the care family members are providing for free. And the need is only growing—the same report projects that by 2035, Americans will have (on average) more elderly relatives and friends than children to care for.

We know that all these factors—financial stress, social isolation, depression—increase a person's risk for adverse health outcomes such as cardiovascular disease, diabetes, hypertension, and stroke. (One notable study quantified the impact of social isolation as being equivalent to smoking fifteen cigarettes a day and being twice as harmful as obesity.[500]) Caregivers report increased stress and depression as well as lower levels of well-being and self-efficacy (that is, a sense of agency and empowerment over one's own life).[501, 502, 503, 504, 505] One study found that caregivers had higher levels of C-reactive protein[506]—a marker of systemic inflammation that is a risk factor for many chronic diseases—while a review article found that caregivers show changes in blood coagulation and cell aging as well as inflammation.[507] An Alzheimer's Association report notes that the chronic stress of caregiving is associated with impaired immune function and slow wound healing[508] (a combination of symptoms whose underlying biology you now understand a bit about after reading the material in this book about the autonomic nervous system, mitochondria, and inflammation). Caregivers' sleep quality and duration suffer,[509, 510] and research has shown that caring for a spouse with dementia accelerates one's own cognitive decline[511, 512, 513, 514, 515] and physical decline.[516, 517] In fact, one study found that people caring for a spouse with dementia had a sixfold increase in their risk of a new diagnosis of dementia compared to subjects whose spouses did not have dementia.[518]

Returning to the earlier concept of allostatic load offers one way to quantify the effects of caregiver stress. One study of spousal caregivers of adults with Alzheimer's disease found that their allostatic load (measured for the purpose of this study by assessing blood pressure, blood lipids, body mass index, and hormonal markers) was significantly higher than non-caregiver controls; many other studies have found similar results.[519] Research has also shown that caregiver burden is greater when caring for someone with dementia than when serving as a caregiver for someone with a different chronic illness.[520]

It's worth noting that the recipe for healing presented in this book can provide relief not just for the person with cognitive decline but for their caregiver. I've published work to promote greater awareness among health professionals of the importance of caregivers taking care of their own health,[521] and this book is designed to build that same awareness with a broader audience. In my research paper "Rapid Reversal of Cognitive Decline," we saw that as the patient became better able to perform the activities of daily living, this reduced the burden on the caregiver.[522] Someone with advanced dementia needs a caregiver to attend to them 24/7 in order to survive. If the person can regain some independent function, they wean themselves off of this "human life support." *Caregiver* is its own diagnosis, and I used to say it had no treatment—but now I realize the treatment is the approach captured in this book.

Turn to the back of the book for the PROQOL assessment, a questionnaire designed to help you evaluate your own level of burnout as a caregiver. Self-care is always worth taking time for, but your questionnaire results might highlight an urgent need to take action. My self-care advice for caregivers is the same as for anyone else; we just need to bring it into focus because it so easily gets swallowed up in the endlessly demanding endeavor of caregiving. Remember to take some "me time" and seek out the lighter side of life. Don't let your own preventive care appointments slide, and enlist support for your mental health as needed. Above all, remember to show yourself compassion. Caregiving has plenty of rewarding and fulfilling moments, but it's also inherently stressful, and acknowledging that doesn't make you a bad person.

Providing a more robust social safety net, with funding to support caregivers in helping their loved ones remain safely at home as they age, would go a long way toward easing the burden. But better funding can't erase the strain entirely. If more caregivers were aware of the importance of self-care, it could drastically improve their quality of life—and, consequently, the quality of life of the loved ones for whom they're caring since the caregiver's emotional state also affects the care they give.

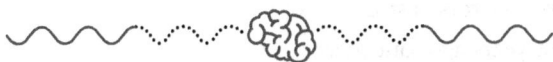

My mother left this earth on August 31, 2019, less than two months shy of her ninetieth birthday. The official cause was sepsis, but dementia had taken her from us long before that.

She managed her condition relatively well—she was always leaving herself notes because she knew she wouldn't remember anything otherwise—but toward the end, she had aphasia, meaning she was unable to speak. The disease took her from us even while she was physically still here.

Dr. Bernie Siegel, a surgeon whose books include *Love, Medicine & Miracles: Lessons Learned about Self-Healing from a Surgeon's Experience with Exceptional Patients* and *Faith, Hope & Healing: Inspiring Lessons Learned from People Living with Cancer*, would always say that when he asked his patients if they wanted to live to be a hundred years old, they would answer, "If I'm healthy"—as if they have no role or agency in determining that. He believed we have a tendency to give away much of our control over the course of our own health, and I agree. Instead I might suggest answering the question by saying something like, "If I use lifestyle changes to not get cancer like my mother did, or heart disease like my father did, or the diabetes that runs in my family."

By following elements of the approach described in this book, my mother was able to become more cognizant and more present in the last decade of her life. She was able to get back some of the functions that neuropathy and dementia were trying to steal from her and to give us a few moments of heartfelt conversation and seeing her there, present again.

The good news is that the sooner we start practicing these habits, the more time they will have to make an impact on our health—and the more established they will become as habits. What we do on a daily basis adds up over the course of a lifetime. When cognitive decline begins to take over, we retreat into what is familiar—so it's best to start now with establishing habits we hope will last a lifetime.

I sometimes wonder how things might have been different if Howard had been able to engage in a more robust self-care regimen. Knowledge of all these protective factors is still developing, and we know more now than we did even a few years ago. But there's also the matter of stigma. Howard was nothing if not stoic, and he never would have wanted to suggest he saw it as a burden to take care of my mom. People from his generation saw needing help as a sign of weakness—and that stigma persists to some extent today.

Caregiving can be joyful at times, in the quiet, small moments and the deep connection you experience with a loved one—but it is an all-consuming job. You don't sleep enough. Your social ties diminish. You lose time for doing the activities you enjoy. Caregiving becomes your whole life.

Neurodegeneration has impacted my life in so many ways—and I know my story really isn't all that extraordinary. I often say that we all end up in one of three "buckets" impacted by this issue—dealing with a neurodegenerative condition ourselves, caring for someone with a neurodegenerative condition, or paying for the care—and many of us find ourselves in more than one of the buckets, either simultaneously or subsequently across the life course.

As it turns out, many of the recommendations I've made for taking care of your brain at any age are the same behaviors that are important to keep practicing as we age. Setting up good habits early in life will set us up for healthy aging. The sooner the better—but it's never too late to start.

The ingredients of the brain health recipe you've learned so far—Photobiomodulation, Repair, Optimize, Nourish—will not only help your brain recover from acute and chronic damage. They will also help your brain stay healthy as you get older—and as you'll learn in the next chapter, that's not really a separate and distinct endeavor from healing brain damage. Rather, it's the other side of the same coin.

CHAPTER EIGHT

Aging Is Inevitable ... Or Is It?

"Age isn't how old you are but how old you feel."

—Gabriel García Márquez

Alzheimer's disease is the sixth-leading cause of death in the United States. One in three seniors dies of Alzheimer's or another type of dementia (although the numbers are difficult to quantify exactly because the official cause of death is often listed as something else, such as complications from a fall or pneumonia due to the way neurodegenerative disease affects the muscles that control swallowing).[523] One recent study projected that the incidence of dementia would triple from current levels to more than 150 million people worldwide with dementia by 2050.[524] Around the globe, someone new is diagnosed with Alzheimer's disease every three seconds.[525] Quite simply, there is a tsunami of caregiver burden and health care burden coming our way.

Health care costs related to Alzheimer's disease amount to $321 billion annually in the United States—and that's just the official number. When we factor in uncompensated care, the total cost to society nearly doubles. More than eleven million Americans provide unpaid care for people with dementia—amounting to sixteen billion hours of care, worth $272 billion in all, on an annual basis.[526] A looming shortage of providers will result in long delays if the ranks of Alzheimer's patients grow in line with the current trajectory,[527, 528] potentially leaving patients and their families to figure out treatment on their own while they wait for an appointment. But if more people educate themselves about prevention and implement what they learn, we may be able to shift the trajectory.

As large as these cost estimates are, they still don't capture the full impact of Alzheimer's.[529] For example, they don't account for the impact on caregivers' health—and that, too, has a cost. This disease has a massive impact on our society, and it grows even larger when you consider the emotional toll. Seeing a parent go through this is agonizing—as is the fear that due to hereditary factors, you yourself are on a path to the same fate.

There's a joke in the medical field that Alzheimer's can be explained by the acronym TMB—Too Many Birthdays—but I'm here to tell you that it's much more complex than that. In this chapter and the next, we'll take a look at what goes wrong in the brain and nervous system to lead to dementia and Alzheimer's. The most important thing to understand is that getting older *does not* mean an inevitable progression into Alzheimer's. Not all old people get dementia, and it is not a foregone conclusion for anyone.

Unfortunately, many doctors treat Alzheimer's and other types of dementia as though the disease's progression is inexorable. They approach treatment through a lens of coping, telling patients and their families to learn to live with the symptoms. I cannot emphasize enough: *This is a huge mistake.* A growing body of evidence is showing us how we can slow down and even reverse the course of Alzheimer's disease. What's more, research is elucidating the early warning signs. Whether a person is headed toward Alzheimer's or another type of dementia, the slow decline begins many years before the symptoms become pronounced enough to interfere with daily living. It is my hope that this book can not only help readers support their loved ones who are dealing with dementia but also help readers change the course of their own health and prevent Alzheimer's and dementia from developing in the first place—be it for themselves or for their loved ones.

As you saw from the story of my mother and Howard—and as you may have seen in your own life—Alzheimer's is a terrible disease. By learning how it operates and how to stop it in its tracks, you may just be saving your own loved ones from having to endure that suffering. (Once again, this goes in both directions: You might be helping a loved one avoid disease, or you might be saving them from the suffering of watching *you* deal with a neurodegenerative disease.)

Cognitive Decline

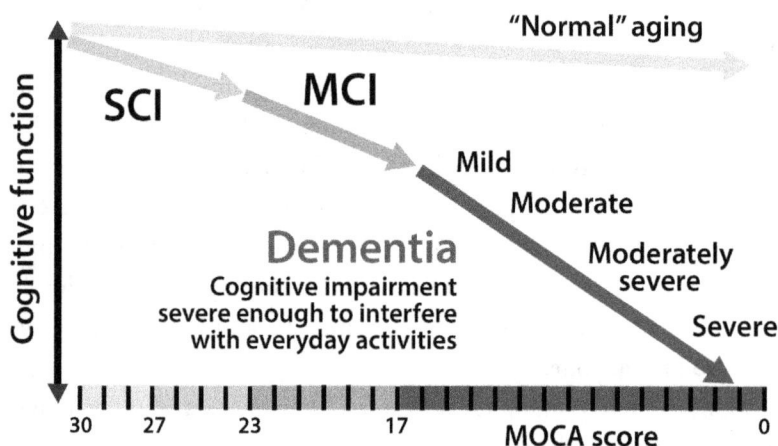

Cognitive function

"Normal" aging

SCI

MCI

Mild

Moderate

Dementia

Cognitive impairment
severe enough to interfere
with everyday activities

Moderately
severe

Severe

| | | | | | | | | | | | | | | | | | | | | | | | | | | | |
30   27   23   17   MOCA score   0

While cognitive function declines slightly even in healthy aging, the decline
is much steeper for people with dementia. The trajectory begins with subjective cognitive impairment, in which the person knows something is wrong
but nobody else can tell, and moves into mild cognitive impairment and,
from there, into the mild, moderate, and severe phases of dementia. However,
this progression is not inexorable. It can be slowed and even reversed.

What I find fascinating is that many of the early changes are similar
to the damage caused by a traumatic brain injury—which is exactly why
I went into detail about the consequences of TBI in the second section of
this book. That type of brain damage tends to happen earlier in life when
people are more active and taking more risks—and if not addressed, it
can lead to cognitive decline later. The good news is that, as you saw in
our discussion of TBI, these symptoms can be healed.

People tend to have a sense of resignation about age-related cognitive decline and Alzheimer's, like "Oh well, what can you do?" I want to
say that this is unequivocally wrong. You *can* turn it around.

Let's take a look at the changes in the brain that lead to Alzheimer's
and other types of dementia. Our exploration of these changes and how
to reverse them starts with an entity called the glymphatic system.

THE GLYMPHATIC SYSTEM:
TRASH COLLECTION FOR THE BRAIN

If you don't remember the word *glymphatic* from your high school biology textbook, it's not because you're losing your memory. It wasn't until the twenty-first century that this system was discovered and given an official name. The word, a combination of *glial* (as in brain cells) and *lymphatic* (as in the system that plays a critical role in detoxification and immune function), describes how the body clears out waste products and toxins from the brain. This cleaning function is largely disengaged while we're awake and active while we are sleeping. Aside from its cleaning function, the glymphatic system also distributes glucose, lipids, amino acids, and neurotransmitters throughout the brain.[530]

Throughout the body, your blood delivers nutrients, but not all of the fluid that goes out from the heart through the circulatory system is returned. The fluid that seeps out through the capillaries into the body's tissues is rounded up by the lymphatic system and returned to circulation, thus restoring fluid balance and preventing excess fluid from accumulating. (This is why people often develop edema, or swelling, in nearby body parts after having lymph nodes removed—for example, during cancer surgery.) The lymphatic system clears out waste products and delivers immune system cells wherever they are needed to help fight infection. Separated from the lymphatic system by the blood-brain barrier, the glymphatic system performs similar functions within the brain. In contrast to the circulation of blood and lymph, which are most active when we are awake and moving, the glymphatic system is most active while we sleep.

Why humans (and other animals, for that matter) need to sleep has been a long-standing mystery to scientists. After all, we are exquisitely vulnerable to predators while we sleep, so something crucially important must be happening that offers an even greater evolutionary benefit—otherwise, animals that don't need to sleep would have won the Darwinian race, right? The answer to this riddle may be that sleep allows the glymphatic system to perform its important work.

Waste Removal in the Brain

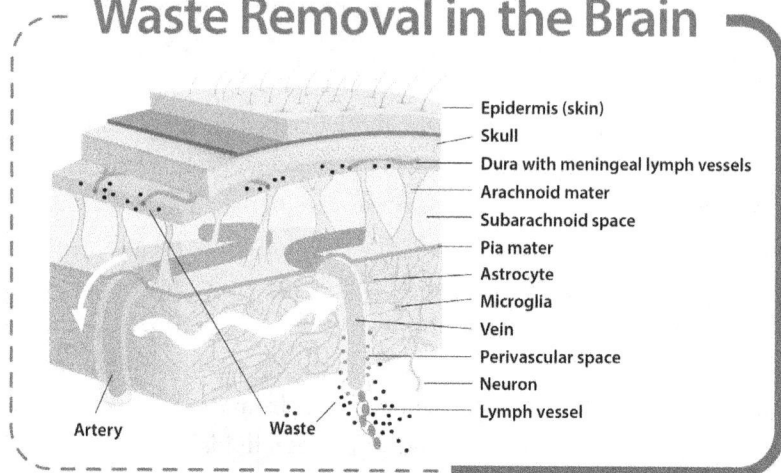

- Epidermis (skin)
- Skull
- Dura with meningeal lymph vessels
- Arachnoid mater
- Subarachnoid space
- Pia mater
- Astrocyte
- Microglia
- Vein
- Perivascular space
- Neuron
- Lymph vessel

Artery   Waste

While neurons might be the most well-known type of brain cell (since they're responsible for cognition, memory, and movement), other types of brain cells called astrocytes and microglia play key roles in the brain's waste removal system, known as the glymphatic system. In this system, the rhythmic pulses of the arterial walls draw cerebrospinal fluid from the subarachnoid space (between the dura mater, or tough outer lining, and the pia mater, or inner lining) deep into the brain. Astrocytes surround the perivascular spaces— open, fluid-filled tunnels that offer little resistance to flow—and act as gates for fluid influx into the brain tissue. As shown by the white arrows, waste is flushed out through the lymph vessels and perivascular spaces along veins as well as through the meningeal lymph vessels along the brain's outer lining. Microglia, the immune cells of the central nervous system, also act as waste collectors—including, importantly, the uptake and clearance of amyloid beta. This exquisitely designed and calibrated system is what protects the health of the neurons and allows them to keep working—or, when conditions tip out of balance, fails to protect them, resulting in neurodegeneration.

Up until the glymphatic system's discovery, it was considered a paradox that the lymphatic vessels that help to clear infection throughout the rest of the body were absent from the central nervous system. Scientists assumed the fact that this system did not extend to the brain meant the brain was a sterile environment—but in fact, this isn't true. The brain just has its own unique system for clearing infection. Within the last decade, scientists have observed the meningeal lymphatic vessels that carry out this clearing function, removing substances such as the amyloid beta and tau proteins known for their role in Alzheimer's disease via the nasal passages and cervical lymph nodes.[531] New paths of research are elucidating exactly how the body carries this out—for example, identifying a "helper protein" that assists with clearing these substances and even a genetic variant that affects levels of this protein and, fascinatingly, is associated with Alzheimer's patients maintaining their cognitive faculties longer than those with the other variant.[532] This research area is rapidly developing, and scientists are also learning that many more substances are able to cross the blood-brain barrier than previously thought—and that the brain has its own microbiome, which some have dubbed the *neurobiome*. More on this later—but for now, just know that the glymphatic system plays a key role in maintaining a healthy neurobiome. Glymphatic clearance also acts to keep inflammation of the brain at healthy, low levels—and when glymphatic clearance is impaired, pro-inflammatory substances build up and a state of neuroinflammation results.[533]

As the glymphatic system does its work while we sleep, cerebrospinal fluid mixes with interstitial fluid, delivering what's needed and removing what the brain needs to get rid of. What's fascinating is that the interstitial space (the space between the cells) increases during slow-wave sleep, the deepest and most physically restorative sleep phase. Picture the narrow streets of Manhattan or an old European city, where space is at a premium, and if a car double-parks, it prevents anyone else from passing. Now imagine if, during the night while people slept, the buildings would actually recede so the streets became wider, making it easier for vehicles to pass—delivering mail and packages, collecting the garbage, and power-washing the sidewalks to leave them freshly cleaned for the new day. This is exactly what happens in the brain while we are sleeping. The space between the cells widens *by more than sixty percent* to allow more space for fluid to move through.[534]

A 2019 study by researchers including Boston University's Laura Lewis captured the nighttime "brain wash" with functional magnetic resonance imaging (fMRI), observing the pulses of cerebrospinal fluid that pump into the brain like ocean waves at high tide, surging and receding in sync with the delta frequency brain waves of deep sleep.[535] Intriguingly,

Components of the Glymphatic System

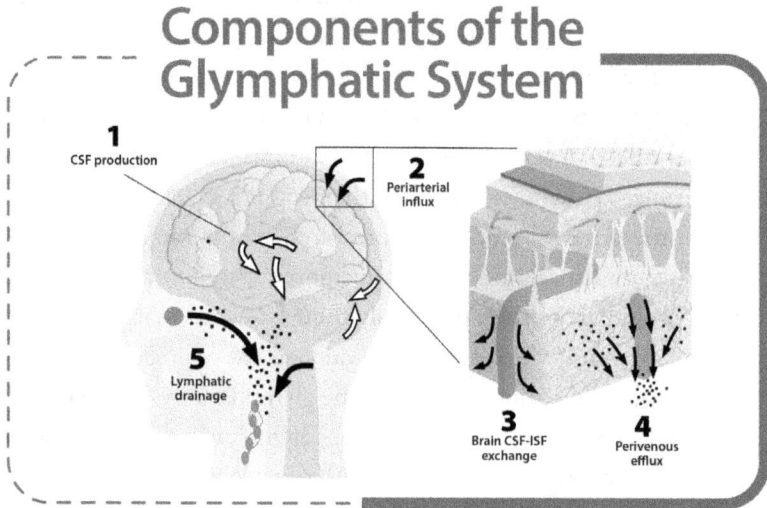

1 CSF production

2 Periarterial influx

5 Lymphatic drainage

3 Brain CSF-ISF exchange

4 Perivenous efflux

The glymphatic system has five main functional components, each of which facilitates waste clearance via the movement of cerebrospinal fluid (CSF) and interstitial fluid (ISF). (1) The CSF that accumulates in the brain as a product of cellular processes and via influx from the capillaries flows out to the meningeal lymph vessels, and from there, (2) arterial wall pulsatility drives the fluid deep into the brain via the perivascular spaces. (3) CSF and ISF mingle as part of this cleaning process. (4) This mixed fluid accumulates in the perivenous space and (5) drains out of the brain via meningeal and cervical lymph vessels, which empty into the lymphatic system.

engineers at Rice University have developed a "sleeping cap" that measures glymphatic system activity and are evaluating the device's potential for future use in assessing sleep quality and diagnosing sleep disorders.

A 2021 study observed that the cerebrospinal fluid waves were uncoupled from slow-wave rhythms in subjects with Alzheimer's disease,[536] demonstrating a link between the disease and abnormal functioning of the glymphatic system. Although more research is needed to determine if this is correlation or causation, this association tells us something important: In Alzheimer's patients, the "brain wash" function breaks down and doesn't work anymore. A 2022 study found that uncoupling of "sleep spindles" (bursts of brain activity that occur during deep sleep and are thought to be part of learning and memory consolidation) from the slow-wave patterns characteristic of deep sleep was linked to early amyloid beta burden and was predictive of memory decline—indicating that declining sleep quality is at least associated with early cognitive decline, if not playing a causal role.[537]

If we're not getting high-quality sleep, the brain can't clean itself—predisposing us to neurodegeneration. Remember that part of what's being cleaned out are the proteins that are hallmarks of Alzheimer's disease. As these proteins accumulate in larger and larger amounts, it grows even harder for the brain to clean itself. That is to say, the problem compounds itself in another example of a vicious cycle that escalates.[538]

In recent years, scientists have begun to understand Alzheimer's not as a problem with the brain per se, but rather as a problem with the brain's clearance system—i.e., the glymphatic system.[539] What's more, researchers have proposed in recent years that much of the research seeking to understand Alzheimer's since it was first described in 1907 has been approaching the problem from the wrong angle, asking why the body produces too much amyloid beta instead of asking the more pertinent question: Why doesn't the body clear amyloid beta from the brain as well as it should?[540]

Research with mice has verified the importance of the meningeal lymphatic vessels (those that drain fluid and waste products from the brain) for the development of Alzheimer's. Mice given a growth factor that enhances the meningeal lymphatic vessels' function displayed improved memory—and conversely, disruption of those vessels' function led to increased amyloid beta deposition (or perhaps more to the point, decreased clearance).[541] Impaired glymphatic clearance is also believed to play a role in the development of Parkinson's disease[542] and in the accumulation of tau proteins as a downstream effect of TBI.[543] In fact, some researchers propose that the glymphatic system's failure is a "final common pathway" in the development of Alzheimer's and other neurodegenerative dementia conditions.[544]

What's more, dysfunction of the glymphatic system after TBI is believed to be one of the reasons headaches often plague TBI sufferers (and especially those also experiencing sleep disruption).[545] What's interesting is that a treatment you're quite familiar with, if you've read this far in the book—photobiomodulation—has shown the ability to stimulate lymphatic

Conditions Affecting the Glymphatic System

Lifestyle
Sedentary
Obesity
Circadian disturbance
Sleep quality
Aging
Stress
Substance abuse

Genetics

Decreased glymphatic output
Fluid stagnation

Pathology
Hypertension
Small vessel disease
Traumatic brain injury
Cardiac disease
Cardiovascular disorders
Apnea

Neuroinflammation and neurodegenerative diseases

Increased protein concentration and aggregation

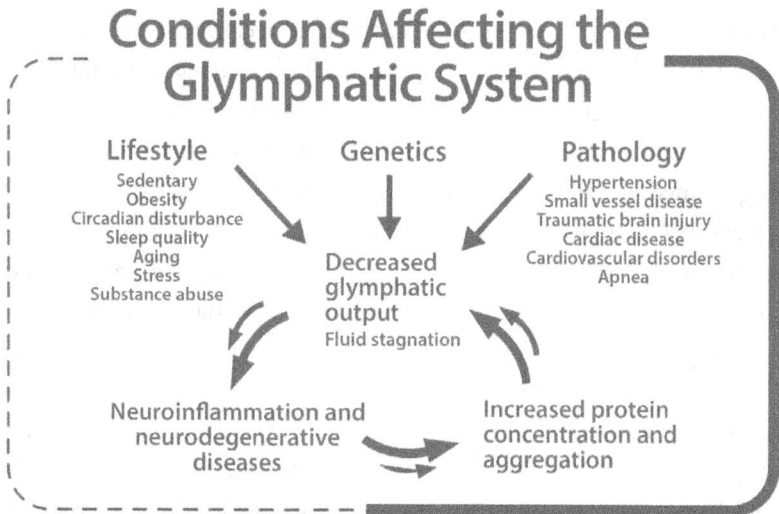

A combination of factors including lifestyle, genetics, and pathology influences how effectively a person's glymphatic system works. Once glymphatic output is impaired, this sets off a vicious cycle in which neuroinflammation and neurodegeneration cause increased protein concentration and aggregation, which, in turn, further decreases glymphatic output.

drainage.[546] We will come back to look more deeply at why and how that works, but for now, just know that effects on the lymphatic and glymphatic systems can be added to the list of ways photobiomodulation is beneficial.

LOSING SLEEP OVER NEURODEGENERATION

As you learned in Chapter Five, sleep is one of the most important factors for a healthy brain. Insomnia is correlated with elevated dementia risk, and although it's not entirely clear which direction the arrow of causation points, there is some evidence that trouble sleeping actually causes dementia and not the other way around. At least in mice, researchers have shown that restricting sleep leads to the buildup of amyloid beta[547] and dementia symptoms.[548] People with normal cognitive function but poor sleep quality have elevated amyloid beta levels,[549] suggesting that impaired sleep may play a causative role or at least be an early symptom of something going wrong.

One study found that people who reported they had trouble falling asleep "most nights" had a forty-four percent increased risk of early death. Those who reported that they often woke in the night and struggled to get back to sleep had a fifty-six percent increased risk of early death. The same sleep problems were also risk factors for dementia: The group that had trouble falling asleep "most nights" had a forty-nine percent increased risk of dementia, and those who reported they often woke in the night and struggled to get back to sleep had a thirty-nine percent increased risk of dementia. The group that had *both* risk factors—trouble falling asleep *and* waking up and having trouble falling back asleep—had an eighty percent greater risk of early death and fifty-six percent greater risk of dementia compared to the subjects who had neither of these problems.[550]

A 2021 paper from British researchers (based on a longitudinal study of nearly eight thousand people) reported that sleep duration of six hours or less was correlated with higher dementia risk than getting at least seven hours of sleep per night.[551] Sleep differences are already apparent in the middle-aged (and cognitively healthy) children of late-onset Alzheimer's disease patients relative to a control group with no family history of Alzheimer's,[552] giving a clue to one of the early warning signs and perhaps a causative factor in the heredity of Alzheimer's disease.

The glymphatic system's waste clearance function is primarily active during non-REM sleep (i.e., deep sleep),[553] yet people typically get less and less deep sleep as they age. In fact, it's common for people over age sixty to not get much deep sleep at all—but this isn't healthy and there is no reason we need to accept it.

Just one night of sleep deprivation is enough to increase amyloid beta levels in the brain.[554] This signature protein of Alzheimer's disease is a sticky compound that disrupts communication between brain cells, eventually killing the cells as it accumulates in the brain. One week of disrupted sleep increases the amount of tau, another protein responsible for the tangles associated with Alzheimer's, frontal lobe dementia, and Lewy body disease.[555] In both mice and humans, tau levels increase in the interstitial fluid of the hippocampus following sleep deprivation, indicating one of the ways sleep deprivation can lead to memory problems.[556]

Although scientists once believed Alzheimer's disease could only be definitively diagnosed after death—and this misconception, unfortunately, persists as conventional wisdom—methods for diagnosing Alzheimer's sufferers and people at risk of it have advanced significantly in recent years. Amyloid beta accumulation and plaques, tau pathology, inflammation, and brain cell damage can be detected via markers in a sample of cerebrospinal fluid. One 2017 study from Wisconsin analyzed these markers in light of subjects' sleep quality and found that subjects who slept poorly were more likely to have the dementia markers, even when controlling for other dementia risk factors such as obesity and cardiovascular disease.[557] Another study found that slow-wave sleep disruptions, in particular, were correlated with elevated amyloid beta levels in cerebrospinal fluid; if this disruption persisted over several days, an increase in tau protein levels was also found.[558] A study of older adults (ages fifty-five to seventy) found that insomnia was associated with a stress signal from the mitochondria in the form of a mitokine response—indicating one of the ways sleep deprivation can set off a detrimental chain of events in the body (recall the *cell danger response* theory explored in Chapter Five).[559] Once they build up in the brain, amyloid beta and tau seem to cause further trouble with getting high-quality sleep, leading some scientists to posit that disrupted sleep could even be used as a diagnostic marker for Alzheimer's disease.[560]

We have already addressed the fact that the brain is not a sterile environment (a disproven claim that you nevertheless still often hear repeated today); scientists are also realizing that, just as "leaky gut" can cause an autoimmune response and inflammation when substances from the digestive tract leak through the intestinal wall, there is also a condition that could be called "leaky brain" when the blood-brain barrier becomes permeable. Studies with mice tell us this condition is exacerbated with hypertension and that a leaky blood-brain barrier sets off a cascade of consequences including neuroinflammation and cognitive decline. (Intriguingly, a study using cardiac magnetic resonance imaging in humans found that subtle changes in heart muscle function lead to changes in cognitive function—and the researchers suggested that this decline might come about because the changes in how the heart muscle works cause problems with the blood-brain barrier.[561]) A fascinating line of research has found that bacteria colonize the brain in Alzheimer's disease, leading to neurotoxicity and pointing to the role the neurobiome plays in the course of disease.[562] This helps to explain why hypertension is a risk factor for Alzheimer's and is yet another example of the way the body's protective mechanisms can spin out of control to cause damage—and an opportunity for us to bring the mechanisms back into balance and create the conditions for healing.

RED ALERT: MILD COGNITIVE IMPAIRMENT

One of the risk factors for Alzheimer's and early warning signs of dementia is a condition called mild cognitive impairment (MCI). The degree of severity is evaluated with the help of neurological and cognitive tests as well as an interview to determine the patient's own perception of how much the condition affects the activities of daily life. The assessment often follows a patient's own (or a relative's) noticing that they are experiencing problems with memory or another aspect of cognition such as language.

In the words of one set of study authors, MCI "is characterized by slight cognitive impairment, greater than expected for an individual's age and education but not severe enough to warrant a diagnosis of dementia, that does not substantially interfere with functional independence, although there may be some minimal deficits in the more complex instrumental activities of daily living." It stands out as a public health problem because it is increasingly recognized to be the prodromal stage of dementia, with an annual conversion rate ranging from five to fifteen percent across different studies, and it affects a consistent portion of the population.[563]

Out of every thousand people aged sixty-five or older, MCI is estimated to affect between twelve and fifteen of those people. Nearly half of MCI patients develop dementia within five years. As it stands, MCI is relatively loosely defined and potentially widely underdiagnosed; we would be well served to get clearer about the clinical criteria that define it and about which specific factors predispose people to faster or more severe cognitive decline. (As with dementia, there is also a caregiver burden associated with MCI that is not yet well quantified or understood.[564]) That being said, there are many intriguing connections between MCI and the other conditions explored in this book, indicating that MCI may be a bridge from risk factors to neurodegenerative conditions and an early warning sign we should be testing for more widely and monitoring more closely.

As research advances, it may become possible to identify who is at risk of neurodegeneration sooner in the progression of symptoms. In a study of the middle-aged children of people with late-onset Alzheimer's disease, Carolina Abulafia and colleagues were able to identify alterations in executive function, despite the fact that the children were still considered cognitively normal by all the standard measures.[565] In a separate study, the same research group found that relative to a control group, the children of late-onset Alzheimer's disease patients displayed subtle but significant deficits in verbal episodic memory and language as well as disturbances in their sleep-wake rhythm.[566] The children of late-onset Alzheimer's patients also were slower to recover after a cognitive stress test, and the severity of the delay was correlated with the level of amyloid deposition and compromised gray matter integrity as observed on brain scans.[567] Furthermore, the children of the late-onset Alzheimer's patients displayed thinning of specific brain areas relevant to Alzheimer's disease.[568] Depressive symptoms affect cognitive performance differently in the children of late-onset Alzheimer's disease patients, a finding that has implications for caregiver stress if those children are the caregivers for the parents affected by Alzheimer's.[569]

By the time MCI develops, it's a "red alert" that danger is high. There's still time to act, but we must not delay or discount the seriousness of the risk. A history of TBI increases one's chances of developing MCI[570] and, among those who do develop MCI, correlates with being diagnosed at a younger age (2.3 years earlier, on average).[571] This makes sense, given what we know about the lingering effects of TBI on brain health.

People with MCI don't sleep as long or as efficiently, and it takes them longer to fall asleep.[572] In particular, their slow-wave sleep (the kind essential for the glymphatic function) is disrupted.[573] People with amnestic MCI (that is, the kind that affects memory) experience more severe sleep disturbances than cognitively normal elderly people.[574] All of this makes sense, given what we know about sleep and dementia—but which came first, the chicken or the egg? Are these people having trouble sleeping because they have MCI or is MCI caused by their sleep troubles? It's likely the answer is both—but in any event, the more important question is: What can we do about it? As we start to explore the answer to this question, let's return to the parasympathetic nervous system and its powerful on/off switch, the vagus nerve.

THE HEART-BRAIN CONNECTION

You already know from Section Two of the book that when we're talking about the autonomic nervous system and moving from sympathetic to parasympathetic activation, the vagus nerve is an important player. To better understand how its operation affects brain health, let's take a closer look at what the vagus nerve is and how it functions.

The vagus nerve extends all the way from the brainstem down to the abdomen (hence the name, which means "wandering" in Latin). The vagus nerve is responsible for parasympathetic activation of the heart (i.e., slowing heart rate down). In general, this nerve plays a crucial role in activating the "rest and digest" parasympathetic functions and notifying our bodies that it's safe to relax because there is no immediate threat in our environment. Stimulation of the vagus nerve with electrical impulses (using a device that's implanted under the skin of the chest) has been relatively well studied and has been shown to be a beneficial treatment for conditions including inflammatory bowel disease, depression, epilepsy, chronic pain, cluster headaches, and PTSD. Vagus nerve stimulation using an electrode on the neck, approved three decades ago for patients with epilepsy, has also yielded significant cognitive-enhancing effects in experiments with Alzheimer's patients.[575, 576, 577, 578] In addition to cognitive enhancement and influence on inflammation, vagus nerve stimulation may impact the coagulant-anticoagulant balance.[579] Because of these multifaceted benefits, vagus nerve stimulation has also been proposed as a therapeutic approach for severe COVID-19 infection.[580]

Short of implanting an electrode underneath your skin, there are plenty of ways to stimulate the vagus nerve, including many that are outlined in the "recipe" chapters of this book. Examples include everything from maintaining a healthy gut microbiome through the foods you eat to splashing cold water on your face, practicing tai chi[581] or qi gong,[582] meditation,[583] and even some yoga poses (that's right, headstand has long been reported to stimulate the vagus nerve, and research has indeed observed increases in HRV after practicing this pose[584]).

You could say that vagus nerve activation is a proxy for overall parasympathetic activation. In that sense, what we're discussing here is not so much different from everything you learned about the autonomic nervous system in Section Two. The point I want to make here, though, is about the anatomy of the vagus nerve. It literally connects the brain, the heart, and the gut to one another. Given that reality—and what we know about what happens when the vagus nerve is stimulated—how could you ever say that a problem in the brain is just about the brain, or a problem in the gut is just about the gut, or a problem with the heart is just about the heart? You can't.

One particularly fascinating finding is that the gut microbiome influences mood and anxiety through its effects on the vagus nerve.[585] Interestingly, although we typically think of depression as a problem of *not enough energy*, science is coming to understand it as a problem of *overdrive* of the HPA axis. When the body is under too much stress for too long and never gets the chance to downregulate and restore, the result is depression. It may manifest as not enough gas in the tank, but it's not because of an innate shortage; rather, it happens because someone's nervous system has been *overfunctioning* for too long. The high churn rate leads to burnout; healing comes from rest and bringing the system into balance.

The gut affects the brain, and the heart affects the gut, but for our primary concern in this book of preventing or reversing neurodegeneration, the *heart-brain connection* is key. If you want to have a healthy brain into old age, you must have a healthy cardiovascular system—without too much hardening or narrowing of the blood vessels. The heart itself is highly affected by the body's overall level of mitochondrial function since mitochondria make up thirty percent of the human heart's cell volume.[586] When the heart lacks sufficient ATP to carry out the work that's being asked of it, this leads to heart failure. You can't have a healthy brain without a healthy heart—and so, mitochondrial health affects the brain not only via the mitochondria within the brain but indirectly via the mitochondria in the heart.

A healthy brain also relies on a healthy and balanced nervous system—as reflected by the metric of HRV. One team of researchers used the term "brain-heart axis" to capture the interdependence of the two organs and the nervous system activity that influences their interactions, with HRV serving as a kind of feedback loop in which low HRV is both an outcome of and a risk factor for cognitive decline.[587] Considered in these terms, it's easy to understand why a dysregulated autonomic nervous system resulting from TBI, as described in the previous section of the book, is a risk factor for further cognitive decline as the heart loses its ability to efficiently provide blood flow to the parts of the brain that need it.[588]

In 1865, French physiologist Claude Bernard delivered a lecture at the Sorbonne about the heart-brain connection[589]—so these ideas are not new, but Bernard was ahead of his time. With our recently developed (and still developing) ability to measure HRV and its components precisely, we are able to explore in greater detail the ideas Bernard first proposed more than 150 years ago and move toward a greater understanding of why chronic illnesses such as heart disease and dementia often go hand in hand—and what we can do about it.

The connection between blood pressure and brain function is well studied and widely accepted at this point—but awareness is just beginning to grow about low HRV as a risk factor for cognitive decline.[590] As one team of scientists noted, "decreased HRV indexes indicate low vagal activity that is associated with the development of several diseases, such as diabetes, cardiovascular disease, cancers, and Alzheimer's disease."[591]

You know from Chapter Three that HRV can be thought of as your joy score—but it's connected to thinking as well as feeling. Low HRV is associated with impaired performance on tasks that measure various dimensions of cognitive function.[592] In a study of sailors with the Royal Norwegian Navy, subjects with higher HRV displayed greater accuracy, faster reaction time, and better working memory on a cognitive performance test.[593] A study of more than two hundred pairs of twins found an association between HRV and verbal skills: Within each pair of twins, the one with lower HRV performed worse (on average) on a word recall test, and a history of PTSD also predicted poorer performance.[594] HRV changes (specifically, depressed parasympathetic activity) have been observed in neurological conditions including Guillain-Barré syndrome and the acute recovery period following a stroke.[595]

Low HRV is associated with reduced executive function, a capacity some scientists characterize as the ability to tune out distractions. If we think about the ability to focus as not so much letting the right information in (seeing what's in front of you) but rather excluding the wrong information (ignoring or suppressing everything else), this, too, can be seen through a model of inhibition. Higher vagal activity (as measured by HRV) indicates suppression of the sympathetic activation that keeps us in fight-or-flight—and only when this is suppressed do we have the laser-pointed focus needed to complete complex cognitive tasks quickly.[596] A wide-ranging review of the research found that increased sympathetic activity and decreased parasympathetic activity (two sides of the same coin) were associated with worse cognitive performance.[597] Analyzing data collected for the Coronary Artery Risk Development in Young Adults Study, one team of researchers concluded that low HRV was a risk factor for diminished executive function in midlife, separate from the predictive value of cardiovascular risk factors.[598] Researchers have also found that low HRV can predict the progression from MCI to Alzheimer's disease[599, 600] and that measuring patients' HRV may be able to help doctors differentiate among the various types of dementia.[601] What's more, declining HRV is associated with subtle cognitive decline, even in subjects without dementia.[602]

In addition to the link between depression and inflammation noted earlier in the book, recent research has hinted that depression may also be understood as a disorder of the autonomic nervous system: That is, during times of rest and relaxation, vagal activity is abnormally low and sympathetic activation is abnormally high. For a quarter-century now, researchers have noted that people with depression have increased cardiovascular risk that does not seem to be explained by their behavior (e.g., it's not just that people exercise less because they're depressed).[603, 604, 605, 606, 607, 608, 609, 610] The heart-brain connection helps us understand this previously puzzling association. Depression is not just a condition that consists of "feeling low" and which we can will ourselves to snap out of; it has real and quantifiable underlying physiological contributors.

One of the most widely used treatments for depression, SSRI medications, can have negative cardiovascular impacts via their effect on circulating levels of serotonin and noradrenaline, and these medications do nothing to improve the low HRV that accompanies mood disorders;[611] thus, people suffering from mood disorders would be wise to pursue ways of improving their HRV instead of or in addition to taking antidepressant medication.

In a study of more than three thousand senior citizens (median age: seventy-five), participants with lower HRV had worse cognitive function at baseline, including reaction time, processing speed, and immediate and delayed memory recall. As the study continued over several years, subjects with lower HRV at the outset also had steeper annual rates of decline in their cognitive function—specifically, in reaction time and processing speed. (Low HRV was not associated with faster decline for immediate and delayed memory recall.)[612]

One paper that analyzed data from a long-term study found that subjects with low HRV were seven times more likely to develop cognitive impairment.[613] Studies have begun to tease apart the mechanics of how this happens, for example, observing white matter lesions in people with MCI and showing that the severity of these lesions is correlated with autonomic dysfunction as measured by HRV.[614]

In fact, low vagal tone (i.e., decreased vagal activation and the accompanying low HRV) is believed to contribute to processes that affect multiple bodily systems through mechanisms such as releasing inflammatory cytokines.[615] (Recall what you learned in Chapter Five about the cell danger response that ties together multiple mechanisms to affect organs and systems throughout the body.) Reduced parasympathetic activation (i.e., low HRV) means the body's processes that reduce inflammation are inhibited—resulting in elevated levels of systemic inflammation, which are associated with cognitive decline.[616] Low vagal tone is also correlated with increased fasting glucose and glycated hemoglobin levels (i.e., risk factors for diabetes).[617] There are enough correlations like this that some scientists believe the vagus nerve could be a regulator of allostatic load, helping the body turn on or off the cascade of symptoms that tip a person into ill health.[618] Indeed, we see that the arrow of influence points in both directions when it comes to the heart-brain connection: Cognitive impairment increases one's risk of a cardiovascular event such as a heart attack independent of other risk factors.[619]

Some researchers believe HRV is the causal link that explains why certain conditions—such as hypertension, diabetes, depression, and chronic inflammation—carry increased risk of impaired cognitive function.[620] One hypothesis is that the autonomic nervous system fails to properly regulate brain perfusion (the circulation of oxygenated blood)—and, of course, we know the consequences of low HRV for the glymphatic system's clearance function. In the kind of vicious cycle we know all too well from the ground we've already covered in this book, as the brain is unable to clear out waste products, cell death can result, impairing the brain's ability to regulate the autonomic nervous system—further compounding the problem of low HRV. In yet another example of the cascade of symptoms that picks up momentum until it tips a person into ill health, autonomic dysfunction leads to blood pressure dysregulation, which makes people more vulnerable to falls as their bodies' systems of sensory perception and responding to changing conditions in the environment are less finely attuned and respond less rapidly.[621]

In fact, one model characterizes the entire process of aging as one of parasympathetic withdrawal, such that the sympathetic nervous system becomes dominant, leading to outcomes such as hypertension (which, in turn, leads to decreased circulation of oxygenated blood in the brain, white matter lesions, and enlarged ventricles—and, thus, MCI).[622] The frontal lobe, parietal lobe, and hypothalamus, which also play a role in autonomic nervous system function, also show degeneration in Alzheimer's disease—and this is one of the factors that differentiates Alzheimer's from other types of dementia.[623] We need to stop thinking about Alzheimer's disease as a problem of plaques building up in the brain and start thinking about it as a problem of imbalance in the nervous system.

Most of us are well aware of the way a stroke damages the surrounding brain tissue, but less well known is the hypoperfusion (lack of oxygenated blood) that results from damage to the small blood vessels with hypertension. This common type of damage is associated with reduced cognitive test performance and detrimental changes to the brain's white matter.[624] As *hyper*tension (high pressure) causes damage to small vessels in the brain, the result is *hypo*perfusion (low passage of blood) into those small vessels—and autonomic dysfunction and low HRV are increasingly being recognized as a cause of this.[625]

(We see similar changes in people recovering from TBI, with the circulation of oxygenated blood to the brain being reduced for them as well[626]—not surprising given what we know about heart rate variability following TBI. Interestingly, our good friend near-infrared light is the tool used to measure this in a technique called near-infrared spectroscopy that uses the chromophoric property of hemoglobin and cytochrome c oxidase to monitor the flow of blood in various areas throughout the brain.[627] This technique may actually prove to be a more precise diagnostic method for concussion and the lasting effects of TBI than some of the more widely used methods, such as testing a person's balance.[628])

If you've ever taken a stress test to evaluate your cardiovascular health, what it was actually measuring was the flexibility and adaptability of your nervous system: How quickly does your vagus nerve send the signal to adapt to changing conditions? Stress tests assess the autonomic nervous system's ability to recover (and how quickly it can do so) after an episode of sympathetic activation.[629] Another way to measure the autonomic nervous system's flexibility and adaptability is what's called the "head-up tilt"—measuring how quickly blood pressure adjusts to changes in body orientation (such as moving

Loss of structure leads to loss of function

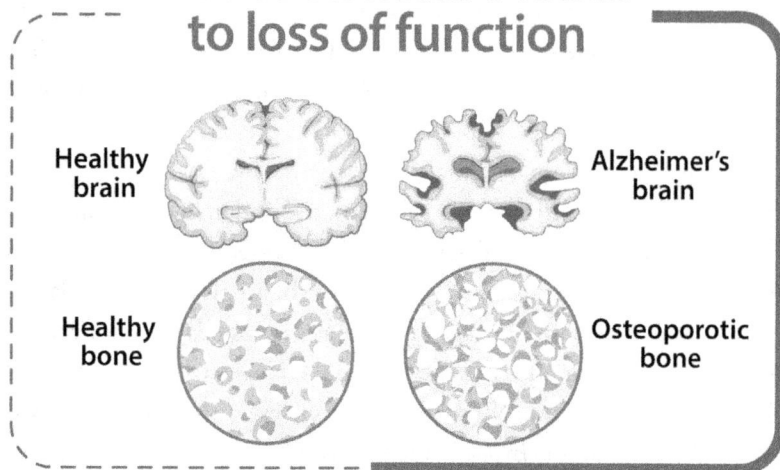

Healthy brain

Alzheimer's brain

Healthy bone

Osteoporotic bone

Most of us are familiar with the concept of loss of bone density in osteoporosis; we see remarkable similarity in the way Alzheimer's disease affects the brain, causing degeneration of structure that leads to compromised function. In the brain, enlarged perivascular spaces impair the ability of the glymphatic system to work properly and clear waste products from the brain during sleep.

from standing to lying down). Indeed, this response is impaired in people with MCI as well as Alzheimer's disease.[630, 631] Here lies the connection between the responsiveness of the nervous system and circulation of oxygenated blood in the brain: The less well-calibrated a person's nervous system, the less it will be able to meet the brain's needs for oxygenated blood in a timely fashion. This is a crucial outcome of the heart-brain connection, and we'll explore it more deeply in the next chapter.

One very interesting aspect of dysautonomia (i.e., dysfunction of the autonomic nervous system) is that it is sometimes referred to as *autonomic neuropathy*. That's right—it constitutes damage to the nerves that govern the autonomic nervous system and, as such, control the internal organs. Just as neuropathy in the feet is not just about loss of sensation but about the downstream effects such as fall risk, *autonomic* neuropathy is not just about the nerve damage itself but about the downstream effects it causes. Autonomic neuropathy is present in all types of dementia and is especially pronounced in people with Parkinson's disease.[632] One study found that dysautonomia was present in two-thirds of subjects with Alzheimer's disease.[633] (Interestingly, researchers have proposed that autonomic dysregulation is one of the mechanisms that trips severe cases of illness from COVID-19 into a life-threatening situation and suggest that stimulating the vagus nerve may be a way to interrupt this reaction and move the body back toward balance[634]—but that's a topic for another book.)

The correlation between reduced HRV, on the one hand, and MCI and dementia, on the other, is becoming relatively well established, but because HRV is not yet a widely accepted vital statistic, it is not routinely measured, and more widespread usage of HRV as a metric will help us better understand the nature and causality of this connection.[635]

We know that people, on average, do less well on cognitive tests as they get older—and we also know that for the average person, HRV decreases with age. Declining HRV is associated with declining cognitive abilities—and although this, too, may be a vicious cycle, with the autonomic nervous system working less well *because* the brain is working less well, we know that declining HRV compounds the problem, leading to additional loss of brain function.

However, age-related decline of HRV is not inevitable.[636] We know that anything we can do to boost HRV will interrupt that cycle or at least help slow it down. Although many clinical studies investigate direct stimulation of the vagus nerve with an electrode, practices such as yoga and breathwork can have a similar effect. If you have a fitness tracker that measures HRV, you can observe this for yourself. Measure your HRV before and after a session of yoga, meditation, or biofeedback resonance breathing, and you'll easily be able to see that it's having the desired effect.

PREFRONTAL CORTEX: THE BRAIN'S DISPATCH CENTER

In addition to hypoperfusion, another element of the all-important heart-brain connection when it comes to the brain and aging is prefrontal cortex activity. Like a dispatch center signaling trains to switch tracks to avoid a collision, this brain region (which you first met in Chapter Six) routes signals into the parts of the brain that govern executive function and complex thinking—or shuts down those signals and keeps them in the parts of the brain that are more focused on physical survival if the nervous system is signaling that resources are needed there instead.

When you're relaxed and calm, you can engage in higher-order thinking. Part of what the prefrontal cortex does is inhibit activity of the amygdala, the part of the brain most closely associated with the fear response. When your amygdala is active and you're stuck in fight-or-flight, higher-order thinking is not available to you. This is sympathetic overdrive; HRV is the symptom and the cause. Lower HRV means you don't perform as well on tasks that require executive function, and people with lower HRV have an exaggerated startle response—a telltale sign of sympathetic overdrive and the inability to relax.[637]

It's not just an overactive sympathetic nervous system that's the problem—it's the inability of the prefrontal cortex to *inhibit* the sympathetic nervous system that really causes problems.[638] This might seem confusing and convoluted—like when someone uses a double negative in a sentence—but it's important. The sympathetic nervous system is programmed to respond to threats in the environment, and this is as it should be. Fear is built into us as a survival instinct—but what enables us to live a peaceful, grateful life is the *inhibition* of that fear. When this inhibitory response is impaired, the system veers off balance.

It's the prefrontal cortex that inhibits the sympathetic nervous system so the frontal lobe can engage in complex thought or, conversely, keeps the frontal lobe dormant so the sympathetic nervous system receives the energy it needs to help us respond to threats in our environment.[639] The prefrontal cortex routes the signals to the appropriate track—but with an overactive sympathetic nervous system, the trains stay on the overused track of the limbic system.

As advances in imaging technology allow us to observe the brain with ever greater precision, we are learning some fascinating things about the prefrontal cortex. Recall what you read in Chapter Five about the prefrontal cortex being less active during a memory retrieval task for subjects with PTSD. In a study of survivors of the 2015 Tianjin explosions in China, examining blood flow to *different areas of* the prefrontal cortex revealed differences between people with PTSD and those whose study intake questionnaires, on the other hand, indicated that they'd experienced *post-traumatic growth*—that is, being shaped in a positive way by a difficult experience instead of being haunted by it. When shown pictures designed to elicit an emotional response, the subjects with PTSD had increased activation in their *right* dorsolateral prefrontal cortex, while those with post-traumatic growth had increased activation in the same area on the *left* side.[640] Findings like this provide comforting validation of a biological basis for the difference between post-traumatic stress and post-traumatic growth while also offering clues for more effective treatments.

In healthy adults, higher resting vagal activity is correlated with a thicker prefrontal cortex.[641, 642] Depression patients had been observed to have a thinner prefrontal cortex, on average,[643, 644, 645, 646, 647] and a 2018 study connected the dots (at least in the adolescent survey population) that the differences in cortex thickness seem to be mediated by vagal activity[648]—that is, a nervous system stuck in fight-or-flight mode leads to changes in brain structure associated with depression.

When it comes to brain activity, we tend to think of it as bottom-up (with the base urges of the limbic system overriding the analysis of our rational mind) rather than top-down but, in fact, influence moves in both directions—yet another feedback loop in the body. HRV affects prefrontal cortex activity, but prefrontal cortex activity also affects HRV.[649] There are ways to target the prefrontal cortex for activation, such as with brain-stimulating techniques and specific types of cognitive tasks, but mainly what I want you to remember is that human beings are not just trapped in a loop of stimulus and response; when things escalate, we have more control over deescalating them than we often realize.

If we can activate the parasympathetic nervous system and get out of fight-or-flight, we can create the conditions for a thicker prefrontal cortex that more effectively inhibits fearful, hypervigilant tendencies when they're not needed—and enjoy improved cognition and good feelings as a result. This appears to be at least part of how higher HRV supports improved brain function as we age. With a nimble nervous system that is responsive and able to relax after times of stress, the prefrontal cortex gets plenty of oxygenated blood—resulting in greater activity in the parts of the brain responsible for higher-order thinking.[650] Here, too, studies that have their subjects view film clips designed to elicit specific emotions have proven informative: We can see how subjects with higher high-frequency HRV scores display greater cerebral blood flow (observed with a PET scan) after viewing movie clips that induce strong emotions such as sadness and disgust.[651] Anger causes blood flow to the prefrontal cortex to decline[652]—and when a person spends a lot of time feeling angry, this can result in structural changes to the brain.

There is increasing evidence that this, too, is an inhibitory model—that high HRV is not an absence of stress but rather an indicator of the body's ability to *inhibit* sympathetic activity by mounting a parasympathetic response. For example, the high-frequency domain of HRV (also known as the vagal component of HRV) predicts likelihood of survival in patients who have suffered a heart attack:[653] The more effective the body is at using vagal activity to inhibit sympathetic activity, the more effectively it can create the conditions necessary for healing, and the more likely the patient is to survive. In one study by German and American researchers, subjects with higher high-frequency HRV scores at the beginning of the study had an easier time coming down from a state of emotional arousal (e.g., an easier time regulating their emotions) after viewing emotionally charged images.[654]

It's clear that with high HRV, more signals get routed to the parts of the brain that handle executive function, whereas with low HRV, the signals stay in the limbic system and don't pass through to the regions responsible for higher-order thinking.[655] (With sufficiently sensitive and accurate monitoring, it has even been suggested that HRV and prefrontal cortex blood flow could be used to detect mental overload and avoid errors in high-pressure and high-stakes occupations such as air traffic control.[656]) This also affects emotion regulation. When all the trains are running on the tracks of our stress response, our behavior will be reactive and impulsive. If we're going to act in a way that is calm and considered, we've got to get some of those trains through to the other set of tracks via the prefrontal cortex—and anything that boosts our HRV can help us do that.

As you've seen in this chapter, the relationship between HRV and brain perfusion (the amount of oxygenated blood supplied to the brain) is well established.[657] Hypoperfusion (reduced cerebral blood flow) occurs early in Alzheimer's disease, inducing lesions to the brain's white matter that correlate with dementia.[658] In other words, hypoperfusion leads to loss of *structure* as neurons die; this, in turn, leads to additional loss of *function*, and the cycle continues. The reduced blood flow is the first step and can be observed prior to the development of symptoms (which only show up once parts of the brain begin to atrophy). What's more, a pharmaceutical approach to treating hypertension can actually lead to cerebral hypoperfusion, as improving the blood pressure for the sake of other organs (such as the kidneys) has negative consequences for brain health.

Some brain regions may overcompensate for the deficits in other areas, explaining the delay in loss of function; this would show up as hyperperfusion (extra delivery of oxygenated blood) to the areas that are overcompensating.[659] This effect was directly observed with near infrared spectroscopy (NIRS) in a study that found abnormally high activation of the right prefrontal cortex (a brain area involved in the formation of new episodic memories) in the earliest stages of MCI.[660] But when the brain reaches a *critically attained threshold of cerebral hypoperfusion*, or CATCH (a phrase and concept coined by Jack de la Torre), the compensatory mechanisms cannot keep up; a chain of events leads to loss of structure and function as cells die off and neurodegeneration occurs.[661]

The association between hypertension and decreased cognitive function is well established, and yet too many of us still view heart problems and brain problems as unrelated phenomena. Scientists have long known that people suffering from Alzheimer's disease have increased sympathetic and decreased parasympathetic activity[662] but have been slower to assemble the puzzle pieces of what that means and what to do about it. Keeping oxygenated blood flowing throughout the brain is important for preserving cognitive function, and taking the brakes off of the prefrontal cortex by boosting HRV is a crucial part of this.

One therapeutic method that has been suggested is electroacupuncture to the trigeminal nerve, which has been observed to increase blood flow to the prefrontal cortex, reduce heart rate, and increase HRV and parasympathetic activity.[663] But anything you can do to increase HRV is going to be beneficial, so I'd recommend you use methods you can practice at home—yoga, meditation, breathing techniques, and (of course) photobiomodulation. (As it turns out, photobiomodulation may be especially beneficial for types of cognitive function that involve the prefrontal cortex![664])

The next chapter will delve into the research findings on photobiomodulation and neurodegeneration, but first, it's important to understand why and how photobiomodulation helps the brain. Not only does it enhance HRV and thus contribute to sleep, healing, and glymphatic clearance—but through its effects on mitochondria and circulation, photobiomodulation also boosts the brain's energy systems. In the next chapter, we'll explore how the brain gets its energy, what interferes with the energy supply, and how to literally boost your brain power.

CHAPTER NINE

A New Definition of Metabolism

"A sad soul can kill you quicker, far quicker,
than a germ."

—John Steinbeck, *Travels with
Charley: In Search of America*

The next time you read that Alzheimer's is caused by a buildup of amyloid-beta plaques and tau tangles in the brain, I hope that it stops you in your tracks based on what you learned in the last chapter. We now know these plaques and tangles are merely a symptom of the underlying problem—yet too many doctors, scientists, and journalists still perpetuate the old way of viewing the disease.

If we have any hope of staving off the tidal wave of dementia and Alzheimer's that is threatening to overwhelm the caregiving capacity of our medical system and entire societies, we have to look at addressing the root problem. That means interrupting the body's vicious cycles of chronic inflammation and sympathetic overdrive to allow our brains to rest, heal, and take out the trash. Another way to look at slowing, stopping, and reversing neurodegeneration is through the lens of metabolism—that is, the metabolism of the brain.

The way we view Alzheimer's disease is undergoing a sea change, and this shift has to do with the energy systems of the body. Alzheimer's is sometimes referred to as "type 3 diabetes" because of how it affects circulation and energy supply to the brain. In type 1 and 2 diabetes, the body loses its ability to regulate blood sugar and the supply of energy to the muscles and organs when the pancreas fails. Although Alzheimer's does not involve the pancreas, we can nevertheless view it through the lens of energy supply. Due to underlying problems with the nervous system and cardiovascular system, the brain gets less circulation of oxygenated blood (which, of course, also carries other substances the brain needs to work its best—such as glucose, lipids, and neurotransmitters). Neurons—whether motor, sensory, or cognitive—need a constant supply of energy to carry on the work they do in our bodies. When the blood supply to the brain is compromised, so is the energy supply on which these neurons rely.[665] As the vicious cycle compounds itself and the plaques and tangles accumulate, the supply of energy only becomes further impaired.[666] Recall that the material presented in this book is a *neurometabolic solution*. When the mitochondria in the brain aren't working well, this, too, is a disorder of the body's energy systems.

Viewing neurodegenerative conditions as metabolic disorders makes sense when we consider that the brain makes up only two percent of our body weight but consumes twenty percent of our energy. Our brains need a strong and continuous supply of energy to work their best. Let's return to the waste collection analogy from the last chapter but add another one: Think of the brain as an engine. When the engine has lots of fuel, it will have lots of power. If the fuel supply is throttled, it will be unable to accelerate as fast. And if it's clogged by waste products, it will "burn dirty," falling short of its full capacity and kicking out some junk along with the desired output. If you never clean it and the waste products build up, eventually, it will just stop working completely. This is exactly what happens in the brain: Damaged mitochondria produce greater amounts of reactive oxygen species, leading to more damage and, eventually, cell death.[667]

In this engine, the blood is the fuel coming in, and the lymph is the oil that collects waste products and clears them out (and perhaps also the coolant that keeps everything from overheating). Arteries (bringing in fresh oxygenated blood) are the fuel injectors, and veins (returning blood to the heart and lungs to be reoxygenated) are the exhaust system. This analogy is not just a hypothesis: Patterns of cerebral blood flow can tell us which people are most at risk of progressing from MCI to Alzheimer's disease.[668] (Diminished cerebral blood flow to certain brain regions, by the way, is also a factor in the aftereffects of TBI;[669] as brain imaging becomes faster, more powerful, and more widely accessible, it can help us to identify who is most at risk for long-term symptoms and who most urgently needs treatment.)

Amyloid beta accumulation is "necessary but not sufficient" for the development of Alzheimer's disease; high blood pressure plays a role as well, driving the amyloid beta into spaces outside of the blood vessels where it interferes with memory.[670] In addition to causing this leakage, hypertension seems to interfere with the body's built-in cleaning abilities, affecting the way the cerebrospinal fluid pulses during sleep to clear out waste products.[671]

With this framework, even the genetic risk factors for Alzheimer's can be understood in a new way. For instance, many of the gene variants that predispose someone to early-onset forms of the disease influence the way the body produces or processes amyloid beta. In the engine analogy, these people have engines that produce more waste products or that clear them less efficiently. It's not about the amyloid beta per se; it's about the body's inability to clear it efficiently enough to prevent it from building up. Seen through this lens, genes are not destiny; even someone with the worst risk factors can keep the engine running cleanly by consciously creating a lifestyle that promotes optimal circulatory, lymphatic, and nervous system health.

By the way, type 1 and 2 diabetes are not *just* about the pancreas, either. Type 1 diabetes is an autoimmune disease that often goes hand in hand with other autoimmune conditions in the same person. For type 2 diabetes, cardiovascular risk factors are a major contributing cause, and more than just blood sugar levels are affected: Type 2 diabetes affects the whole autonomic nervous system as well as mitochondrial function. In the first case, the immune system goes haywire, attacking and doing damage through some of the same mechanisms we've covered in our discussions of vicious cycles and the cell danger response; in the second, energy regulation and supply all throughout the body are affected, with implications for every single process that requires energy, from organ function and tissue healing to cell metabolism. I'm not the only one who's connecting these dots to argue for a broader definition of metabolic disorders; to take just one intriguing example, research has recently found that people with insulin resistance (a metabolic disorder in the traditional, narrow sense) have significantly diminished mitochondrial function in their skeletal muscle (an association that ties in to a broader view of the body's energy systems, including the mitochondria, as defined in this book).[672]

Dementia and diabetes are not the only conditions that benefit from viewing through the lens of this new definition of metabolism. As it turns out, we can also add depression to this list: Scientists have long understood that symptoms of major depression are linked to significantly reduced regional blood flow to the brain—yet the antidepressant medications currently in use have the effect of *decreasing* the brain's blood flow.[673] Why we've focused for so long on serotonin, to the exclusion of foundational bodily processes such as circulation and nervous system balance, is anyone's guess—but now that we know better, we can do better.

MITOCHONDRIA: KEY PLAYERS IN THE BRAIN'S ENERGY SYSTEM

In addition to the plaques and tangles and cardiovascular risk factors, recent research is elucidating how mitochondrial function also plays a role in the development of neurodegenerative conditions.[674] Of the one hundred four identified genes that have an association with adult-onset neurodegenerative conditions, at least thirty-six are associated with mitochondrial function.[675] As one study noted, "Mitochondrial dysfunction, inadequate supplies of ATP, and oxidative stress are contributory factors in almost all forms of brain disease."[676] There was a reason I spent so much time introducing the mitochondria in Section One. They hold the key to understanding how to optimize and heal so many different types of processes in the body.

The mitochondria play a critical role in the body's processes of balancing energy needs with nutrient supply, and when these metabolic processes are not properly balanced, they can lead to the development of disease in the system in question—be it the heart[677] or the brain. In fact, within our bodies, our brains are among the organs most densely populated with mitochondria.

Of all the organs and systems in the body, "the brain appears most vulnerable to mitochondrial defects, suggesting that neurons are particularly sensitive to bioenergetic fluctuations," Martin Picard and Bruce McEwen wrote in their commentary summarizing research in this area, titled "Mitochondria impact brain function and cognition."[678]

Generally speaking, when our mitochondria are working well, this is a recipe for healthier aging. Upleveling autophagy—in which sluggish or unhealthy cells are targeted for destruction—increases both lifespan and healthspan.[679] In other words, it's not just more years lived, but the fact that those years are healthy. This increase in the body's reduce-reuse-recycle function also results in better mitochondrial function, as the mitochondria that don't work as well are culled from the herd. (The way they tested this is pretty interesting: Lithium can be used to upregulate autophagy in C. elegans, a soil-dwelling nematode that, like the fruit fly, is often used in lab experiments. Since these organisms have a much shorter life expectancy than humans, results observed in the lab over a short period of time can be extrapolated to the human lifespan. At the end of the day, nobody is proposing to dose humans with lithium on a wide scale to lengthen our lifespan—but we do know of some other ways to increase autophagy, such as intermittent fasting.)

Mitochondrial dysfunction in neurons is one of the earliest and most prominent features of Alzheimer's disease. Defects in mitochondrial respiration—a process that is highly dependent on vascular function in the brain—are well known, but other types of mitochondrial dysfunction are being revealed to play a role in neurodegeneration.[680] One of the things that goes awry is the balance between fission and fusion.[681] As explained in Chapter Two, this process allows cells to preserve the best-working and most efficient mitochondria while culling the ones that are sluggish; when this process isn't working properly, overall efficiency of the mitochondria suffers. The chronic oxidative stress that accompanies Alzheimer's disease also influences mitochondrial abnormalities, and the brains of people with Alzheimer's have fewer healthy mitochondria.[682]

Damaged mitochondria produce increased amounts of reactive oxygen species, leading to more damage.[683] In addition, reduced cytochrome c oxidase activity makes the tissue vulnerable to excitotoxicity and reduced oxygen availability.[684]

The prefrontal cortex is especially susceptible to age-related mitochondrial dysfunction.[685] This may help to explain why emotion regulation becomes more difficult the worse a person's dementia gets. Their signaling system isn't working, so they can't get out of an emotionally reactive state and into their higher-order, rational mind.

In Alzheimer's disease, when the delicate balance of mitochondrial fission and fusion is disrupted, the balance tips toward fission, resulting in an abundance of damaged mitochondria—a disruption of the body's innate wisdom that, in a healthy brain, culls underperforming mitochondria and maximizes the efficiency of the ones that remain.[686] This decline in mitochondrial "quality control" also happens to be an underlying cause of sarcopenia, the age-related loss of skeletal muscle mass that leads to frailty, disability, and mortality.[687]

Some researchers have even cast changes in mitochondrial function as "a global metabolic disturbance" that operates in a similar way to cancer—suppressing glucose oxidation, upregulating glycolysis, and making cells resistant to apoptosis that should be marked to cull from the herd.[688] Both circulation and mitochondrial function play a role in making the "engine" of the brain run as it should.

(Incidentally, Alzheimer's disease isn't the only neurodegenerative condition for which that is true. We know that autophagy is dysregulated in the brains of people with Parkinson's disease,[689] and there is evidence that changes in mitochondrial function play a role in Parkinson's disease.[690] Research is also pointing toward mitochondrial dysfunction as a significant causative factor in the development of Parkinson's disease, as defects in mitochondrial signaling and quality control lead to the death of dopaminergic neurons that defines the disease.[691])

In their paper noting the contribution of mitochondrial dysfunction to the development of Alzheimer's disease, one team of researchers writes, "There is now compelling evidence" that the brains of people with

Alzheimer's disease "are bioenergetically impaired, that this metabolic deficiency appears early in the clinical evolution of Alzheimer's disease, that it worsens with clinical deterioration, and that it is associated with mitochondrial enzymatic impairments" in the electron transport chain.[692] "That the personal and societal tragedy of loss of self in Alzheimer's disease should arise, in part, from deficient functioning of this primitive organelle," they write, "testifies to the exquisite biological vulnerability of that which defines us as humans."

The mitochondrial deficiencies that are present in Alzheimer's disease have also been observed in people with MCI.[693, 694] Researchers believe that a bioenergetic approach that focuses on improving mitochondrial function—as well as the related functions of glucose metabolism, reducing levels of reactive oxygen species, and balancing apoptosis and autophagy so cells are neither killed too soon nor allowed to continue living when they aren't working well—can prevent MCI from progressing into Alzheimer's or, if Alzheimer's has already developed, from becoming more severe.[695]

To the extent that hormones play a role in the development of Alzheimer's, this also comes back to a bioenergetic perspective. Women's risk of Alzheimer's disease is almost twice that of men. Meanwhile, Parkinson's disease and Lewy body dementia are more common in men than in women.[696] Regarding the role of estrogen, we know that declining mitochondrial function leads to a decline in the production of estrogen—meaning that menopause, too, is a bioenergetic phenomenon.[697] Estrogen, in turn, promotes brain plasticity and also has a neuroprotective effect (and in fact, estrogen is thought to be part of the reason women live longer than men on average since it has antioxidant effects and acts to upregulate longevity-related genes).[698] What this means is that for women, the more you can protect and boost your mitochondrial function, the longer your body will keep making its own estrogen—and once you do reach menopause, consulting with a qualified provider about estrogen replacement can help protect your mitochondria and keep your body out of the vicious cycle in which diminished energy production leads to the loss of a neuroprotective factor that then accelerates the decline in energy production.

As it turns out, this new definition of metabolism has some links to the conventional definition of metabolic disorders (all the more reason it's insane that the prevailing discussion of metabolic disorders pretty much ignores the mitochondria entirely). For example, research has shown mitochondrial dysfunction can contribute to the development of insulin resistance by leading insulin target tissues such as skeletal muscle and liver not to carry out sufficient autophagy, which, in turn, leads to the release of a mitokine that promotes insulin resistance.[699] Or consider this finding: A peptide called humanin is a well-known neuroprotective factor whose circulating levels decline as we age; researchers have identified six other peptides (known as small humanin-like peptides) encoded in the same mitochondrial DNA region that work together to reduce apoptosis and the generation of reactive oxygen species and improve mitochondrial metabolism. They also suppress glucose production in the liver and increase glucose uptake, meaning they have an insulin-sensitizing function—once again demonstrating the connection between mitochondria and metabolism.[700]

Although mutations in mitochondrial DNA were once believed to be responsible for the dysfunction of the mitochondria in the brains of people with Alzheimer's, research has shown otherwise. When mitochondrial DNA samples were collected from the brain tissue of Alzheimer's patients, those mitochondria were able to function at the same level as mitochondria collected from subjects the same age without Alzheimer's.[701] Thus, the decline in function is not due to deleterious mutations that build up over time; rather, the mitochondria in the brains of people with Alzheimer's still have the potential to work well if we can remove the interference.

Mitochondria in blood cells reflect the alterations of mitochondria in the central nervous system, so as the science develops further, it's possible that one day we could all get bloodwork to examine our mitochondria for early signs of dementia.[702] This is still in the realm of sci-fi for now, but we can act on what we do know: Protecting and enhancing our mitochondrial function promotes a healthier brain. When amyloid beta accumulates in the brain, it interferes with mitochondrial function.[703] Thus, it is important to enable the body to clear out this protein efficiently—and that requires effective operation of the glymphatic system and the vascular system.

THE VASCULAR SYSTEM: FUEL LINES FOR THE BRAIN

The brain has a high energy demand compared to other organs, and neurons do not have sizable surplus energy reserves the way some other cell types (such as muscle) do. This energy demand also changes rapidly, requiring the supply system to be flexible and adaptable from moment to moment. Humans already have unusually large brains for our overall size, and yet space inside the head is so limited—hence the limits placed on energy stores and the need to maintain pressure within a narrowly defined range via precisely calibrated inflow and outflow in response to changing conditions.[704]

The total length of capillaries in the human brain is more than six hundred kilometers, and virtually every neuron is supplied by its own capillary. These tiny blood vessels are particularly vulnerable to damage by hypoperfusion or hyperperfusion when the body's systems of regulating pulse and flow don't work effectively at maintaining pressure within the optimal range.[705] As we go about the activities of daily life, our nervous systems are constantly regulating blood pressure and the fluid balance in the brain. When you lift a heavy box or blow your nose or play a wind instrument or get startled—all of these lead to sudden changes in blood pressure. The human nervous system is remarkably skilled at adapting to these changes, but when these adaptive mechanisms break down, the consequences can be dire.

Cerebral perfusion typically declines as we age and declines even more in people with Alzheimer's disease. Once this decline crosses a critical threshold, it causes degeneration of the capillaries in the brain, such that it actually becomes impossible to deliver energy supply widely throughout the brain.[706] (This degeneration is reversible and the capillaries can be regrown, which researchers including Ivan Maksimovich of Russia have shown.[707]) When the brain cells do not have the fuel they need, the brain's energy demand outstrips supply, resulting in a "metabolic cascade" of mitochondrial dysfunction, oxidative stress, decreased ATP production, and more.

We've known for a quarter-century now that amyloid beta is not the whole story. In 1997, researchers published their findings from a longitudinal study of Catholic nuns who agreed to have their brains examined after their death as part of the study. Among the nuns whose brains displayed the plaques and tangles characteristic of Alzheimer's disease, only some of them had exhibited symptoms of cognitive decline or dementia while alive. So, what was the difference between the nuns who displayed symptoms and those who had the plaques and tangles but maintained normal levels of cognitive function? Circulation. For the nuns who'd experienced cognitive decline, their brains displayed not only the plaques and tangles but also infarcts (evidence of strokes resulting from damage to the blood vessels supplying the brain, caused by factors such as hypertension, high cholesterol, and metabolic disorders).[708] Damage to the vascular system, not the plaques and tangles themselves, was the determining factor in who developed disease.

Microinfarcts—small lesions of dead tissue commonly found in the brains of people with dementia—are thought to occur when both arterioles (small offshoots of arteries that deliver blood to capillaries) and venules (small blood vessels that collect blood from capillaries and deliver it to larger veins) are blocked.[709] The engine isn't getting enough motor oil to lubricate the parts, and the oil isn't free to return to the source and take waste products with it. Your brain becomes like a car that needs an oil change; when things aren't flowing freely, sludge builds up—and if it goes on long enough, engine damage occurs. I consider this its own sort of *acquired brain injury*; I like that framing because of the parallels it draws between this type of neurodegeneration and the damage that results from TBI as discussed in the previous section. Not all brain damage results from trauma.

As we age, what's known as *oxygen extraction fraction*—the ratio of oxygen a tissue takes up from the local blood supply to maintain its function and structural integrity—increases in the frontal and parietal cortices (except for the primary motor and somatosensory regions) and in the temporal cortex. This is one more way our bodies become less efficient—more oxygenated blood is needed to maintain the same level of functioning. There is an inverse relationship between oxygen extraction fraction and capillary oxygen tension, meaning that as one increases, the other declines—and given this, increased oxygen extraction fraction can compromise oxygen delivery to neurons.[710]

A study of more than one thousand adults without dementia, followed for two years, found that risk factors including diabetes, hypertension, heart disease, and smoking predicted their likelihood of developing Alzheimer's disease by the end of the study. If they had three or more of these factors, their risk tripled compared to subjects who had none of the risk factors.[711] The common denominator among these risk factors is their effect on the vascular system—suggesting that vascular health (or lack thereof) is a key factor in assessing Alzheimer's risk. Buildup of amyloid beta is a symptom of the problem—not the problem itself.

Alzheimer's disease and vascular dementia are not as different as they've been made out to be. Vascular dementia is attributed to cerebral hypoperfusion and ischemia, leading to excitotoxicity and neuronal apoptosis. Whereas Alzheimer's disease had been thought to be a result of amyloid beta depositions, research over the last two decades has been giving us clues that vascular factors play a role in who gets Alzheimer's and who doesn't.[712] Practically all of the risk factors for Alzheimer's disease—diabetes, hypertension, heart disease—have a vascular component that reduces cerebral perfusion.[713] Hypoxia in the brain has a series of devastating downstream effects, including a compromised blood-brain barrier, neuroinflammation, dysautonomia, and the formation of tau proteins that are toxic to surrounding neurons and glial cells.[714] New research using MRI and PET scanning to observe blood flow patterns in the brain demonstrates that subjects with the most severe symptoms of

Alzheimer's and dementia have both vascular dysfunction and a buildup of tau proteins in key brain regions.[715]

One very interesting study found that carriers of the APOE-ε4 gene have reduced capillary coverage in the brain and half the number of pericytes[716]—cells embedded in the capillary walls that control interactions between neurons and the cerebral vasculature to meet the brain's energy demands—showing how even genetic factors may exert their influence via the vascular system.

(Incidentally, Alzheimer's disease is a major risk factor for severe symptoms and death when infected with COVID-19, and greater severity of COVID-19 infection is also correlated with the APOE-ε4 genotype, one of the major genetic risk factors for Alzheimer's.[717] Given what we know about COVID-19's effects on the cardiovascular, circulatory, and nervous systems, this is a fascinating correlation that only adds more weight to the argument that Alzheimer's is not just all about buildup of proteins in the brain.)

As with so many disease processes in the body, a vicious cycle takes hold with a cascade of downstream effects. Vascular risk factors lead to thickening of the blood vessel walls, dysfunction of the blood vessels, oxidative stress, hypoperfusion, and increased risk of stroke. Increased production of reactive oxygen species leads to a reduction in nitric oxide, leading to vasoconstriction over time.[718] This creates a chronic hypoxic environment within the deep white matter of the brain, resulting in a loss of interregional connectivity. Hyperphosphorylation of tau protein, a crucial step in tangle formation and plaque accumulation, occurs.[719] Our old friend, the HPA axis, also gets involved: This system becomes dysregulated in people with Alzheimer's disease, and they have higher levels of cortisol in their plasma and cerebrospinal fluid than people the same age who do not have Alzheimer's.[720] In people with dementia, the specific brain regions that govern HRV are impacted; if they aren't functioning well, the autonomic nervous system becomes less flexible and adaptable.[721] HRV, in turn, declines; hypoperfusion worsens; and the downward spiral continues.

The vascular hypothesis of Alzheimer's disease was postulated in 1993 by de la Torre and Mussivand after they noticed the reductions in blood flow, glucose metabolism, and oxygen consumption were proportional to disease severity. Amyloid beta deposition, meanwhile, does not correlate with disease severity and has also been found in the brains of healthy people (such as the nuns in the study mentioned earlier in this chapter).[722] Buildup of proteins can contribute to and/or precipitate post-ischemic brain neurodegeneration,[723] but this is far from the whole story.

As you learned in the last chapter, if you're not sleeping long enough, the glymphatic system has less time to do its work—but shorter sleep duration is also associated with lower oxygen levels in the brain.[724] Reduced cerebral blood flow is a risk factor for early death, independently of the conditions that can cause this decreased blood flow, such as cardiovascular disease, diabetes, and hypertension. In other words, if we can increase the blood flow to the brain, it helps to reduce your risk even if you don't address the other risk factors (although, of course, you'd see even more benefit if you do both). Letting the brain clear itself out during sleep via the glymphatic system is key, but blood pressure and cerebral oxygenation while we are awake are also crucial factors in the brain health equation.

In particular, a type of cell called microglia may play a crucial role in removing amyloid beta from the brain. You first met these cells back in Section One, but as a reminder: Microglia are the chief innate immune cells in the brain and are sometimes called the macrophages of the central nervous system (making an analogy to cells outside of the brain that perform a similar function). Inflammation can hold the microglia back from carrying out this important task—and as we would expect, cognitive decline happens faster in people with Alzheimer's disease who have acute systemic inflammation.[725]

When our bodies are in sympathetic overdrive, everything is affected. Blood pressure and circulation are among the biological systems regulated by the autonomic nervous system. This is why the aftereffects of TBI (as described in Chapter Five), driven by the heart-brain connection, have an impact on circulation and oxygenation in the brain. The body's chemoreceptors (sensitive to chemicals—both those from external sources, such as medications, and those produced by the body, such as neurotransmitters) and baroreceptors (sensitive to pressure) don't work as well, and the exquisitely sensitive nervous system does not adjust as quickly or accurately as usual. As it turns out, hypoperfusion might be responsible for some of the neurological symptoms that are part of post-concussion syndrome—such as headaches, dizziness, and blurred vision.[726]

When it comes to chronic kidney disease—a condition that affects more than ten percent of the global population and *more than half* of those over age seventy (and which poses a downstream risk of cardiovascular disease and cognitive impairment)—arterial stiffness has been identified as an indicator of those most at risk for the downstream effects and also as a proxy for microcirculation in the brain.[727] In other words, the status of your circulatory system has the power to predict whether this common affliction is likely to have negative cardiovascular and cognitive outcomes.

Arterial stiffness, which accompanies aging in many people, contributes to the autonomic nervous system's decline in flexibility—in this case, literally, as the stiffness of the blood vessels limits the precision of the body's adjustments to blood flow strength and speed.[728] This is not a new concept—Hippocrates once said, "A man is as old as his arteries"—but we seem to have underestimated its significance. (We could add an even more modern version of this: A person is as old as their HRV, which we might say is a measure of the nervous system's flexibility.) In addition to being less nimble and responsive to fluctuations in sympathetic/parasympathetic balance, stiffness makes the blood vessels more brittle and susceptible to damage—like the leakage of amyloid beta into the brain and reduced effectiveness of clearance mechanisms. Indeed, stiffness of the carotid artery, specifically, was shown to be associated with amyloid beta accumulation in the brain in seniors with MCI.[729]

Pulse wave velocity (specifically, in the carotid-femoral artery) is another proxy for arterial aging and a marker of cardiovascular disease—and another indicator of the link between circulation and cognition. The greater the pulse wave velocity (an indicator that the body is overcompensating for restriction in the blood vessels), the lower the cognitive performance.[730]

The brain regulates its own pressure, helping to protect it against blood pressure fluctuations, but this mechanism is impaired in mice with Alzheimer's disease. The same phenomenon has not been observed in humans with Alzheimer's disease, even though it would help to explain why high blood pressure is a risk factor for Alzheimer's disease. However, advancements in research methods and imaging technology may open up new avenues for exploring whether the findings in mice play out in human subjects.[731]

We do know that neurodegeneration results from a breakdown in what's known as neurovascular coupling—the ability of the vascular system to support the energy needs of the neurons in a well-coordinated fashion—and new methods are enabling us to observe this with greater precision.[732, 733] Brain function breaks down as a result of factors including chronic hypoperfusion (reduced blood supply) and ischemia, endothelial dysfunction, arterial stiffening, and reduced flexibility and responsiveness of cerebral blood vessels.[734]

In adults with MCI, cerebral blood flow is more affected by changes in mean arterial pressure, meaning the nervous system has become less efficient at maintaining the steady state of blood flow and constant pressure the brain needs to function at its best.[735] This is another indicator that reduced flow of oxygenated blood in certain brain regions isn't just due to reduced demand (which we might expect if cells in those regions aren't working like they used to)—but rather, that coordination of energy supply with demand has become less well calibrated.[736] Research with mice has shown that just as stiffening of the arteries impairs circulation and brain perfusion, it also adversely affects glymphatic function[737]—meaning that the brain's waste clearance system is breaking down at a time it's needed more than ever.

Looking back on my life and career, I find clues that the vascular system was somehow connected to age-related decline. One of my aunts had Marfan syndrome, in which a genetic mutation interferes with the body's synthesis of fibrillin-1, a key protein for the formulation of collagen. Collagen production declines with age for most people, leading to

NeuroMetabolic Cascade

Subclinical changes in the systemic vascular health	Heart	Diminished cardiac function	Arterial stiffness	Low HRV
Cerebral blood flow alterations	Brain	Disturbed hemodynamics, cerebral hypoperfusion	Reduced total blood flow and dysmetabolism	Less NO
Supply-demand mismatch	Mitochondria	Bioenergetic decline	Reduced energy substrate delivery	Reduced ATP production, loss of mitochondrial energy
Microvascular damage, inflammatory cascades	Neurometabolic brake	Oxidative stress	Neuro-inflammation	Capillary degeneration, microvascular inflammation
Alzheimer's disease pathology accumulation	Glymphatic	Impaired waste clearance	Enlarged perivascular spaces	BBB breakdown, toxic accumulation
Loss of brain structure	Neurodegeneration	Neuronal damage	Synaptic dysfunction	White matter damage, low HRV
Loss of cognitive function	Cognitive decline	Impaired executive function and verbal fluency	Decreased psychomotor speed and memory	Physical dysfunction · Gait speed · Falls · Balance

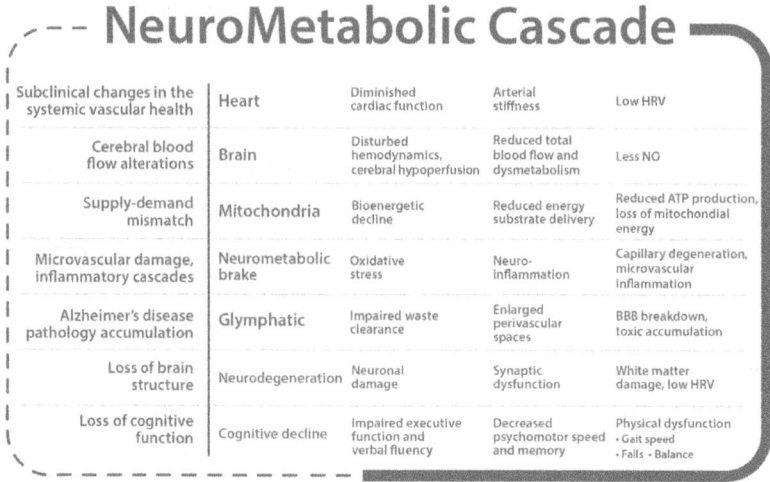

This diagram captures parallel processes that affect various organs and systems of the body. Within each body system, a downward spiral gathers momentum (moving horizontally within the chart) as damage accumulates, and the deleterious effects also spill over from one body system to impact others (moving vertically within the chart). For example, subclinical changes in systemic vascular health manifest as diminished cardiac function, arterial stiffness, and low HRV—which, in turn, have effects on cerebral blood flow, mitochondrial function in the brain, the workings of the glymphatic system, and, ultimately, brain structure and cognitive function. The **PRONEURO** approach aims to reverse the downward spiral in all of these systems so the brain and body can heal and regenerate.

wrinkles as the skin loses its elasticity—but for people with Marfan syndrome, collagen synthesis is impaired from the start. Then in my chiropractic practice, I saw patients with Ehlers-Danlos syndrome, a condition (also genetic in origin) that causes hypermobile joints and fragile skin that doesn't heal well. Because of this vulnerability, people with Ehlers-Danlos are more likely to suffer spontaneous dissections, or tears of the small blood vessels in the upper neck that feed the brain; this emerged as a risk factor in my research on how chiropractors can avoid injuring their patients.

These syndromes (in which symptoms that typically accompany aging instead happen in younger people) help us understand what mechanisms contribute to age-related decline and see connections between symptoms.

Any problem with the blood vessels and the endothelial cells that line them affects every body system, as the blood supply to that system is affected. (People with Ehlers-Danlos also have a higher incidence of depression and other mental health conditions, a connection I found intriguing since it points to the role the vascular system may play in conditions typically thought to be caused by imbalances of neurotransmitters.)

Seeing connections like these can help us move beyond an overly narrow focus (like amyloid beta in Alzheimer's or serotonin in depression) and take a broader view that leads to new insights. Indeed, although having at least one copy of the APOE-ε4 gene does raise one's risk of Alzheimer's disease, recent analysis of data from a longitudinal study found that a healthy lifestyle (assessed using a metric from the American Heart Association that considers smoking, diet, physical activity, body mass index, blood pressure, cholesterol, and fasting glucose) dramatically reduced subjects' odds of developing dementia even if they were genetically at risk.[738] When we focus myopically on a single molecule or allele, we lose sight of the big picture and the ways factors are interrelated.

As researchers have "zoomed out" to consider Alzheimer's disease as not just an excess of proteins and peptides in the brain but also of conditions in the vascular system, this big picture view points toward a completely different approach to treatment[739]—one that offers reasons for both hope and alarm.

Turning to the negative first, people with high blood pressure have reduced structural and functional connectivity in their brains[740]— and hypertension is an epidemic! It affects an estimated two-thirds to three-quarters of senior citizens worldwide. This is an emergency!

All the same, some researchers maintain that cerebral blood flow does not have to decline in healthy aging and, in fact, does not in people who don't have MCI.[741] This means "engine failure" as we age is not inevitable.

Whatever we can do to improve vascular function and allow our brain's "fuel lines" to operate at full capacity is going to have a protective effect. Improving circulation is one more among the many benefits of photobiomodulation; let us now turn to the evidence of how and why that works.

PHOTOBIOMODULATION AND CIRCULATION: INCREASING YOUR HORSEPOWER

If we consider that hypoperfusion results in changes that progress into MCI and, in the most severe cases, Alzheimer's disease, then photobiomodulation holds enormous therapeutic potential due to its power to enhance cerebral perfusion and mitochondrial activity.[742]

Neurodegenerative conditions tend to worsen with any condition that affects circulation, such as hypertension, heart disease, or diabetes. Using photobiomodulation, we can increase the circulation of oxygenated blood in the brain, thus allowing the mitochondria in the brain to do their job and providing the energy supply needed for all the various aspects of brain function. The longer in our life course the mitochondria in the brain remain efficient at producing energy, the longer we will be able to stave off neurodegenerative conditions and their deleterious effects.

Photobiomodulation's effect of increasing circulation in the area where the light is applied is well documented.[743,744,745,746] Using functional near-infrared spectroscopy (or fNIRS, a non-invasive technique for monitoring the supply of oxygenated blood to the brain) and other methods, we see a clear increase in the supply of oxygenated blood when photobiomodulation is applied.[747,748] Even brief photobiomodulation treatments can have both acute and lasting effects, increasing the flow of oxygenated blood by one-fifth to one-third.[749]

And the improvement in oxygenation translates to an improvement of function: Using fNIRS to monitor hemodynamics, a team of researchers found that photobiomodulation had a large effect on oxygenation of the prefrontal cortex when the treatment was applied while subjects were performing tasks that required sustained attention and working memory performance.[750] (In an intriguing finding, improved cerebral perfusion as well as improvement of symptoms have also been seen in patients in a persistent vegetative state who receive photobiomodulation treatments.[751])

In healthy elderly women who received transcranial photobiomodulation treatments twice a week for four weeks, ultrasounds showed an increase in both systolic and diastolic velocity of the left middle cerebral artery as well as a decrease in the pulsatility index and resistance index values. That is, the treatment seems to have reversed (at least partially) some of the vascular effects typically seen in the brain with aging.[752] A Moscow-based scientist, Ivan Maksimovich, has shown improved cerebral microcirculation—along with reduction or reversal of cognitive decline symptoms—in his subjects with Alzheimer's disease using an intravascular catheter to deliver photobiomodulation to blood circulating to specific brain regions, with mechanisms for this improvement including increased capillary blood supply, improved tissue metabolism, stimulation of neurogenesis, and the clearance of amyloid beta.[753, 754]

We also know that thanks to abscopal (indirect) effects, we don't have to apply the light directly to the brain region we want to reach. One study found that within thirty minutes of intranasal photobiomodulation, blood flow increases by twenty to thirty-five percent—globally (throughout the whole brain) and specifically to the prefrontal cortex (which is, incidentally, quite close to where the light hits from either transcranial or intranasal photobiomodulation).[755] In another study that combined transcranial photobiomodulation with fMRI, brain imaging showed that blood-oxygen-level-dependent signals increased by as much as thirty-one percent in the prefrontal cortex after the subjects received photobiomodulation treatment, an effect consistent with rapid inflow of blood to the region and an increase in oxidative metabolism.[756]

In fact, abscopal effects may be even *more* important when it comes to the brain since they allow for reaching all regions of the brain (via systemic factors that affect the whole body) and not just the areas close to the surface of the skull.[757] Research in animals has shown that mesenchymal stem cells can cross the blood-brain barrier[758] and that this phenomenon helps to explain how photobiomodulation reduces amyloid beta deposition in Alzheimer's disease.[759]

If you don't feel like wearing a helmet, intranasal photobiomodulation (with a device that clips the lights inside your nostrils) is another good option for shining light on the brain and the blood and fluids that supply it, due to the nose's proximity to the brain and the thin, translucent skin and abundant capillaries in the nasal cavity.[760] Researchers are beginning to acknowledge the power of abscopal effects and that photobiomodulation anywhere on the body (e.g., on the abdomen with a body pad) can have a protective effect for the brain.[761, 762] A number of animal

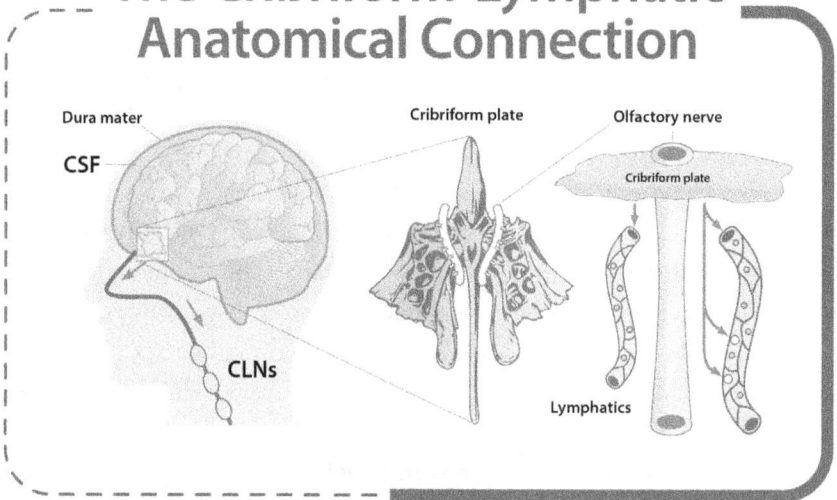

The Cribriform-Lymphatic Anatomical Connection

The cribriform plate is a spongy, lightweight bone that separates the brain from the nasal cavity. The proximity of the brain to immune system components in this location illustrates not only why intranasal photobiomodulation is a powerful way to influence cell-free mitochondria and other components of blood flow proximal to the brain but also why loss of the sense of smell (via inflammation and damage to the olfactory nerve) commonly accompanies neurodegenerative conditions. In fact, the lymphatic vessels that facilitate immune function and waste clearance in the area are intertwined with the branches of the olfactory nerve. Glymphatic drainage of cerebrospinal fluid (CSF) that originates in the space between the dura mater and the brain tissue exits via these lymphatic vessels, traveling down through the neck along a route that passes the cervical lymph nodes (CLNs), which play a role in trapping and filtering invaders such as viruses and bacteria.

studies have found benefits for Alzheimer's disease[763, 764] and Parkinson's disease[765, 766, 767] via abscopal effects (i.e., via photobiomodulation not directly applied to the head). Because of the density of mitochondria in the brain, it is one of the organs that can benefit most from the indirect effects of photobiomodulation. Even if you're using a body pad instead of a helmet or an intranasal device, your brain is getting the benefits.

Intranasal photobiomodulation has been demonstrated to increase cerebral blood flow, decrease blood viscosity,[768] and otherwise alter the blood's properties in ways that are linked to improved cognitive function[769] and mood.[770] Researchers also believe intranasal photobiomodulation may improve glymphatic drainage behind the cribriform plate, the thin, spongy bone at the back of the nasal cavity.[771, 772]

More research is underway to determine how exactly these abscopal neuroprotective effects come about, but likely candidates include impacts on cell-free mitochondria; vasodilation via nitric oxide release; the activation of mesenchymal stem cells; and, intriguingly, effects on the gut microbiome that, in turn, have a protective effect for the brain.[773] The remainder of this chapter will examine some of the evidence for these mechanisms, walking you through research findings that shed light on how and why photobiomodulation helps prevent neurodegeneration and promote neuroregeneration.

NITRIC OXIDE: THE CARBURETOR

Continuing with our engine analogy, we can consider nitric oxide to be the carburetor—and here I'm showing my age. New cars haven't had carburetors since the 1990s, when modern fuel injection systems replaced them to fulfill the same function: creating the proper balance of air and fuel for efficient combustion. Carburetors were replaced by better technology because their jets (small holes that air and fuel flow through) often became clogged—and this is why I'm using the carburetor analogy instead of just saying "fuel injection system." When photobiomodulation prompts the release of nitric oxide and, consequently, vasodilation results, you get that bump in brain power similar to a carburetor that's working well. Your engine will feel powerful and responsive, like you can go from zero to sixty on a dime.

As oxygenated blood travels throughout the body, it's nitric oxide that gives the cue for oxygen molecules to release from the hemoglobin that transports them. Nitric oxide is sometimes called a "miracle molecule" for the chain of effects it sets off—vasodilation, pain relief, angiogenesis, neurogenesis, reducing inflammation, and preventing the oxidation of cholesterol that would then build up on blood vessel walls, among others. Robert Furchgott, Louis Ignarro, and Ferid Murad received the Nobel Prize for Medicine and Physiology in 1998 for their work illuminating nitric oxide's mechanisms and the signaling role it plays in the cardiovascular system. In the brain, nitric oxide plays a role in neurovascular coupling, helping to mediate the supply of oxygenated blood to the locations where it's needed throughout the brain. As activated neurons release nitric oxide, the surrounding blood vessels dilate, drawing oxygenated blood into the area.[774] Perhaps relatedly, nitric oxide has a protective effect against hypoxic damage, and populations that live at high altitudes have been observed to have higher nitric oxide levels in their blood. Nitric oxide is also a retrograde neurotransmitter, meaning that the messages travel backward relative to the usual direction neurotransmitter signals follow, creating a kind of feedback loop in the brain so the "upstream" neuron can sense the conditions "downstream."[775]

Nitric oxide is a type of free radical, highlighting the way this category of molecules can play either a positive or a negative role in our physiology, depending on the type, location, and amount. As it turns out, nitric oxide plays a role in coordinating the balance of reactive oxygen species in organisms[776]—so it is a key player! It also is part of how phagocytes (cells that devour pathogens as well as dead or dying cells marked for autophagy) carry out their immune system role of killing foreign invaders. This miracle molecule is versatile!

It is well established that photobiomodulation has the effect of dilating the blood vessels due to the release of nitric oxide it prompts,[777, 778, 779, 780] and thus it has the potential to mitigate the impaired cerebral perfusion that compromises cognitive function and leads to further neurodegeneration. As one team of researchers wrote: "In hypoxic/compromised cells, cytochrome c oxidase is inhibited by non-covalently bound nitric oxide. When the mitochondria are exposed to red/near-infrared photons, nitric oxide is released and diffused outside the cell wall, promoting local vasodilation and increased blood flow."[781]

So, we know that nitric oxide can help once a problem arises—but as it turns out, low levels of nitric oxide may also be at least partly to blame for the problem and, thus, implicated in the cause as well as the solution. One intriguing line of research suggests that depletion of nitric oxide in the body leads to impaired circulation[782]—and if that's the case, using photobiomodulation to encourage the release of nitric oxide can address one of the root causes of poor circulation that underlies Alzheimer's and cardiovascular disease.

If your head is starting to spin with all the ways photobiomodulation is beneficial, just know that these effects are interrelated. It's thought to be because of nitric oxide that photobiomodulation can make sluggish mitochondria work better without having the effect of making the healthy ones overactive (the Goldilocks effect). Hypoxic cells are likely to have too much nitric oxide; when photobiomodulation enables its release by uncoupling it from cytochrome c oxidase, the result is an immediate influx of oxygen and, thus, the resumption of cell respiration.[783] Looking at this interaction from a different angle, healthy functioning of cytochrome c oxidase is essential for maintaining an optimal balance of reactive oxygen species; as we age, cytochrome c oxidase decreases its function, and as a result, reactive oxygen species can build up and oxidative stress results. Because photobiomodulation can convert cytochrome c oxidase from its reduced state into its oxidized state, it can help combat this buildup and the resulting stress.[784, 785] What's more, in healthy cells, photobiomodulation may cause hypoxic conditions when it dissociates nitric oxide from cytochrome c oxidase—which, if the theory bears out, would explain how photobiomodulation has a hormetic effect, building cells' capacity to withstand hypoxic conditions and recover.[786]

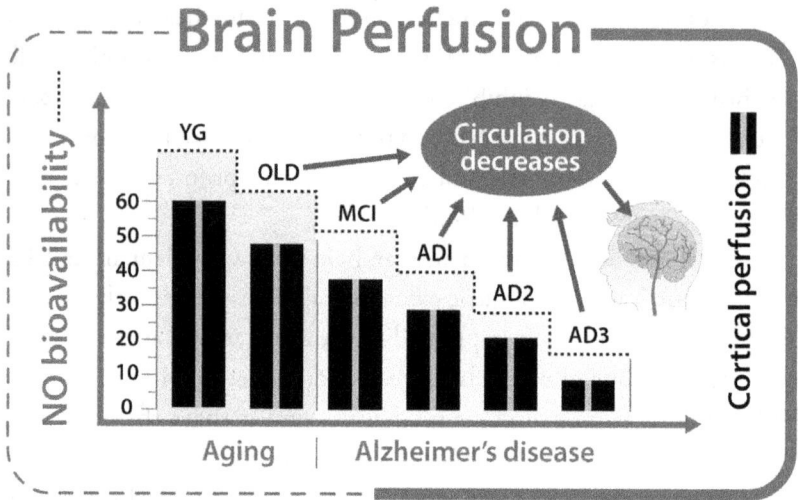

Brain Perfusion

In this image, we have superimposed one chart on top of another to demonstrate the similarity in the way bioavailability of nitric oxide declines with age, on the one hand, and cortical perfusion declines with age, on the other. This makes sense since reduced availability of nitric oxide leads to a decline in circulation throughout the body. Both of these factors decline further in Alzheimer's disease, which is why treatments such as photobiomodulation that stimulate the release of nitric oxide can help with circulation and cortical perfusion.

BRAIN DETOX: PHOTOBIOMODULATION AND THE GLYMPHATIC SYSTEM

Now that we've covered photobiomodulation's effect of enhancing the flow of oxygenated blood to key brain regions, let's recall that there are two sides to the equation. Just as important as supplying your engine with fuel is the efficient removal of waste. Here, too, photobiomodulation has demonstrated benefits.

Photobiomodulation has been shown to promote the clearance of both amyloid beta and tau proteins in rat and mouse models of Alzheimer's disease.[787, 788, 789] In the brains of mice with Alzheimer's disease that received four photobiomodulation treatments, spaced two days apart, amyloid beta levels decreased, and the mice also showed improvement in cognitive, memory, and neurological measures. Using an imaging technique called optical coherence tomography, the research team was able to observe clearance from the brain via the glymphatic system and the neck.[790] In addition, a study in mice by a Russian research group has found that photobiomodulation enhances glymphatic clearance of amyloid beta through the meningeal lymphatic vessels.[791]

When used with mice at risk of Alzheimer's disease, the mice that received photobiomodulation three times a week for six months had significantly reduced levels of amyloid beta plaques and were also less likely to display the behaviors associated with advanced amyloid deposition. The mice that received photobiomodulation also had higher ATP levels and mitochondrial function.[792] Another study found that daily photobiomodulation treatments for nine days improved the neurocognitive status of mice with Alzheimer's disease due to increased clearance of amyloid beta from the brain via the meningeal lymphatic vessels and increased blood oxygen saturation of the brain tissues (measured via pulse oximetry).[793] And yet another found that photobiomodulation disassembled amyloid beta in the brains of rats with Alzheimer's disease, allowing it to be cleared—a process enhanced by the light's effect of improving the flow of interstitial fluid in the rats' brains—resulting in the improvement of function in the rats' brains, as measured in the Morris water maze test.[794]

A study with mice documented photobiomodulation's ability to enhance the lymphatic clearance of red blood cells from the brain after an intraventricular hemorrhage, one of the most commonly fatal forms of brain injury.[795] This finding shows not only the potential of photobiomodulation to help reduce the severity of the worst types of brain injuries but its broader potential to help the brain heal itself by removing the substances that cause damage in the wake of an injury.

Photobiomodulation attenuates memory and neurological deficits in mice with Alzheimer's disease based on their observed behavior; lower amyloid beta levels in the brain, accompanied by higher amyloid beta levels in the mice's cervical lymph nodes, confirm that the body is clearing the amyloid beta deposits via the glymphatic system. A team of researchers from Russia, China, and Germany showed that photobio-modulation decreases transendothelial resistance, allowing fluid to travel in both directions (in and out of the brain) more freely to assist in flushing out harmful substances.[796] Another study by the same research team substantiated the role vasodilation plays[797]—so, going with our street cleaning metaphor, the streets become wider as the astrocytes shrink and the space between cells increases; vasodilation is like pressure washers coming down the street and giving everything a good flush.

Although glymphatic clearance in humans is less easily observed, we can infer from the improvement of symptoms that the same mechanisms seen in animals probably apply to humans, too. In humans, case studies have found that Alzheimer's and dementia symptoms improve significantly with regular photobiomodulation treatments.[798, 799, 800, 801, 802, 803] Subjects see improvements such as better sleep, reduced anxiety, fewer angry outbursts, and less wandering behavior. A small double-blind, placebo-controlled trial that gave some subjects with dementia twenty-eight sessions of transcranial photobiomodulation (six minutes a day) found that the group that received the treatment instead of the placebo showed improvements in executive function, immediate recall, the ability to draw a clock face, visual attention, and task switching, among other measures.[804]

And in my own research study, a case study published in 2019, we achieved incredible results with four weeks of twice-daily home photobiomodulation treatments (transcranial, intranasal, and body pad). The subject, a sixty-four-year-old woman with an Alzheimer's diagnosis, went from 18 to 24 on the Montreal Cognitive Assessment (from the Alzheimer's range to the upper end of the MCI range of 19-25, and very close to a score that's considered normal). The subject's olfactory dysfunction was also reversed, as measured by the Alberta Smell Test and the peanut butter test—the first documented recovery of olfaction in a neurodegenerative condition to our knowledge. The subject noticed changes in mental clarity almost right away after starting the treatments: During the first week, when she was only using the light helmet, she told us, "Things are better... I notice that my mind seems clearer. I know things now that I didn't know."[805]

----Optimal Brain Power----

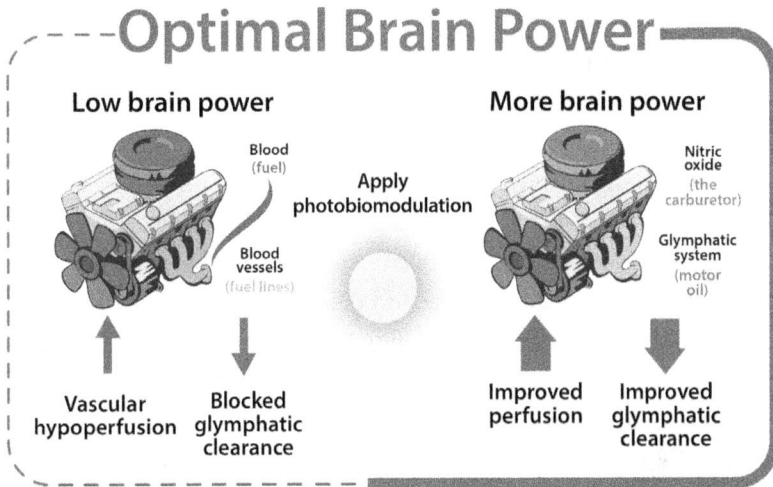

Low brain power

Blood (fuel)

Blood vessels (fuel lines)

Apply photobiomodulation

Vascular hypoperfusion

Blocked glymphatic clearance

More brain power

Nitric oxide (the carburetor)

Glymphatic system (motor oil)

Improved perfusion

Improved glymphatic clearance

In our analogy of the brain as an engine, the blood vessels are like the fuel lines supplying the energy the engine needs to run properly. Nitric oxide is the carburetor, providing a bump in brain power via vasodilation and increased circulation—just like the carburetor can influence engine power by adjusting the amount of air injected into the fuel. The glymphatic system acts like motor oil, clearing out waste products as the fluid circulates to keep the engine running at its full power. If the brain as an engine is not working well (left), hypoperfusion results in a scarce supply of energy, and blocked glymphatic clearance inhibits the removal of waste products. We call this the *neurometabolic brake*: When both influx and efflux are restricted, it's like driving around with your parking brake partially engaged. You can't generate maximum power with that kind of drag on the engine. We can improve how the "engine" runs (that is, increase our brain power) by enhancing perfusion and glymphatic clearance (right).

Of course, as noted earlier in this chapter and throughout the book, glymphatic clearance is not the only contributing factor to neurodegeneration and neuroregeneration, and photobiomodulation acts on multiple aspects of the brain's energy system. Thus, it is not surprising that— separately from the studies of specific mechanisms—we see symptoms improve for animals with Alzheimer's disease, dementia, and cognitive impairment, just as we do for humans. In one study, mice with mitochondrial dysfunction, apoptosis, and cognitive impairment showed improvements in all three of these areas when they received transcranial photobiomodulation three times a week for six weeks.[806] Another study that involved injecting rats' brains with amyloid beta found that after three weeks of photobiomodulation, the rats had better spatial memory and neurobehavioral and motor skills.[807]

An intriguing line of research claims that one way photobiomodulation improves the operation of the glymphatic system is by increasing the permeability of the blood-brain barrier to allow better access for immune system cells such as macrophages and enhanced clearance of substances like amyloid beta as well as blood left over after a hemorrhage (which can cause further damage to the brain if it isn't cleared).[808, 809] Recent research has indicated that the level of permeability changes with our circadian rhythms;[810] still, it's not fully clear what distinguishes beneficial permeability of the blood-brain barrier from the so-called "leaky brain" condition that allows bad stuff to get in, and this will certainly be an area of scientific inquiry to watch as it develops. We do know that a key component of the blood-brain barrier is endothelial cells, which have a concentration of mitochondria five to six times greater than in other cell types[811]—so if mitochondrial function is compromised throughout the body, we would expect that to have pronounced repercussions for tissues plentiful in endothelial cells, including the blood-brain barrier.

PHOTOBIOMODULATION: ROUTINE MAINTENANCE FOR YOUR ENGINE

At this point in the book, photobiomodulation has been mentioned in just about every chapter, so I thought it might help to pause and synthesize how and why it works. By summarizing one last time all the ways photobiomodulation helps the "engine" of your brain run more cleanly and powerfully, I hope to pull together all the evidence in a way that will be memorable and motivating—so you'll never miss a day of photobiomodulation and will tell everyone you love about this life-changing and health-changing treatment!

In the brain, photobiomodulation is generally accepted to promote healing through five mechanisms:

+ Increasing ATP production (which you know all about from Chapter Three)
+ Increasing cerebral blood flow in the regions to which the light is applied
+ Activating anti-inflammatory and antioxidant effects
+ Activating transcription factors that cause changes in protein expression
+ Increasing neurogenesis and synaptogenesis[812]

However, the complete picture is even more detailed than that. Applying photobiomodulation to the head and neck boosts HRV, reduces blood viscosity so the blood flows more easily, bolsters the function of mitochondria in the brain, increases cerebral blood flow (as well as blood and lymph flow to the meningeal vessels), and creates a "heat sink" as the body responds to the gentle temperature increase by increasing circulation and drainage.[813] Linking back to the importance of nitric oxide, research has pointed to this "miracle molecule" as the reason photobiomodulation increases circulation—and has also identified reduced blood flow and brain oxygenation as important features in Alzheimer's disease.[814]

Photobiomodulation is well established to improve cerebral hemo-dynamics and metabolism of the human brain in both young and older adults.[815] As one study notes, "more than twenty-five years of experience" has shown that this treatment "directly influences the parameters of all cells in the blood, blood plasma, the coagulation process, and all the structural components of the vascular wall." It also "directly or indirectly affects the cells of the immune system, hormones, and exchange processes in an organism, thereby not only improving the function of the vascular system but also the other systems of an organism."[816] Photobiomodulation improves cerebral metabolic activity and blood flow and provides neuroprotection via anti-inflammatory and antioxidant pathways. Intranasal photobiomodulation devices in particular have shown promise for treating MCI, Alzheimer's disease, Parkinson's disease, cerebrovascular diseases, depression and anxiety, and insomnia.

Photobiomodulation works to raise levels of brain-derived neurotrophic factor (BDNF), a protein that helps to maintain existing neurons and encourage the growth of new neurons and synapses (an underlying mechanism of the neurogenesis and synaptogenesis benefit listed in the bullet points).[817] Among other reasons, this mechanism is relevant because a deficiency of BDNF contributes to neurotoxicity and dendrite atrophy in Alzheimer's disease. Dendrites are the tree branch–like structures at the tip of each neuron through which the neuron receives input from other cells. Dendrite atrophy happens due to a combination of amyloid beta accumulation and BDNF deficiency; photobiomodulation has the ability to preserve these structures (and their very important function) by upregulating BDNF.[818] This has implications for healing after TBI and stroke as well as staving off neurodegeneration—and all the mechanisms outlined here are ways in which photobiomodulation affects brain bioenergetics.

For Alzheimer's and Parkinson's, the two most common neurodegenerative disorders, even if certain symptoms are treatable, the progression of the disease continues as more neurons die off.[819] This is why photobiomodulation's protective effect against cell death is so promising and so needed. (Incidentally, research in animals and humans has found that photobiomodulation helps improve symptoms of Parkinson's disease, with more studies currently underway;[820, 821] in a laboratory model of Parkinson's, applying photobiomodulation to cells in culture can keep the cells from dying in conditions when they otherwise would have.[822, 823]) When the brain's energy demands outstrip the available supply due to hypoperfusion, mitochondrial stimulation via photobiomodulation can help fill the gap, not only leading to improved cognitive performance but also avoiding the toxicity that occurs with an overabundance of reactive oxygen species.[824]

In neurodegenerative conditions, widespread mitochondrial dysfunction, increased levels of aluminum and heavy metals, and neuroinflammation produce significant levels of oxidative stress—which, in turn, cause amyloid beta deposition, tau hyperphosphorylation, and the subsequent loss of synapses and neurons.[825] Thus, the amyloid beta and tau are the symptom, not the cause—as we saw with clear contrast in the Nun Study of Aging and Alzheimer's Disease.

Animal studies have helped to elucidate the molecular mechanisms of action. In the brains of elderly rats, transcranial photobiomodulation treatments applied daily for ten days led to the activation of intracellular signaling proteins linked to vascular function and cell survival in the aging brain (and also had anti-inflammatory effects).[826] In rats whose brains were injected with amyloid beta, photobiomodulation ameliorated neurodegeneration and improved the rats' spatial memory and recognition; molecular studies showed that photobiomodulation improved mitochondrial dynamics, raised mitochondrial membrane potential, boosted cytochrome c oxidase activity and ATP levels, reduced oxidized mitochondrial DNA, inhibited apoptosis, increased mitochondrial antioxidant expression, and suppressed inflammation, among other mechanisms.[827] In addition to aiding with amyloid beta clearance, photobiomodulation has been shown (at least in mice) to protect against the accumulation of tau oligomers that are toxic to neurons.[828, 829] A team of researchers in Ukraine and China found that mouse cells injected with toxic oligomeric amyloid beta produced lower amounts of inflammation-promoting cytokines when photobiomodulation was applied, pointing to the treatment's ability to protect cells from the toxic effects of these substances' buildup.[830] Another study with mice confirmed the treatment's effect of protecting neurons from oxidative stress, inflammation, and toxicity.[831] And yet another found that five months of whole-body infrared photobiomodulation treatments increased the production of proteins that typically decline as we age.[832] This decline (typical of aging, but reversed with photobiomodulation in this study) contributes to abnormal protein folding—a hallmark of Alzheimer's disease, as the misfolded proteins accumulate and form amyloid plaques.[833] As we get older, the number of glial cells in our brains tends to increase as the number of neurons decreases—but at least in animals, photobiomodulation can protect against this hallmark of aging.[834]

Because photobiomodulation addresses the underlying contributors to neurodegeneration, it also impacts the symptoms. Photobiomodulation has shown the ability to reduce amyloid beta levels in a human cell culture,[835] and in rat cells, it suppresses the oxidative and inflammatory response induced by amyloid beta.[836] A study in rats connected photobiomodulation's memory-enhancing effects to its influence on cerebral perfusion and metabolic capacity in the prefrontal cortex.[837]

One particularly interesting study in humans reported that photobiomodulation's effect of increasing oxidized cytochrome c oxidase (which, in turn, increases production of ATP) seems to be amplified with age, perhaps indicating that photobiomodulation fills in to compensate when mitochondria aren't working so well (versus a "broad brush" approach of simply upregulating all mitochondrial function).[838]

As Michael Hamblin notes in his 2019 paper "Photobiomodulation for Alzheimer's disease: Has the light dawned?" the treatment "has demonstrated the rather unique property of affecting cells in different states of health in different ways, essentially modifying the cell in whatever way might be necessary to promote its survival."[839] In normal cells, when cytochrome c oxidase absorbs light, this leads to an increase in mitochondrial membrane potential and a short surge of reactive oxygen species production. But in cells where mitochondrial membrane potential is low (for example, due to oxidative stress or excitotoxicity), the absorption of light by cytochrome c oxidase leads to an increase in mitochondrial membrane potential—which, in this case, results in a *decrease* of reactive oxygen species production,[840] signaling that the state of stress the cell was in before the application of light has resolved. In a similar example of the Goldilocks principle—in which photobiomodulation takes conditions that are too high or too low and makes them *juuuust* right—the treatment leads to an increase in intracellular ionized calcium (denoted as $Ca2+$, this signaling molecule participates in nearly every essential process in the body) in healthy cells,[841] but in cells that already have too much $Ca2+$, photobiomodulation reduces the amount of ionized calcium, promoting cell survival, reducing oxidative stress, and raising mitochondrial membrane potential back up to a normal level.[842] In other words, photobiomodulation is acceleratory, not excitatory.

Under normal conditions, the uptake of Ca2+ enhances mitochondrial respiratory function and tunes mitochondrial function to synaptic activity. However, excessive reactive oxygen species generation can disturb Ca2+ homeostasis and induce Ca2+ overload, leading to changes in the mitochondria that induce further production of reactive oxygen species and causing the mitochondrial membrane to become permeable, a "point of no return" that leads to cellular apoptosis. This "calcium overload" is seen in both Alzheimer's and Parkinson's disease as well as TBI.[843]

While our main focus in this book is the improvement of symptoms and underlying causes of neurodegenerative conditions, part of the reason I say photobiomodulation should be part of "routine maintenance" for a healthy brain is its ability to enhance cognitive function even in healthy people with no evidence of neurodegeneration. One study found that when photobiomodulation was applied to the foreheads of healthy subjects, their reaction time and performance improved on cognitive tasks, and their mood also improved after the treatment.[844] Another study by the same researchers noted that "transcranial infrared laser stimulation produces beneficial effects on frontal cortex functions such as sustained attention, working memory, and affective state."[845] A different research group also found the treatment had benefits for attentional performance.[846] A small study of transcranial photobiomodulation with a helmet at home found that subjects who received the treatment displayed significant improvement in motor function, memory performance, and processing speed, while the placebo group did not.[847] (Animal studies point toward similar conclusions; while many photobiomodulation studies induce neurodegenerative conditions as part of their methods, one that gave photobiomodulation treatments to year-old mice—considered "middle-aged" in the lifespan of a mouse—found that the treatments improved the mice's cognitive performance, bringing it up to the level of "young" mice that were just three months of age.[848])

In a study of older adults, a single session of transcranial photobiomodulation (less than ten minutes long) led to improved performance on tests of frontal lobe function—for example, when prompted with a letter, the subjects could name three times the number of animals whose names start with that letter compared to before the photobiomodulation treatment.[849] A single photobiomodulation treatment just four minutes in length improved subjects' performance (relative to controls) on what's known as the Wisconsin Card Sorting Task, a test that involves attention, working memory, and visual processing, among other aspects of cognition.[850] In a study of older adults with subjective cognitive decline but no diagnosis of dementia, the subjects displayed improvement on every cognitive test administered after receiving five weekly transcranial photobiomodulation sessions of eight minutes each.[851] In a study with case reports from three patients with MCI, all three showed improvement in cognitive function after receiving photobiomodulation treatments twice a week for nine weeks. One subject's verbal memory improved from the first to the sixty-seventh percentile, another from the fourth to the twenty-sixth percentile, and the third from the eleventh to the fifty-fourth percentile.[852] Another study of eighteen adults with MCI found that those who received photobiomodulation demonstrated significant improvement in visual memory performance and that blood flow patterns indicated they were expending less mental effort with the same tasks relative to the control group.[853] Research indicates that photobiomodulation may be especially beneficial for types of cognitive function that involve the prefrontal cortex.[854]

Our knowledge of how exactly photobiomodulation works is still evolving, with new mechanisms being evaluated and theories tested as we are preparing this book for publication.[855] But regardless of which mechanisms of action are producing these effects, the fact remains that photobiomodulation has the power to improve cognitive function—but cutting-edge monitoring and imaging techniques allow us to get some idea of the mechanisms involved. Although not new, electroencephalography (EEG)—a way of measuring electrical activity in the brain via electrodes attached to the scalp—is being used in new ways and new high-density formats that enable new kinds of observation. One recent study used EEG to observe photobiomodulation's influence on gamma band neural activity in the human brain—a type of brain activity linked to performance on complex and attention-demanding tasks.[856]

Using fNIRS, researchers found that a single eight-minute transcranial photobiomodulation treatment enhanced information-processing speed and efficiency of the brain network and increased functional connectivity significantly in the frontal-parietal network.[857] In one particularly intriguing study, subjects who received an eight-minute photobiomodulation treatment before performing a challenging cognitive test showed less frontal lobe activation on brain scans than subjects who completed the same test without photobiomodulation.[858] Our bodies direct the flow of oxygenated blood to the brain regions that demand it; a lower level of activation means the subjects who received photobiomodulation were able to complete the same task more efficiently without needing as much oxygenated blood to get it done. Their brains were less stressed and better able to meet the demand without a surge in energy supply.

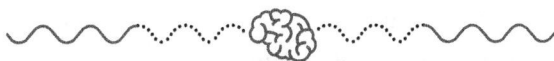

Lao Tzu said in the Tao Te Ching that "The flame that burns twice as bright burns half as long"—but I prefer a different perspective. I say each of us should aspire to burn brightly all the way to the end of our burn time. If your pancreas dies at forty, your kidneys die at fifty, your liver dies at sixty, and your brain dies at seventy—you might still be alive, but that's no way to live if you ask me. The goal isn't to opt out of aging completely and live forever. (After all, who really wants to be alive a hundred years from now?) The goal is to maintain vitality and resilience for as long as we are alive.

The current model of Alzheimer's disease research—with inadequate overall funding and pharmaceuticals strongly preferred over other avenues for treatment and prevention[859]—is not helping with this, but fortunately, the tide is beginning to turn. Pfizer made headlines in 2018 when it announced the suspension of its research program for drugs to treat Alzheimer's and Parkinson's diseases and laid off three hundred employees. Researchers have long reported how hard it was to get published and get research funding for any hypothesis other than treating Alzheimer's by targeting amyloid beta, but that seems to be changing slowly amid failures of drugs that were once considered promising. Also contributing to the desire to cast a wider net in the search for a cure is the recent revelation that an influential researcher in the field allegedly used doctored images that overstated the association between dementia symptoms and amyloid beta oligomers in mouse brains. (We seem to keep learning the same lesson over and over; recall the nuns study from a quarter-century ago in which some subjects who never showed symptoms of dementia had brains that were revealed to be full of plaques and tangles after they died.)

As the scientific establishment is increasingly acknowledging that amyloid beta is not the whole story and is not the only acceptable treatment target, openness is growing to other lines of investigation and other theories of the disease's causes and contributors. Incidentally, there would be a role for photobiomodulation even if getting pharmaceuticals into the brain were an effective mode of treatment. Due to its ability to improve circulation, oxygenation, and glymphatic clearance, photobiomodulation could help drugs reach their targets in a brain that's blocked up with plaques and tangles or where circulation is less than optimal.

Personally, I like the picture Paolo Cassano (as of this writing, assistant professor of psychiatry at Harvard Medical School and director of photobiomodulation at the Massachusetts General Hospital Depression and Clinical Research Program) painted in his 2019 article "Photomedicine and Pharmaceuticals: A Brain New Deal." Cassano proposes that the medical field should stop giving photobiomodulation a backseat in favor of pharmaceutical approaches to treating neurological disorders. "To be more explicit, these two industries should together explore how their respective treatment modalities should complement each other. The key is that photomedicine is promoting a new intervention in need of large trials to adequately test its potential; pharmaceuticals, a more established industry, could share resources and clinical trials' knowhow with photomedicine," Cassano writes. "A brain new deal, where the two industries integrate their efforts to innovate, would benefit both industries—and the patients most of all."[860]

CHAPTER TEN

The Recipe: Exercise, Unwind, Restore, Oneness

"We don't stop playing because we grow old. We grow old because we stop playing."

—George Bernard Shaw

We know that a significant proportion of dementia cases are never diagnosed and that in some cases where a provider makes a diagnosis, the patient is not told;[861] the percentage of cases that go undiagnosed is probably even higher for MCI. If people aren't aware these conditions are affecting them, they are less likely to take actions that prevent the condition from getting worse. Fortunately, by this point in the book, you know how many of us are affected by these conditions—and how we can all benefit from behaviors to prevent them from worsening or from developing in the first place.

In the previous recipe chapters, you have already started to see how certain behaviors and lifestyle habits can influence the risk factors for neurodegeneration. This chapter will introduce even more ingredients to our recipe for brain health. The list of risk factors for dementia includes some non-modifiable ones (age, gender, family history, genetics, past head trauma) but also plenty that are modifiable (educational attainment, socioeconomic status, social engagement, blood sugar levels, physical activity, nutrition, use of alcohol and tobacco).[862]

If you are going to give your body what it needs to repair—and achieve neuroregeneration instead of neurodegeneration—then the **PRONEURO** approach provides a framework to do that. You've already seen how photobiomodulation can reverse some of the structural and functional changes to the brain that come with aging. In Chapter Six, you learned about the importance of getting your body into Repair mode—and that same approach applies for the brain. The right amount of stress (not too little, not too much, but *juuuust* right) trains the body and brain to build back stronger than before. In Chapter Eight, you learned about the parasympathetic nervous system and how activating it can help your body and brain get out of fight-or-flight and into repair mode. Many of the suggestions given in the Optimize and Nourish sections of Chapter Six also support your body's repair functions and the process of training your body to respond better to stress.

In this chapter, we'll go through the last four ingredients of our ice cream sundae—that is, the last four letters of the **PRONEURO** approach. (Remember, when making our sundae, we started with the foundation. You can't have a sundae without ice cream. If, out of the entire recipe given in this book, you only adopt one new behavior—Photobiomodulation—you will still be doing yourself a world of good.) Plain ice cream is great on its own, but it gets even better when you add toppings you love. In this chapter, you'll learn about some additional "toppings" you can layer on top of your sundae. If you've already made a solid habit of using your light pad or helmet, it's best to focus next on the "ingredients" that were presented in Chapter Six: Repair, Optimize, and Nourish (including hydration). Read through the present chapter to know what comes next, but remember: It's best not to try to take on too much at once. If you try to adopt eight new habits simultaneously, you might succeed for a few days, but ultimately you'll probably fail at all of them. It's nothing personal—that's just how habit change works. You'll have a much better chance of success if you move through the **PRONEURO** approach one letter at a time. And you may be amazed at where you find yourself after, say, one year.

By that time, you'll have had a chance to address all eight areas, or ingredients in our recipe. You'll be experiencing the benefits of daily photobiomodulation treatments. You'll be eating better and sleeping better. You'll feel more capable of detaching from stress and not letting it affect you—and of recovering when it does affect you. Above all, you'll notice how much better you are feeling (and thinking) as a result of all these changes. Visualize your success—and then dive into this chapter to learn more about the steps to make that vision a reality.

E: EXERCISE (MOVE IN THE RIGHT WAY)

One widely cited study found that age, sex, education, hypertension, high cholesterol, and obesity predicted dementia risk over a twenty-year follow-up period. (These risk factors are mostly applicable in middle age; the relevant risk factors change for older adults.)[863] You obviously can't help your age or your sex, but when it comes to the factors you *can* change, there is one behavior that's practically a magic pill, influencing blood pressure, cholesterol, and weight (along with many other beneficial effects). That behavior is exercise—getting your body moving on a regular basis.

In this chapter, we'll dig into the science (which is probably what you're expecting from me at this point)—but before we do, I want to emphasize one thing: Broadly speaking, getting moving is better than not getting moving. If you're a science geek or a biohacker, go ahead and nerd out on all the details shared below about how to optimize your physiology and get the most out of your time spent exercising. But if all this detail feels more overwhelming than fascinating, then just know that exercise is something you don't need to do perfectly. Something is better than nothing. There will be time to fine-tune the details once your exercise habit is solid and steady. Focus on creating the habit first. (And if creating that habit is your main challenge, please do reach out to my team about the coaching we offer; we specialize in guiding people to successfully create new habits!)

That being said, here is the official guidance: The CDC recommends 150 minutes of moderate-intensity exercise each week—so, for example, a half-hour workout five days a week is enough to meet this requirement, and three hour-long walks is also more than enough. An alternative is seventy-five minutes of vigorous (higher-intensity) aerobic activity each week. So, you could also use three intense high-intensity interval training (HIIT) workouts of twenty-five minutes each to meet the guideline.

These levels of activity have a host of benefits for many different aspects of health—energy, mood, sleep, heart health, blood pressure, metabolism, and body composition, to name a few.

Of all the ingredients in our sundae, exercise may be the closest to a magic pill. It requires more time and effort than photobiomodulation and stress reduction. We discussed nutrition and supplements earlier in the book because all of us need to eat—so we might as well make some healthy tweaks while we're at it. But if exercise is not yet part of your routine, I can't emphasize emphatically enough how much of a difference it can make for you to create this new habit.

Although there are many ways to improve cognitive function, exercise is one of the most powerful. Regular exercise results in enhanced performance on a wide variety of cognitive tasks.[864] In one study that compared the influence of various factors on the rates of neurogenesis (creation of new brain cells) in the hippocampi of mice, exercise came out ahead of activities specifically designed to challenge the animals' minds.[865] In a study of humans (specifically, formerly sedentary seniors), regular walking increased the size of the hippocampus and improved memory performance.[866] A 2020 study found that seniors at risk of dementia who engaged in regular physical exercise over the course of a year had increased blood flow to the hippocampus and the anterior cingulate cortex, both key brain regions for memory.[867] A 2022 study found that subjects who averaged a daily step count of approximately four thousand reduced their risk of dementia by twenty-five percent relative to sedentary subjects, and the risk of a dementia diagnosis dropped further with a step count approaching ten thousand.[868] Higher levels of physical fitness are correlated with better cognitive performance and a lower incidence of central arterial stiffness.[869] Exercise's benefit of improving insulin sensitivity (and thus reducing diabetes risk) is also crucial for brain function since the body's insulin response plays a key role in supplying the brain with the glucose it needs to function properly.[870] Exercise causes muscle cells to release a protein called irisin, which can act to convert white fat into metabolically active, thermogenic brown fat and also can enter the brain and upregulate expression of BDNF (the protein that helps to maintain existing neurons and encourage the growth of new neurons and synapses, and whose deficiency is a contributing factor in Alzheimer's disease).[871]

Most people are familiar with the concept of an "endorphin rush" that we experience after exercising, but the feel-good chemicals exercise releases within the body also include endocannabinoids—and these, in turn, act to increase dopamine levels. Aside from its relevance for Parkinson's disease, dopamine is a key player in the brain's reward system and also increases the pleasure we derive from being around other people.[872, 873] In other words, exercise doesn't just act directly on our health; it also has an indirect benefit of improving the yield of other health-promoting activities such as social connection.

Exercise also influences serotonin, the neurotransmitter whose deficiency is linked to depression (and which is also important for memory). During exercise, the muscles take up amino acids that compete with serotonin's precursor, tryptophan, to be carried across the blood-brain barrier.[874] With these amino acids taken out of circulation, more tryptophan can cross the barrier—meaning more serotonin in the brain.

Moderate activity during midlife is associated with a thirty-nine percent reduction in risk of developing MCI later in life, compared to being sedentary;[875] one study of pairs of twins in Sweden found that regular exercise involving sports had even greater benefit for preventing dementia than light exercise such as gardening or walking (although both types of exercise had significant benefits).[876] The Canadian Health and Aging Study found that physical activity was associated with a forty-two percent reduction in risk of cognitive impairment.[877] A meta-analysis that covered more than one hundred sixty thousand subjects found a forty-five percent reduction in the likelihood of developing Alzheimer's disease for people who exercised.[878] A study that analyzed twenty-two different genetic datasets related to Alzheimer's concluded that exercise has a "striking" ability to downregulate the genes associated with developing the disease and to upregulate the genes that prevent it.[879]

Once someone does have MCI, exercise can help mitigate the symptoms and slow its progression. It has been shown to improve cognitive function,[880, 881] memory performance,[882] attention,[883] and executive function[884, 885] in people with MCI. Aerobic exercise led to improvement in cognition after short and long-term treatment in MCI subjects and, thus, has potential as a therapy for MCI.[886] In addition, MCI is less likely to progress into dementia in people who are physically active.[887] A 2021 study found that people with MCI who exercised three or four times a week for a year (taking a brisk walk of at least twenty-five minutes for each exercise session) had improved cerebral blood flow, memory, and executive function (as well as cardiorespiratory fitness) compared to the control group.[888] In people in the early stages of Alzheimer's disease, higher fitness levels are associated with larger brain volume (i.e., less brain atrophy).[889]

Regular aerobic exercise preserves the structural integrity of the brain's white matter.[890, 891] It also improves cerebral blood flow and capillary density[892]—factors whose importance you understand after reading the previous chapter. At least in rodents, exercise has been shown to improve glymphatic function.[893, 894] What's more, among people with higher Alzheimer's risk due to the APOE-ε4 gene, regular aerobic exercise is associated with lower levels of amyloid beta deposition.[895] Regular aerobic exercise also has the effect of ameliorating endothelial dysfunction and central arterial stiffness.[896] Exercise has the ability to reverse some of the vascular changes that have been seen to lead to dementia and Alzheimer's disease.[897] Middle-aged adults with a regular practice of endurance exercise have improved function, reactivity, and adaptability of the vascular system compared to their peers who don't engage in this type of exercise, and these differences are associated with better cognitive performance.[898] A study in which sedentary older women started exercising and continued to exercise for three years found that exercise was effective at reversing or at least slowing the age-related declines in motor performance and speed of cognitive processing.[899] Exercise has also shown promise for ameliorating the symptoms of Parkinson's disease.[900] Cutting-edge analysis techniques are allowing scientists to zero in on the mechanisms—such as a 2022 study that compared analysis of brain tissue after death to subjects' activity levels during life and found that exercise seems to affect the activation of microglia (immune cells in the brain that have the power to promote conditions of health or disease depending on their surrounding conditions and which tend to become dysregulated in old age and in neurodegenerative conditions).[901] So, you can see why, for all these reasons, exercise has protective benefits when it comes to neurodegeneration.[902]

Exercise also wields an indirect influence on brain health via its benefits for other body systems and functions. Exercise helps preserve mitochondrial function as we age[903] (and you know the importance of that from Chapter Two). It has powerful anti-inflammatory effects.[904] Exercise generally seems to improve sleep quality and duration,[905] although more research is needed about the most effective types of exercise for these desired outcomes.[906] Exercise also enhances the number of beneficial bacteria in your gut and enriches microbial diversity—completely independent of the effects of your diet![907, 908] Regular physical activity protects us against cancer, diabetes, and cardiovascular and coronary heart disease—as well as dementia—especially when maintained throughout the life course.[909]

Some studies have found that exercise is not as effective at improving cognitive function in seniors with advanced Alzheimer's; therefore, it's imperative to start *now*, not after the diagnosis occurs. Once you've got a routine in place to hit the minimum requirement, there are ways to tweak your habits even more to maximize the health benefits. Although not all these benefits directly relate to the brain, remember that many other types of health benefits—e.g., better sleep quality and improved cardiovascular health—benefit brain health as well.

There is some evidence that strength training can have benefits above and beyond those conferred by aerobic exercise (such as improved balance and injury prevention as well as cognitive benefits),[910] and thus, an ideal exercise program for an older person (or, really, any person) would include both. Strength training may have specific benefits for cognitive function separate from aerobic exercise.[911] Strength training has also been shown to be beneficial for raising the HRV of people with fibromyalgia, a condition in which autonomic dysfunction is suspected to play a key role.[912] In a study of people with MCI, following a strength training routine for six months led to improvements in memory, attention, and executive function.[913] It seems that a program combining aerobic and resistance training is most beneficial for preserving cognitive function as we age.[914] Both strength training[915] and balance training[916] have the benefit of reducing fall risk—which (as you know from our discussion of neuropathy and my mother's story) is something that can lead to a major decline in physical health, cognitive health, and quality of life for an elderly person.

I hope you're seeing by now that the benefits of exercise extend far beyond building muscle mass and helping maintain a healthy weight. Exercise tips off a cascade of cellular and molecular processes with effects throughout the body—and the brain. These processes include angiogenesis (the formation of new blood vessels), neurogenesis (the formation of new neurons), and synaptogenesis (the formation of the connections between neurons).[917]

Part of the reason exercise is so good for us is because of how it affects the mitochondria. Both strength training and endurance training increase fatty acid oxidation and therefore mitochondrial density.[918] HIIT workouts have been shown to enhance mitochondrial biogenesis.[919] In people with metabolic syndrome, exercise has been shown to reduce the markers of mitochondrial dysfunction, indicating that the mitochondria may be a key mediator in how exercise protects against metabolic disorders.[920] Another part of the way exercise wields its benefits is by improving nitric oxide function, and therefore endothelial function and cerebral blood flow.[921]

Aerobic exercise increases dopamine levels in the brain and also enhances the sensitivity of the receptors for this neurotransmitter, which plays a key role in the brain's reward system.[922] Incidentally, dopamine levels and sensitivity both decline as we age, but exercise can help preserve the capacity of this system[923]—helping us to hang on to pleasure, enjoyment, and zest for life. (Not to mention that the death of the specific type of brain cell that produces dopamine is the underlying cause of Parkinson's disease.)

Different kinds of exercise may affect the brain in different ways, perhaps pointing to the value of a training regimen that includes more than one type of activity at varying intensity levels. One intriguing recent study found that low-intensity exercise triggers brain networks involved in cognition control and attention processing, while high-intensity exercise primarily activates networks involved in the processing of emotion.[924]

Aerobic exercise also increases our levels of growth factors such as BDNF, insulin-like growth factor 1 (IGF-1), and vascular endothelial growth factor (VEGF), molecules that stimulate neurogenesis (the growth of new neurons) and angiogenesis (the growth of new blood vessels).[925, 926, 927, 928] Fascinatingly, a new theory proposes that one of these molecules, BDNF—a protein whose main function is nerve growth—contributes to depression when levels are low and that part of how antidepressant drugs work is by increasing BDNF. So, in addition to neuroregeneration, increasing someone's BDNF levels may also help them feel less depressed.[929] We have known for a long time that exercise acts as a mood booster, and this new finding helps to explain why. (As you've read earlier in the book, photobiomodulation has also been shown to increase BDNF levels[930]—one of the reasons we say it gives you the benefits of exercise without actually having to exercise.)

EXERCISE AND HRV: A POSITIVE FEEDBACK LOOP

As more people recognize the importance of HRV and what it means for our health, we can expect that more emphasis will be placed on the types of behaviors we know affect HRV positively. This has implications for specific groups that lead a sedentary lifestyle due to their occupation—for instance, in a study of sailors from the Royal Norwegian Navy, a four-week exercise training program was shown to improve HRV and cognitive performance scores[931]—but also for the vast numbers of people globally who by default lead sedentary lives.

There is some evidence that higher resting HRV is correlated with cardiorespiratory fitness,[932] and this makes sense. After all, it is well established that how quickly your heart rate returns to its normal level after you stop exercising is one measure of your fitness level: The faster your heart rate normalizes, the more fit you are. What is actually happening as your heart rate returns to normal is that the sympathetic nervous system (activated during exercise) is retreating, while the parasympathetic nervous system is becoming more active to balance out sympathetic activity.

When we exercise, the parasympathetic nervous system withdraws and the sympathetic nervous system takes over—and then when we are done exercising, the opposite happens. If we've been stuck in a state of sympathetic overactivity, exercise can act like a circuit breaker. (This mechanism is not as well-calibrated as usual after a TBI,[933] which is why HRV is emerging as a metric to monitor to determine how soon post-concussion athletes should return to regular practice and play.[934] The fact remains that exercise is beneficial for everyone—including people recovering from TBI—but those in the recovery phase should not push their bodies to the level professional athletes do.)

Our HRV typically takes a dive during a challenging cognitive task, but physical fitness has an impact on this: The higher our fitness level, the more resilient our autonomic nervous system, keeping HRV high even when our brains are being challenged.[935] We know that physical fitness helps us recover from stressful conditions (such as first responders whose jobs require working for twenty-four hours at a stretch).[936] Thus, being physically fit can help our brains stay fit as we age, giving us the cognitive resilience to keep on rising to the challenge and then recovering afterward.

When it comes to effects on HRV, aerobic exercise appears to be preferable to flexibility exercises that don't provide the same kind of cardiopulmonary challenge. In one study of seniors, the group that engaged in aerobic exercise (as opposed to stretching) for twelve weeks improved their HRV scores and also their performance on a cognitive task.[937] Some studies have shown that strength training in particular is helpful for increasing HRV[938] (over the long term, that is, as opposed to during a given exercise session).

In a study of "pre-obese" people with a body mass index (BMI) between twenty-four and thirty, these people had lower HRV in a resting state than the control group with lower BMI; during and after exercise, the "pre-obese" group displayed a blunted autonomic response (their sympathetic nervous systems not ramping up as quickly during, nor down as quickly after, exercise). However, it's not clear which is cause and which is effect.[939]

Exercise is beneficial all throughout the life course, and this doesn't change as people get older—or even once their cognitive health starts to decline. One study found that seniors with clinical depression (a risk factor for dementia) had greater improvements in their HRV with exercise than with antidepressant medication alone.[940] Exercise has been shown to be helpful in boosting HRV for seniors with heart failure.[941] High-intensity interval training has been shown to be successful for this purpose with this population[942]—placing the body's systems under stress (of the beneficial kind) so those systems can adapt and become more resilient.

The results of one meta-analysis showed a significant effect of exercise training on RR interval and HF power. This supports the current theory that aerobic exercise training can alter neuroregulatory control over the heart.[943]

All these observations about HRV and fitness point us toward a different approach to exercise. If you use a fitness tracker, the biggest number on your display after your workout is probably the calories burned. In my opinion, we've been going about this all wrong. Focusing primarily on the calories burned implies that more is better. It's not just about quantity; it's about quality. It's as much about the recovery as it is about the workout.

Fortunately, short HIIT workouts seem to be trendy right now, and I don't hear as often from people who are spending hours a day in the gym, trying to fill all their spare time with steady-state cardio (and flooding their bodies with stress hormones in the process). While we don't have specific findings just yet regarding what type of exercise is best for boosting HRV, I suspect that HIIT—pushing your body hard for a little while and then giving it plenty of time to recover—may ultimately prove to be the most beneficial. This type of exercise matches our concept of hormesis—revving up your engine with an intense challenge and then allowing it to rest and repair—and indeed, we have at least some evidence that HIIT can activate mitochondrial biogenesis within the muscles.[944] Of course, that type of intense exercise is not advisable or even possible for everyone; you need a baseline level of fitness before you ramp up the intensity. Remember that, ultimately, the best kind of exercise is the one you're able to do and will do consistently.

PHOTOBIOMODULATION AND EXERCISE: A WINNING COMBINATION

Given all that you've learned about photobiomodulation so far, it probably won't surprise you to learn that photobiomodulation can have beneficial effects for sports performance and can help you reap even more benefits from your exercise regimen. Both transcranial photobiomodulation and intense exercise enhance mitochondrial respiration and cerebral oxygen consumption; combining them magnifies these effects.[945]

Photobiomodulation has been found to increase the performance outcomes of recreational runners during running tests,[946] soccer players during isokinetic tests,[947] and cyclists in incremental tests until exhaustion.[948] Studies of young men have demonstrated that photobiomodulation maximizes the strength gain and the hypertrophic response to resistance training.[949, 950, 951] One study found that applying photobiomodulation to the quadriceps and gastrocnemius muscles (of the thigh and calf, respectively) ten minutes before exercise improved peak oxygen uptake and performance on a cardiopulmonary exercise test, or CPET.[952] Other studies have found that applying photobiomodulation to major muscles before exercise increases the number of repetitions subjects are able to do.[953, 954, 955] Research in rats has specifically found that photobiomodulation can enhance performance and stamina on an anaerobic exercise test requiring short bursts of intense strength.[956] Another study in rats found that combining photobiomodulation with exercise led to increased muscle fiber density as well as decreased glycogen depletion and less build-up of lactate in their muscles (markers of fatigue) compared to exercise alone.[957]

This points to another benefit of combining photobiomodulation with exercise: It appears to help the body recover better after exertion. In a study of young women, photobiomodulation was effective at reducing fatigue levels and increasing muscle performance when applied prior to exercising their quadriceps muscles.[958] This makes sense due to photobiomodulation's bioenergetic effects (it literally makes more energy available to the muscles, so it makes sense they'd get fatigued less easily). Thus, photobiomodulation might represent a preventive approach at avoiding injury, whereas sports medicine often focuses on dealing with the aftermath.

One study found that applying photobiomodulation to the biceps muscles of volleyball players had the effect of increasing their endurance for repeated elbow flexion movements and decreased their post-exercise markers of fatigue (blood lactate, creatine kinase, and C-reactive protein).[959] In a study of runners, photobiomodulation was found to reduce the intensity of delayed-onset muscle soreness.[960] A study of forty healthy men (staff and students at a university in Brazil) found that photobiomodulation improved exercise recovery and reduced delayed onset muscle soreness for the subjects who received it, relative to the control group.[961] Photobiomodulation has been found to increase the maximal load in exercise and reduce fatigue, creatine kinase, and visual analog scale (a subjective measure of pain level). Gene expression analyses show decreases in markers of inflammation and muscle atrophy with photobiomodulation; protein synthesis and oxidative stress defense are upregulated with photobiomodulation.[962]

Many of the studies cited thus far in this chapter have involved athletes or at least physically healthy individuals, but those aren't the only people who can benefit from photobiomodulation in combination with exercise—far from it. Exercise has beneficial effects for people with type 2 diabetes, and the blood sugar–regulating effect was enhanced by using photobiomodulation before exercise.[963] In a trial involving a twelve-week aerobic exercise program, elderly subjects who received photobiomodulation treatments in addition to exercising showed even more improvement in their cognitive function than the subjects who only exercised.[964] For healthy elderly men who completed twelve weeks of twice-weekly resistance training with application of real or placebo photobiomodulation to their quadriceps muscles before each training session, the group that received real photobiomodulation experienced better recovery between training sessions, contributing to better performance in the next session.[965]

Photobiomodulation has the power to improve muscle performance during exercise,[966] reduce fatigue during exercise,[967] accelerate tissue repair[968] and regeneration,[969] reduce inflammation in connective tissue,[970] aid muscle recovery after exercise, and promote cardiovascular health even apart from exercise.[971] Given its effects on mitochondrial health, it's no surprise that photobiomodulation helps the muscles train harder and recover better, so adding it to your exercise routine will help you boost the benefits you reap from being active.

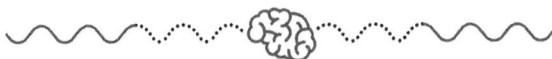

According to the Cleveland Clinic, eighty percent of American adults don't meet the minimum exercise recommendation. What is the reason so many of us miss this target? I think a large part of the explanation is that not enough of us are engaging in mindful and joyful movement. Quite simply, if you have to force yourself to exercise and grit your teeth to get through the workout—it probably won't stick, and you definitely aren't reaping the maximum benefits. So, it's worth taking the time to find a way of moving that actually feels enjoyable while still meeting the health guidelines.

If exercise feels like a grind to you, consider what you can switch up with regard to these three questions:

1. *What do you do?* If your workout routine feels stale, make a point of trying new activities. Sign up for a class or just hunt down a video to follow on YouTube. Trying new kinds of movement also challenges your brain in a positive way.
2. *Where do you do it?* Just taking your regular workout outside can make a world of difference. Switch up the setting: If you usually walk near your home, drive to a state park instead. If you usually run in a flat area, seek out an area with some hills.

If you've done the same gym routine so many times you could do it in your sleep, what about purchasing some free weights so you could do a similar workout at home or outside? If you've walked the same route so many times you're wearing grooves in the sidewalk, how about exploring a new neighborhood that will have interesting details to notice? Also think about combining your interests—for example, if you don't love to exercise but you do love bird watching, perhaps it's worth driving to a nature preserve to get your walk in.

3. *How do you do it?* Something as simple as listening to music you love can make exercise way more fun. Pairing exercise with a favorite hobby can also work well. Save your favorite podcast to listen to on a walk; if you love to watch movies, maybe a treadmill, elliptical, or exercise bike would be a good investment so you can get moving while watching instead of sitting on the couch. Lastly, if you don't love exercising on your own, you could invite a buddy to exercise with you or even look into sports clubs and leagues in your area.

Another important tip is to watch your inner monologue while exercising. Are you acting out of self-love or self-loathing? If you find yourself thinking degrading thoughts—such as "I'm so much weaker than I used to be" or "Wow, my mile time was really slow today. I suck!"—it's time to switch that up ASAP. (And if you hate exercise, this might be part of the reason why. After all, why would you enjoy an activity that involves subjecting yourself to constant self-abuse?)

Exercise has proven anti-inflammatory effects, which is part of how it improves the symptoms for almost every health condition you may already have and reduces your risk of developing others. But remember, if you're thinking negative thoughts the whole time, you're adding to your body's toxic burden, which will only require more work to detoxify.

If you're having trouble fitting in a structured workout, another way to approach it is to start small and build more movement into everyday activities. When shopping, park farther away from the entrance and take the stairs instead of the escalator. Use a standing desk for part of the day. Dance to music you love instead of standing still while cooking dinner. Take a walk with a friend instead of sitting at the coffee shop to catch up.

Fitness trackers and other wearable devices can help encourage you to be more active. Especially for goal-oriented people, seeing hard evidence in the form of numbers can be very rewarding, both positively (in terms of meeting activity goals) and negatively (in terms of avoiding missing a goal). Fitness trackers can also motivate you to push harder in a workout as you strive to get into the "high intensity" activity category—and a workout where you give your all will be more beneficial than a halfhearted one. These trackers also often have reminders to get up from your seat once every hour; you could use these reminders as a prompt to do a little bit more activity, like some stretches or a set of push-ups or a one-minute wall sit, when you get up to walk around.

Plugging into a community also has benefits for accountability. Join an online group following the same workout program, or invite a group of friends to commit to a workout calendar with you and check in after each session. Even checking in with one friend daily can harness this benefit. The idea that you are going to let someone else down if you miss your workout can be a much more powerful motivator than the desire to avoid letting yourself down.

Separately from the benefits of getting moving, cultivating mindfulness throughout your day has its own health benefits—and movement becomes even more beneficial when it is done mindfully. Mindfulness is a skill that's developed over time. The more you practice, the more in tune you will become with your body until eventually you will be able to feel when your body needs to move, and you will want to do it—instead of exercise feeling like a chore. Mindfulness can also help you know whether you are pushing too hard or not hard enough for your body's capabilities on a given day and calibrate your intensity level to work hard enough to be challenging but not so hard you get injured.

You can start right now with this simple exercise. Standing with your feet shoulder width apart, stand still and take a deep breath. Become aware of your body and how it feels. Where is your weight settled? Notice that it may not be evenly distributed. Which parts of your feet feel heaviest on the floor? Lift your chest and roll your shoulders back and down. Become aware of the muscles holding you upright. As you inhale, slowly raise your arms straight in front of you and then stretch them straight up vertically. As you exhale, lower your arms back down by your sides. As you continue to raise and lower your arms along with your breath, notice how your balance may shift along with the arm movement. Also notice the way other parts of your body may adjust and compensate: the pelvis, the abdomen, the ribs, the shoulders, the head and neck. Repeat for at least ten breaths.

If all else fails, just get outside. If you can't get to a nature preserve, take a walk around the block or even just down your driveway. Remember what John Denver said about sunshine on your shoulders. Almost by default, you'll find yourself breathing deeper and stretching once you're surrounded by fresh air and green things. In a study of university students, the act of transferring potted plants significantly increased HRV as well as self-reported feelings of relaxation, relative to the control group that performed a similar task without any plants.[972] The group that touched the plants also showed patterns of blood flow in their prefrontal cortex that indicated they were more relaxed and less stressed than the control group.

U: UNWIND AND UNSTRESS

The next ingredient in your sundae is not so much an activity as a state of mind. There is no device you can buy, no pill you can swallow, no trainer you can hire—this is something you simply have to do on your own. It's an inner transformation, but in this section, I'll outline some practices you can try to start you on the right path for the next letter of **PRONEURO**—U for Unwind and Unstress. This is not something you can add to your to-do list (although you may find practices that help you with it, and you can certainly add *those* to your list). It's an attitude that underlies everything you do. In any moment, you can choose to be stressed or *unstressed*.

Since we've just been talking about exercise, let's use that as an example. While you are in the midst of exercising, you can dwell on how much you hate it. You can focus on how the number on the scale isn't moving as fast as you'd like it to. You can count the minutes until it's over.

That is one way to approach exercise. But let's look at an alternative way. Instead, you can focus on what feels good about it—the wind in your hair as you're biking or running, how strong you feel when doing a push-up, how much you like the songs on your workout playlist. You can anchor into the belief that every rep and every minute of your workout is serving your health and the feeling of pride that accompanies that belief.

With nearly every activity we do, we can choose to do it in a stressed or an unstressed state. Exercise is a natural stress-buster, so let's take a different example. Let's say you're completing an important report for work, and it has a strict deadline that will be challenging for you to meet. In that situation, it makes sense that you'd be a ball of stress while sitting at your computer—shoulders hunched, chest collapsed, jaw clenched. But you still have choices about how to approach this situation. Maybe you dwell on stressful thoughts ("I'll never finish this on time," "This isn't my best work," "I hope I don't get fired"). Can you feel how your body contracts further into the stress posture just by reading those statements?

Now let's make a different choice. Picture yourself in your desk chair, still needing to complete the report and still unsure whether you can produce a quality result by the deadline. What if you focus on thoughts that make the challenge seem less daunting as opposed to more daunting? Some examples: "I'm feeling stressed right now, but in five years I won't even remember this report." "It doesn't need to be perfect; done is good enough." "I'm doing my best, and my colleagues will appreciate that." What do you notice in your body when you read *these* statements? I'm betting that you're sitting up a little straighter, that maybe your body feels less locked in a freeze response, that maybe your breathing is a little deeper and more relaxed.

See what I mean about this being not an activity but a state of mind—not a behavior but a mindset? We have a choice in every moment about how we view our situation. The choice we make affects our physiology.

Think back to the concept of allostatic load from Section One of the book. Higher allostatic load is correlated with more pronounced changes in brain structure as a person ages.[973, 974] Now, we can't do anything about many of the factors that contribute to our allostatic load; we can't go back and erase adverse childhood experiences, and we only have so much control over our exposure to environmental pollution. But mitigating stress—that is, learning to Unwind—is one very powerful way we can increase our bodies' ability to cope and thus help to lessen our allostatic load. Early life adversity is correlated with lower HRV in adulthood,[975] but if we can raise our HRV, perhaps we can break (or at least weaken) the link between childhood trauma and ill health.

There are some behavioral practices that can help. Remember the study from the last section about just being in the presence of plants? When we get out into nature, we can't help but take a deep breath and appreciate the beauty. And if you can't do that, maybe you can get up from your desk for a minute and do some stretches. I guarantee you'll be breathing deeper and feeling just the tiniest bit less stressed. Even looking at a picture of nature on the wall of your office (a shortcut to the practice of "nature bathing" when you don't have time to go outside) can do the trick.

Now that I've made the point of how this applies to everything we do in the course of daily life, let's look at some practices to help you Unwind and Unstress—and to make it your permanent state of mind.

Self-awareness is the simplest and most powerful tool you have in this area. With practice, you will be able to develop the ability to notice your own stress response unfolding. Once you notice the telltale signs of sympathetic activation—rapid heart rate, shallow breathing, muscle tension, the feeling that you are so on edge you can't even blink—you can take a moment to breathe and consciously relax. Just in that small moment, you can alter your heart rate, HRV, blood pressure, and the balance of hormones coursing through your system.

Developing this skill also has the potential to improve your relationships. During difficult conversations, if you can learn to pause in the heat of the moment and take a deep breath, you can avoid saying things you'll later regret. Self-awareness may be simple, but it is not easy. Nevertheless, it's worth focusing on since it holds the key that unlocks our power to change many different kinds of behaviors. It can help us change anything that seems to happen on autopilot—whether it's stress eating, habitual social media or smartphone use, or staying up too late.

One tool that can help with this is naming your emotions. (There are apps that can help with this, including the ones that go along with some fitness trackers.) By putting a name to your emotions and checking in with where they show up in your body (and how you're feeling physically overall), you are building your self-awareness and also getting out of your head and into a fuller, embodied way of living.

Self-awareness will also help you observe which types of relaxing activities benefit you the most. If you relax by watching a movie but the movie is scary or violent, is it just further jacking up your sympathetic nervous system? It may be better to choose a more soothing option when it's time to relax.

To a certain extent, we can choose how we feel. When we have a crummy morning, it's our choice whether we allow those events to continue to impact our mood or whether we instead choose to let go and salvage the day by at least having an enjoyable evening. Holding onto grudges, ruminating on events that upset us, and going over again and again in our minds things we wish we'd done differently are all ways we can choose how we feel—and we can also choose the opposite: to let go and enjoy the present moment regardless of what happened in the past. Try it for yourself, and you'll see what I mean: Next time you find yourself ruminating, make a choice to change gears and think about something in your life you feel grateful for. I suspect you'll notice an immediate and profound physiological change.

Here's a "recipe" for helping you get into the habit of observing your emotions, practicing gratitude, or simply taking a deep breath to release stress (with a hat tip to B.J. Fogg's Tiny Habits method for behavior change). Choose a prompt (such as noticing your shoulders have migrated up to your ears). Then decide what you will do to release stress whenever you notice this prompt. Lastly, choose a small "celebration" that you can complete in a single moment (ideally, at the same time as your behavior that releases stress). The purpose of the celebration is to allow you to really sink into that feeling of satisfaction; this helps you cement your new habit. For example:

When I notice my shoulders are tense, I'll stretch my arms overhead and smile.

When I notice I'm holding my breath, I'll get up from my desk for a quick break and tell myself, "Awesome self-awareness!"

When I catch myself in a negative thought, I'll think of one thing I'm grateful for and then give myself a hug.

When I notice my eyes are strained from looking at the computer screen too long, I'll look out the window and notice one thing I see that makes me happy.

Try it yourself with your own formula. What will your "prompt" be to notice that you're stressed? What will you do to move into a more unstressed state of mind, and how will you celebrate to really feel into your satisfaction with your new habit?

When I notice _____ *I will* _____ *and* _____.
　　　　　　　(anchor)　　　(behavior)　　　　(celebration)

Remember from Chapter Six the "triangle of disease": Trauma, toxins, and auto-suggestion contribute to our toxic load and prevent our bodies from healing. Research has shown how negativity bias (an assumption of negative outcomes and focus on worst-case scenarios) can depress HRV and push the body into sympathetic overdrive.[976] (This may be how negative thoughts contribute to ill health outcomes such as more severe asthma symptoms.[977]) When this happens, essentially, through your own negative thinking, you're impairing that inhibitory response that starts with the prefrontal cortex telling the amygdala to quiet down and cascades through the whole parasympathetic nervous system. By learning not to engage so readily with these negative thoughts, you can help your body come back into balance.

Ruminating thoughts and catastrophizing (dwelling on negative circumstances and worst-case scenarios) have long been known to contribute to the development of depression, and breaking these habits of negative thinking is often a goal of cognitive behavioral therapy. Fascinatingly, recent research points to HRV as the mechanism that links worrying and depression.[978, 979] Another study found that the habit of cognitive reappraisal—that is, purposely shifting one's perspective to find a silver lining or lesson in adversity—was associated with not only higher HRV but longer telomeres (the chromosomal markers of aging discussed in Section One of the book).[980] These findings underscore the importance of choosing what we focus on.

Of course, there are times in life when we experience emotions too big to "choose" our way out of. For the major losses and let-downs in life, we can't force ourselves to immediately move beyond the sense of grief and disappointment we feel. But we can choose to be grateful "in spite of"—to focus on the good friends who are here to comfort us after our loss or the fact that the weather is beautiful and sunny even though we also feel sad. Cultivating the ability to hold both helps us move through the difficult emotions and maintain a sense of hope.

A **meditation** practice is one of the most effective tools that exists for developing mindfulness, self-awareness, and the ability to notice (and choose) your thoughts and feelings. Research shows that meditation reduces stress levels (and brings all the health benefits that go along with that), as well as reducing risk of depression and anxiety. It improves sleep quality and cognitive function. It helps control blood pressure and reduces chronic pain. One fascinating study even found that subjects who practiced meditation had a more pronounced immune response after receiving the flu vaccine;[981] another one found that meditation training could improve immune cell counts in HIV-infected adults.[982] (One study found that meditation matched the effectiveness for stress reduction of both HRV biofeedback and physical activity[983]—further evidence that, when it comes to building healthy habits, it's so much better to do something than nothing, and you shouldn't get too caught up in doing the one right thing but should, rather, take the action that seems most easily within your reach right now.)

With so many meditation videos, apps, and tutorials available at your fingertips (many of them free of charge), I'm not going to make a specific recommendation for which one to use. The most important thing is just to do it—and to show yourself compassion while building the habit. Beginners often quit because they feel they're "not good at" meditation. If you've found yourself saying this, that's a sign you may want to keep an eye on your internal monologue because you might be just a little bit hard on yourself! But the larger point is that nobody feels they are good at meditating when they first start. It's a skill you develop with practice, so stick with it. As with exercise, don't be afraid to try different styles and tools (such as videos that offer you a visual to focus on or audio meditations with guided imagery) until you find something that works for you. Meanwhile, with every session you try, you'll be building your skills as you go.

Meditation does not always involve breathwork, but breathwork can be a form of meditation. There is a natural relationship between heart rate and breathing, such that heart rate slows when you exhale and speeds up when you inhale—so by lengthening your exhalation, you can consciously slow your heart rate down.

Try this breathing exercise now: Breathe in for four counts, then stretch your exhalation to eight counts. Can you feel yourself relaxing as you go? What you are feeling is your parasympathetic nervous system activating and your HRV increasing![984] Yoga breathing practices called *pranayama* have also been shown to increase parasympathetic activity and raise HRV.[985, 986]

Remember, you can always use your breath to influence your physical state. This is a tool that's available to you at any time—even standing in line at the grocery store! And if you have trouble focusing during meditation, counting your breaths out this way can help quiet down distracting thoughts.

There are also some physical practices you can use to quickly hack into a more relaxed physical state. One of these is abdominal foam rolling and self-massage of the abdominal wall. According to a study published in the *International Journal of Neuroscience*, massage therapy decreased cortisol levels by as much as thirty-one percent and increased serotonin by twenty-eight percent and dopamine by thirty-one percent.[987] Massaging the abdominal wall in particular may enhance this effect, given the location of sensory fibers of the vagus nerve there. Bodywork modalities such as craniosacral therapy, myofascial release, and acupuncture have also been shown to have HRV-boosting effects[988, 989, 990, 991]—offering a physiological marker of why these treatments help us feel more relaxed.

Laughing—and not just a superficial laugh, but a deep, genuine belly laugh—can have the same effect of stimulating the vagus nerve and signaling to the body that it's safe to relax. Have you ever experienced a "laugh attack" at the end of a particularly stressful day or after completing a stressful task or conversation? If it seems like things that would ordinarily be only mildly funny are striking you as completely hilarious, this is your body trying to complete a cycle and move back from the stress response into a more relaxed state. We can intentionally cultivate this kind of release as well: There's such a thing as "laughter yoga," and I had a great time sampling this type of class! One theory of how and why this works is that as laughter stimulates the movement of your inner organs, the result is vagus nerve stimulation via a nice, soft belly massage.

Odd as it may sound, gagging also stimulates the vagus nerve. Purposely stimulating your gag reflex (just lightly, nothing too severe) can help you improve vagal tone to more easily tap into these beneficial effects. Tongue scraping and gargling enlist the same muscle group, as does singing—so put on your favorite song, and go ahead and sing your heart out!

Lastly, don't forget to allow yourself time to unwind. Breathing exercises and a five-minute meditation are one thing, but taking time out of your schedule for relaxing activities might not even seem like a plausible option when you're very busy. The thing is, these are the times when it's actually the most important. Remember, it's all about balance. Testing your body with stress isn't a negative thing—as long as you give your nervous system the time and space to counteract the effects of stress. This is why including downtime, restoration, and fun in your schedule is absolutely essential.

Stress affects every body organ and system. Remember, the goal is not to avoid stress; it's to *increase our capacity to withstand stress* and recover from it. If exercise constitutes hormesis training from one angle, the techniques in this section of the chapter come at hormesis training from the opposite angle. We apply stress or a challenge to increase the body's capacity, but we need to "wind down" in order to heal. Just as you couldn't keep running indefinitely (or at least, your body wouldn't do well if you tried), we can't stay in a state of stress indefinitely—as much as it might seem that modern life is asking us to.

Recent research on chronic pain also demonstrates the importance of giving our parasympathetic nervous system the chance to become more active. In our discussion of HRV in Chapter Three, I briefly touched on the new characterization of this condition as not "too much pain," but rather "not enough inhibition." When our pain signals have gone haywire, they no longer serve as useful information to promote survival. When pain is not an indicator of "Take your hand off the hot burner" but, instead, is present all the time, this is a sign that the autonomic nervous system is dysregulated.[992] Catastrophizing thoughts keep us in a constant state of fight-or-flight. If we can focus on the positive and give ourselves a chance to relax, the sympathetic nervous system can settle down, giving the parasympathetic nervous system a chance to inhibit those pain signals. You can apply your light pad and practice your biofeedback breathing as ways to boost your HRV, but you'll do your body and mind a world of good if you incorporate practices throughout your day that keep you in an unstressed state of mind.

R: RESTORE (REENERGIZE AND GET RESTFUL SLEEP)

Persistent short sleep duration in midlife is associated with significantly increased dementia risk, even after controlling for other sociodemographic, behavioral, cardiometabolic, and mental health risk factors.[993] After learning about the glymphatic system in Chapter Eight, you're well aware of the important work our bodies carry out while we are sleeping. Think of sleep as your favorite topping for an ice cream sundae. Whether it's nuts, hot fudge, caramel sauce, or whipped cream that makes your taste buds light up—think about how much more you enjoy a sundae that has that topping. A sundae is still a sundae without it, but your experience of eating the sundae is greatly improved by having it.

Sleep plays a similar role in the **PRONEURO** formula. We could say that it's part of the foundation, but improving your sleep can take some trial and error and often requires serious commitment. Therefore, if you're really suffering with low energy because your brain isn't firing on all cylinders, it's usually better to start with some quick wins like using your light pad and taking some supplements. Then, once you start to feel better as your energy and focus are increasing, you can work on some of the habits that can be tougher nuts to crack, like exercise and sleep. That being said, sleep is almost as much of a magic pill as exercise, with a wide variety of benefits across many different aspects of health—but most importantly for our purposes in this book, preventing and reversing neurodegeneration.

Sleeping after learning a new task substantially improves performance on that task. We don't know exactly why this is, but we can hypothesize that learning challenges our brain to connect in new ways, and these connections are consolidated and streamlined while we sleep, so the connections are made faster and more efficiently the next time we try the task.[994]

While we are sleeping, the autonomic nervous system's activity oscillates rapidly, with the high-frequency components of HRV increasing and low-frequency components decreasing during deep sleep and vice versa during REM sleep.[995] While we sleep, our bodies, brains, and nervous systems are at work on consolidating memories, clearing out waste products from the day just ended, mounting an immune response to any threats detected, balancing hormones, and resetting blood pressure to its lowest daily level.[996] When our sleep suffers, all these functions are affected.

While we sleep, parasympathetic activity is dominant, and HRV is higher than when we are awake. Certain health conditions disrupt this pattern; for example, after a heart attack, parasympathetic activation during sleep is impaired, and analysis of specific components of HRV can help identify which recent sufferers of heart attacks are most at risk of sudden death while sleeping.[997] These findings help to highlight the reason sleep hygiene is especially important in the wake of health events that affect sleep (such as TBI, heart attack, and stroke). Research indicates that disturbed sleep is both a result of having a stroke and a risk factor for having another stroke.[998] After suffering one of these medical incidents, the need to improve your sleep quality takes on even more urgency than under ordinary circumstances.

In recent years, new research methods have shed light (literally) on the reasons sleep deprivation is so damaging. NIRS imaging allows us to see that cerebral blood flow is affected, and the brain receives less oxygenated blood when we don't get enough sleep.[999] Sleep deprivation places us at greater risk of hypertension and metabolic disorders[1000]—both conditions with serious implications for brain health. Persistent short sleep duration is associated with a thirty percent increased risk of dementia when measured at either age fifty, age sixty, or age seventy.[1001] Although this is a correlation and we don't know for sure which way the arrow of causation points, we *do* know that sleep deprivation (whatever the cause) strains the glymphatic system—which in itself is a risk factor for neurodegeneration.

People with MCI display lower HRV during sleep, and those with amnestic MCI (the kind involving memory loss) exhibit a greater reduction in this metric.[1002] If HRV is affected, this means the glymphatic system's ability to prepare the brain for optimal function during waking hours is also impaired. As blood flow to the brain diminishes, neurons are lost and the brain's control over the heart diminishes further in a downward spiral of the heart-brain connection.

Alzheimer's patients spend less time in deep sleep and exhibit decreased slow-wave activity. This means the glymphatic system is less active—which causes a vicious cycle with escalating consequences. Just to name one, suppression of slow-wave sleep markedly reduces insulin sensitivity and leads to impaired glucose tolerance.[1003] Conversely, we see that increases in deep sleep improve several important aspects of cognitive function, including verbal declarative memory,[1004] object location memory,[1005] and picture memory.[1006] Slow-wave sleep can be stimulated using various visual and auditory techniques as well as magnetic and direct current stimulation.[1007] Later in this chapter, I'll offer some of my favorite ways you can easily do this at home.

Numerous aspects of sleep quality are tied to our circadian rhythm. Because of this, it is hard to get high-quality sleep if you work at night and sleep during the day, no matter how solid your routine and sleep hygiene practices are. There certainly are steps you can take to minimize the effect of a schedule that's out of sync with circadian rhythms, but unfortunately, there's no way to completely escape the effect, aside from changing your schedule of working and sleeping. We will probably always need workers who persevere through the nighttime hours—nurses and security guards, law enforcement and hotel clerks—but those workers pay a price with their health. If this is your situation right now, it's best if it's only temporary and you switch back to a day shift when you can.

In Chapter Five, you saw how TBI can lead to insomnia and disrupted sleep cycles, which means the brain is less able to access the healing it needs—in a vicious cycle with symptoms compounding as it continues. The good news is that you can break the cycle with the sleep hacks in this chapter. It will take some time and dedication to implement them—and it may even take some sacrifice if you believe you are a "night person." If your body is out of sync with your circadian rhythms, you can bring it into sync with these practices—and I think you will find that if you do, you'll feel better than you ever thought was possible.

Getting more sleep and better sleep is one of the most powerful things we can do for our health. So, why does our entire modern culture go against this in favor of working longer, staying up later, and sleeping less?

We have to re-learn how to sleep. We know how to sleep as babies, but somewhere along the way, that's replaced with habits of overstimulation and staying up too late. To quote the podcast title of my friend Mollie Eastman, *sleep is a skill*. Don't make difficulty sleeping (or lack of interest in sleep) part of your identity, and don't assume that it can't change. It's just like any other skill you can build with intentional practice. On that note, let's dive in to the **PRONEURO** approach to getting better sleep.

First, **invest in a biodata tracker.** Wearable devices have come a long way just in the last few years in terms of the data they can provide about your sleep quality. I'm not endorsing any brands here—not least because by the time you're reading this book, the market leaders may have changed (that's how quickly this segment is innovating and evolving). But look for a tracker that can accurately measure HRV and blood oxygen saturation as well as heart rate, respiratory rate, body temperature, and movement. As of this writing, those are the metrics that allow devices to determine (with at least decent accuracy) how much time you spend in each sleep phase throughout the night. (Incidentally, we've developed a customized biodata dashboard that we use with our coaching clients in the **PRONEURO** program to help them glean the most powerful insights from the raw data their devices serve up. I just had to toot my own horn a bit because I think our team has created something unique that truly is not available anywhere else!)

Start getting ready for bed as soon as you wake up. People often refer to the last few hours before bedtime as your "runway" in which you wind down and prepare for sleep like an airplane getting ready for takeoff. But your runway really starts as soon as you open your eyes in the morning. That's right—you can consider the entire day your preparation for a good night of sleep ahead. Just try viewing your life this way—I've found it causes people to drastically reevaluate how they are doing things! You may notice that certain ways of eating (too much sugar, too little protein) or having caffeine too late in the day prevent you from sleeping well. You may find it easier to avoid alcohol if you're focused on the prospect of diminished sleep quality later rather than the fun you're having right now.

Gather information and use what you learn to tweak your routine and take action.

Start your day with a gratitude practice and some sunlight in the morning. When the light hits your retinas, that serves as a signal for your body to calibrate your circadian rhythm so that the right hormones will be released at the right times: cortisol to wake you up in the morning and melatonin to help you wind down at night.

Beware of blue light. Once the sun goes down, wear blue blocker glasses and/or install light filtering apps on your devices—or just don't use screens after sunset. We talk about light pollution that prevents us from seeing the stars, and we can also think about bright light (especially blue light) in the evening as a kind of toxin that interferes with our brains' ability to wind down, rest, and repair. Bright light at night boosts alertness, raises your core body temperature, increases your heart rate, and suppresses melatonin[1008]—which, in addition to making us sleepy and acting as a powerful antioxidant, plays a crucial role in regulating autophagy and the ways the process goes awry in neurodegenerative conditions.[1009] Bright light exposure also increases cortisol[1010]—which is not your friend if you are trying to get into rest and repair mode. It's best if you can unplug and do relaxing activities in the evening and detach from thinking about work. If it feels like you can't stop working, just try it for one night (and one night might turn into a few and then forever). By eliminating evening work sessions, you can realign your circadian rhythm to be more productive and efficient in the morning—and ultimately get more done in less time overall.

Avoid weekend jetlag. (This is sometimes called *social jetlag*, but you don't need to be doing anything social to get into the bad habit of staying up too late on the weekends; it's easy enough to do this all on your own at home.) As tempting as it is to stay up late when you don't have to be at work the next morning, this has major effects on your sleep quality. Sleep later in the night (moving toward morning) is generally less restorative than sleep earlier in the night. Your body is used to your own regular routines, and you tend to get most of your deep sleep in the first two to three hours after falling asleep. If you stay up two or three hours beyond your usual bedtime, your body doesn't just start its usual sleep cycles later. It skips the first one or two sleep cycles, meaning you lose out on your deep sleep for that night and go straight into REM. (Try a sleep-tracking device and see for yourself if you don't believe me!) By pushing back your bedtime, you are compromising your body's ability to engage in all the restorative processes that happen during deep sleep. Try to get in bed nine hours before your usual wake-up time, no matter what day of the week it is.

Keep it quiet, cold, and dark. A drop in temperature is a natural signal for your body to wind down (dating to an earlier time before central heating existed). Keeping your bedroom cool and dark will help your body know when it's time to sleep. Especially if you live in an area with a lot of noise or bright streetlights, sleeping with earplugs and an eye mask can also be helpful—as can light-blocking window coverings. Contrary to the popular belief that light that hits the retina is the only way light affects our circadian rhythms, research is increasingly showing that light affects the rest of our bodies too[1011] (so blackout shades on the window might be better than sleeping in a bright, sunny room wearing a mask that covers your eyes). At least one researcher has found that transcranial bright light exposure (applied to the head but not visible to the eyes) helped to reduce jetlag symptoms as well as the symptoms of seasonal affective disorder.[1012] (Interestingly, photobiomodulation was originally categorized as "circadian medicine" rather than recognizing its broader influence in the bioenergetic system.)

Keep it relaxing. For reading before bed, use a dim/soft lamp. (Emerging research even shows that light angle makes a difference in how the receptors in your eyes process the light and the hormones and neurotransmitters that are released as a result—so instead of an overhead light, try a bedside lamp that's close to the "horizon line" and mimics the sunset as closely as possible.) Avoid reading anything stimulating or discussing anxiety-provoking topics such as finances, health problems, or relationship conflicts. Lavender has been linked to increased deep sleep as well as insomnia relief, so bring on the lavender—essential oils, candles, laundry detergent for washing your bedsheets. Invest in high-quality bedding and a comfortable bed, including pillows that allow you to sleep with good body alignment. (Incidentally, you may wish to try sleeping on your right side as often as you can—at least one study has found that this is the position that best promotes robust glymphatic clearance![1013])

Have a routine. With time and practice, all the activities that are part of your bedtime routine will become signals your body understands in their own right—all part of the message that bedtime is coming and it's time to wind down. The most important thing is to set aside time for this routine and to build consistency in doing it. But there are certain items that are grounded in research and will have an impact right away. Chamomile tea contains a certain type of antioxidant (apigenin) that binds to receptors in your brain that decrease anxiety and initiate sleep. Breathwork is a great addition to your bedtime routine for all the reasons mentioned elsewhere in this book. Your gratitude practice can also help you detach from worries at bedtime. And don't forget about your body pad—some photobiomodulation can help provide you with a parasympathetic boost to drift off into dreamland.

Eat for sleep. This one is really about what *not* to do. Finish eating at least three to four hours before bedtime; otherwise, your body will still be putting energy into digestion after you fall asleep and won't be able to shift into deep sleep and repair mode. Large meals and spicy foods should especially be avoided close to bedtime. You should also avoid caffeine-containing beverages late in the day, avoid alcohol for four hours before bedtime, and try to have your workout completed at least four hours before bed as well.

Try binaural beats. This practice of playing two audio tones slightly different in frequency—one into each ear (so you will need to listen with headphones)—is designed to synchronize your brain waves. The difference between the frequencies causes the illusion of a third sound, and the neurons in your brain begin to fire at the same frequency as that imagined third sound—meaning that you can use binaural beats to influence the frequency of your brain activity. There are different ways to use these tones depending on the type of brain activity you want to cultivate—creative, alert and focused, mellow—and you can use them specifically to lull your brain into the delta wave frequency characteristic of sleep. (You can also use binaural beats to enhance the parasympathetic recovery response after exercise.[1014] Pretty cool, right?) Through the different binaural beats apps available, you can listen to pure tones or tones with different kinds of relaxing music layered over the top. Find an app you like and make it part of your bedtime routine.

Stay positive. If you happen to have trouble sleeping, don't catastrophize. Thinking thoughts like "I'm going to be exhausted tomorrow" or "What's the point of staying in bed when I can never get to sleep?" only leads to feelings like frustration and anguish—which do not help you get back to sleep! Replace those thoughts with positive statements like "I will sleep through the night," "I can fall asleep," or even "I am learning to fall asleep easily." You can even just pretend to be asleep! Tell yourself that you *are* asleep. Lie completely still and focus on slow, smooth, regular breathing. In this state, your body will still be able to carry out some restorative functions—and in the process, your thoughts may become your reality. It can also help to keep a notebook next to your bed to write down thoughts or tasks that keep coming to mind. The act of writing them down tells your brain you'll be able to take care of them tomorrow so you don't need to worry about them now.

Be aware. If you are consistently having trouble sleeping for more than a few weeks, consult your health care provider. You may be referred for counseling/therapy, or your doctor may recommend that you get tested for a condition such as allergies, asthma, or sleep apnea. (If you use a sleep tracker, it may already be picking up clues to this.) You can't do anything about these issues unless you know you have them, so don't hesitate to seek a diagnosis if you suspect something is wrong. Coaching can also help you identify what's causing difficulty; if you feel this would be of value, please reach out to me through my website because I have a capable team working to help people in just this way.

Get some supplemental help. In addition to the list of supplements given in the Optimize section of Chapter Six, there are a few I especially like to help with sleep. They're listed in this chapter because they are probably best used as part of an overall effort to improve sleep quality, to be undertaken once you already have some healthy habits in place and therefore have the bandwidth for some trial and error, assessing what is working and what's not as you experiment with various remedies for sounder sleep. As with any supplements, consider the quality and purchase them from a reliable source so you can trust that you're actually getting what's listed on the bottle.

Melatonin is the hormone that regulates our circadian rhythm, triggering that sleepy feeling that signals it's time to turn in after the sun goes down—and its levels decline with age.[1015] Start with a low dose (½ or 1 mg) and work up since even a small dose can raise blood levels to many multiples of your naturally occurring level. Melatonin is relatively quickly absorbed and quickly cleared from the body—which can be fine if your main problem is falling asleep—but if your issue is *staying* asleep, you may want to consider one of the time-release formulas on the market.

5-hydroxytryptophan (5-HTP) is an amino acid that your body naturally produces. It is a precursor to serotonin, a neurotransmitter associated with feelings of well-being. Serotonin is thought to be a major reason behind carb cravings, as people with low levels of the neurotransmitter self-medicate by eating foods that induce serotonin production. As it turns out, serotonin is a precursor to melatonin—so low serotonin might be one reason a person isn't producing enough melatonin to support sound sleep, and supplementing with 5-HTP is another way to overcome that deficiency and help produce more melatonin.

5-HTP is more effective when combined with *gamma-aminobutyric acid (GABA)*, a neurotransmitter that promotes relaxation. This combination has been shown to reduce the time it takes to fall asleep, increase sleep duration, and improve sleep quality.[1016, 1017, 1018]

Taurine is another naturally occurring amino acid. Under ideal conditions, our bodies only need minimal amounts of it, and these amounts can easily be gotten from the food we eat. But we need much more of it under conditions of stress—and if you've been paying attention, you know it's my belief that we are under constant conditions of stress in modern life, and this is the reason our brains can't heal and repair. Taurine works to increase GABA receptor sensitivity, but it can't do its job (and we therefore won't get sleepy) if we don't have enough of it.

Valerian root (sometimes called "nature's Valium") is an herbal remedy that has been used since the Middle Ages to treat insomnia. It is thought to have its effects at least in part by increasing the circulating amount of GABA. A 2020 review of the literature found that valerian does appear to have beneficial effects for sleep problems, although it noted that a lack of quality control and limited shelf life could account for some of the inconsistencies in the findings.[1019]

L-theanine is another amino acid that enhances the production of serotonin and therefore can influence melatonin levels. It has been found to reduce insomnia and improve sleep quality[1020]—and works even better in combination with GABA supplementation.[1021] Green and black tea are natural sources of L-theanine.

Sound sleep was among the benefits of *magnesium* supplements mentioned in Chapter Six. In addition to the general role it plays as a muscle relaxant and activator of the parasympathetic nervous system, magnesium influences levels of melatonin[1022] and GABA.[1023] Our bodies become less efficient at absorbing magnesium as we age, so supplementation is especially important for older adults—and deficiency in this mineral may contribute to age-related sleeping difficulties. (Incidentally, you can also directly supplement with *GABA*.)

You'll notice that many of the above recommendations are geared toward activating the parasympathetic nervous system and soothing the sympathetic branch. Chronic activation of the sympathetic nervous system is a common cause of insomnia,[1024] and fortunately, there are things we can do about this!

I also want to point out that all of the ingredients in your sundae (the letters in **PRONEURO**) that come before this one can help you get sound sleep. Photobiomodulation has been shown to improve sleep quantity and quality in case reports as well as a small number of randomized controlled trials[1025, 1026, 1027, 1028, 1029, 1030, 1031, 1032, 1033, 1034]—not just for TBI sufferers but for everyone (and besides, remember that many more of us have brain damage than we like to think). In addition to the effects of the light, some research has found that transcranial photobiomodulation increases surface temperature on the skull just enough to then create a "heat sink" as the body responds to cool the brain, contributing to the glymphatic system's drainage function when applied just before bed.[1035] In fact, some researchers believe this temperature differential between the brain and the body is a main driver of glymphatic clearance—removing waste products from the brain the way coolant prevents an engine from overheating.[1036]

Getting your body into Repair mode by quieting down your sympathetic nervous system and balancing it with parasympathetic activation is what allows you to relax and sleep deeply. Photobiomodulation can help ameliorate the negative effects of sleep deprivation[1037]—so not only can it help you sleep better, but it can help temper the damage to your health if you're *not* sleeping well. We have already discussed in this chapter how to Optimize your sleep habits with supplements, and the supplements discussed in Chapter Six can help with this, too. Nutrition and Exercise have a strong impact on sleep—and, of course, so does living life in an Unstressed state, as well as the final ingredient that you're about to learn about.

O: ONENESS (SPIRITUAL AND SOCIAL CONNECTION)

All of the ingredients in our sundae thus far have been activities you can undertake by yourself. Sure, attending an exercise class or enlisting an accountability buddy for your new healthy eating regimen can help—but ultimately, the first seven letters of **PRONEURO** are things you do on your own. However, we cannot ignore the importance of connection to something greater than ourselves—and this is what the final letter of **PRONEURO** stands for: Oneness, encompassing both spiritual and social connection.

A key finding of the Harvard Study of Adult Development—a landmark longitudinal study that started following a group of college sophomores in 1938 and continues to follow, to this day, the people from the original study population who are still alive, as well as their children—is that, of all the factors the researchers analyzed, the most powerful influence on physical health (at least for this study population) is the quality of one's relationships. The subjects who reported high levels of satisfaction with their relationships—not just romantic partnerships but also family and friend relationships—at age fifty were the healthiest at age eighty.[1038]

Findings from this study have also shed light on the influence of relationships on brain health specifically. The study was initially limited to men since Harvard College was all male at the time; in 2003, the study was expanded to include the spouses or domestic partners of the remaining living subjects. A 2015 analysis showed that for the women in the sample, those who had harmonious relationships were not only less depressed but had better memory performance than those who reported having frequent marital conflicts.[1039]

A 2018 national survey assessed loneliness levels in twenty thousand American adults; more than half of respondents said they either "sometimes" or "always" feel alone, and forty percent said they feel isolated and that their relationships are not meaningful.[1040] According to a 2006 study, nearly one-quarter of Americans said they didn't have a single friend they felt they could talk to about important matters.[1041] This is just plain sad, but it's also a health crisis. A 2022 study of seniors without the APOE-ε4 allele (i.e., people whose genetic risk of Alzheimer's is lower than those who have the allele) found that subjects who reported feeling lonely had triple the dementia risk of the other subjects.[1042] A 2019 study that analyzed data from more than five hundred eighty thousand adults found that social isolation increased the risk of premature death from every cause for every race.[1043] And a 2015 meta-analytic review of numerous journal articles concluded that loneliness, social isolation, and living alone increased one's mortality risk by twenty-six percent, twenty-nine percent, and thirty-two percent respectively.[1044]

Social isolation is associated with diminished immune function, poor cardiovascular function, impaired sleep quality, and depression, as well as reduced executive function and accelerated cognitive decline, according to a 2015 review article.[1045] Under the tightly controlled conditions that are possible with animal studies, social isolation has been shown to promote more rapid tumor growth in rodents.[1046,1047] Social isolation can be as detrimental to your health as physical inactivity or smoking cigarettes. This is why it's imperative that we consider our relationships and fostering a sense of connectedness as an important part of our self-care regimen. Good times with friends aren't just fun—they're good for you! (As a matter of fact, maybe it's time we stopped trivializing activities that are "just fun"—because having fun, in and of itself, is good for your health!)

Similar to what's mentioned above about self-awareness, when it comes to connection, you can use meditation to help you jump-start the habit. In one study, participants were instructed to sit and think compassionately about others by silently repeating phrases like "May you feel safe, may you feel happy, may you feel healthy, may you live with ease," and keep returning to these thoughts when their minds wandered. This practice led to an increase in positive emotions like joy, interest, amusement, serenity, and hope for these meditators—and these emotional changes were linked to a greater sense of connectedness and an improvement in vagal function, as measured by their HRV.[1048]

But, of course, we want to move from a meditation experience into actual connection with something (and someone) outside of ourselves. You can start by sharing the information in this book with someone you love. Whether it's the benefits of photobiomodulation, the significance of HRV, or the widespread incidence of brain damage and the need to take action—putting what you've learned into your own words creates a deeper level of understanding that will make it more likely you'll retain and implement the information.

Take an inventory of your relationships: Which ones do you value the most? Are you giving those relationships enough of your time and your heart? Are there any relationships in your life where the dynamic feels unhealthy? What actions could you take to find new friends who share your interests and values (for example, your commitment to a healthier lifestyle)? Which of your friends do you feel truly listen to you—and can you spend more time with those friends? Pay attention to how other people's presence makes you feel—there is some evidence that the people we spend time with can even influence our HRV![1049]

What activities do you thoroughly enjoy doing with friends and family? How often are you doing those? What's holding you back from doing them more? (For example, if your spouse doesn't like to go to concerts, but you love going to concerts, what's stopping you from inviting a friend instead and doing different activities with your spouse?) Remember that relationships are a balance of give and take. If you notice that some of your relationships are all about making the other person happy at the expense of your own happiness, it's time to recalibrate that balance.

It's been well established and well documented that seniors who take part in activities such as a church group, a choir, or a book club remain more mentally engaged and take a greater interest in life.[1050, 1051] This makes it easy to understand why social isolation would be a risk factor for early death. Our hearts and minds play an important role in motivating us to move in the direction of goals, whether it be completing a project around the house or living to see a niece's or grandchild's wedding. We've all known an elderly person who's just given up on life; when you lose the motivation to take actions that are good for you, a downward spiral for your health tends to follow.

One particularly interesting paper analyzed the molecular mechanisms by which social isolation seems to affect health negatively. Epigenetics appears to be part of the story: Our genes are expressed differently under conditions of rich and vibrant social connection than they are when we feel isolated. Specifically, loneliness alters gene expression in ways that promote inflammation and influence immune function—as well as alterations that are associated with anxiety, panic disorder, and addiction. One research team documented an "upward spiral" of positive emotions and high HRV in people with strong social connections.[1052] We are also more likely to engage in behaviors with risks to our health, such as smoking and neglecting to exercise, when we feel isolated.[1053]

While digital methods of communication may have helped to preserve social connections amid lockdowns and other pandemic-induced isolation, there are certain aspects of the human connection that cannot be replicated over Zoom—the main one being physical touch. "Pleasant touch" like hugs, snuggles, massages, and holding hands stimulates the vagus nerve, prompting the body to relax via parasympathetic activation.[1054, 1055, 1056] Pleasant touch also stimulates serotonin (the mood-boosting well-being hormone that drives our cravings for carb-rich foods) as well as the bonding and feel-good hormone oxytocin.

Oxytocin makes us feel more generous[1057]—which, in my mind, is an indicator we feel safe. After all, when we're in a scarcity mentality, feeling like we might not have enough to meet our own needs, we don't feel safe to give anything away because we don't believe we have any extra. Generosity is the opposite of this—the feeling that we have more than we need and that more will be coming, so we might as well spread the love. Oxytocin also connects us with feelings of gratitude, which has downstream effects for our heart health and brain health.[1058]

There is actually a condition called *touch starvation* in which the body mounts a stress response due to the absence of physical touch—leading to elevated cortisol levels and, consequently, changes in heart rate, respiratory rate, blood pressure, and muscle tension. Similar to any other time this response is activated by stressful circumstances, you'll have trouble relaxing and your parasympathetic nervous system won't kick in if you aren't getting adequate physical touch.

Getting more pleasant touch in your day is one of the easiest ways there is to improve your sense of connection and overall health. Snuggle up on the couch while watching TV, hold hands over dinner, or take a break from work for a quick hug or backrub. If you live by yourself, other ways of releasing oxytocin include cuddling with a pet, singing, and dancing. Getting yourself pampered with a massage, facial, haircut, or mani/pedi can also provide some of the benefits of pleasant touch.

Thus far in this section, we've focused mostly on social connectedness—but the O in **PRONEURO** also includes *spiritual* connectedness. On average, people who regularly attend religious services live longer.[1059, 1060, 1061] Attending religious services also seems to have a mitigating effect on the factors that otherwise increase one's allostatic load.[1062, 1063, 1064] Without a doubt, this is partly because there is a *social* component to the *spiritual* endeavor of attending church services. You're part of a community, engaging in meaningful social connection—and probably getting some physical touch in the form of hugs and handshakes to boot. But that's not the only reason being part of a spiritual community is beneficial.

Many, if not most, religious traditions build in a practice of gratitude with a ritual of offering thanks for one's blessings—and this, in itself, has health benefits. A feeling of gratitude to a higher power has been associated with stress-buffering health effects in senior women.[1065] One study found a reduction in biomarkers of inflammation in the blood of heart disease patients after they spent eight weeks with a daily gratitude journal practice.[1066] A gratitude practice has also been associated with improved sleep quality[1067, 1068, 1069] and has been found in several studies to have beneficial effects for depression, anxiety, and stress as well as fostering prosocial behavior (the kind that leads to strong and fulfilling relationships).[1070]

The practice of prayer that is typically part of religious observance also has positive health effects. A regular personal practice of prayer has been shown to be beneficial in coping with and recovering from depression.[1071, 1072] Other research has found that engaging in prayer reduces blood pressure (presumably a proxy for its effect on the nervous system and HRV).[1073]

If you don't belong to a religious community, developing your own practice of spirituality and mindfulness can help you reap some of these benefits separately from the social aspect of religious practice. Transcendental meditation has been found to have similar blood pressure–reducing effects to those of prayer.[1074] HIV-positive patients who practiced meditation had a slower decline in their immune cell count.[1075]

Also remember the way worries act like a kind of toxin, preventing our parasympathetic nervous system from kicking in, keeping our HRV low and keeping our bodies from relaxing and getting into repair mode. The ability to place our trust in a higher power means we can hand our worries over; we no longer have to be responsible for everything, control everything, fix everything. For example, research has shown that students who report a spiritually oriented way of seeing the world (whether explicitly religious or not) mount a less intense stress response when preparing to take an exam.[1076] Even if organized religion isn't your jam, it's important to find a way to let go of your worries. With practice, you can learn to trust that it will all work out.

A sense of connectedness is not just about relationships but is also about our connection to something greater than ourselves more generally. How do you feel about your work? Do you have a sense of purpose, and are the ways you spend your time clearly connected to that purpose? The same job can be heaven for one person and hell for another. Holding a job you don't enjoy "just for the money" might be soul-crushing for one person, while for another it strongly serves their purpose of taking care of their family financially. It's all in how you view it. If the view isn't to your liking, you have a choice to change it by either changing what you're seeing or changing the way you see it.

If you're feeling stuck in your current work situation, but changing the view (leaving the job) isn't an option, what choices do you have for changing the way you view it? Can you have conversations with your boss and colleagues to help make it a more pleasant place to work? Can you get better at saying no and setting boundaries (and perhaps set an example for others and influence office culture in the process)? Can you start asking for help, even if it is difficult at first? The simple realization that we have choices often improves our situation greatly. It improves our sense of agency as well as potentially changing the very circumstances that are bothering us.

We can also think about relationships from the perspective of detox. Notice how you feel in the relationships in your life. Maybe it's time to step aside from the ones that make your body tense up and keep you in a constant state of stress in favor of spending more time in the ones that make you feel relaxed, supported, and loved. Of course, if there's the potential to work on a relationship and transform it from the former category into the latter, that could be a great option too—especially when there's significant shared history you'd be losing by ending the relationship—but you can only control one side of the dynamic, and not every relationship can be salvaged and made into something healthy and supportive.

In relationships and otherwise, stress and trauma can become addictive. The drama feels so familiar that we don't know who we would be without it. Our nervous systems are so calibrated to the presence of a threat that relaxation feels foreign. Notice the ways you are making a choice to stay in the "drama" energy. This might be an unhealthy relationship, taking part in vitriolic debates on social media, or even watching movies and TV shows that jack up your nervous system and keep you on high alert. Not just in your relationships but everywhere you place your attention, start to notice what's disturbing your peace—and think about ways you can protect it. A constant feeling that you're under threat is a surefire way to tank your HRV. On the other hand, choosing to focus on gratitude and feelings of being safe and provided for will boost your HRV instantly—and it's a choice you have in any moment. Prayer and trust in a higher power are one way to connect to these feelings, but they are not the only way.

Remember that you can't keep your engine revving at a high RPM forever. If you let yourself stay in a constant state of stress, you'll burn out—and your brain health will suffer. (We saw this in sharp relief with the pandemic as the additional stress piled on top of the usual stressors of life led to an increased prevalence of anxiety and depression.) You can't shield yourself from stress entirely—nor would you want to because then your system becomes out of practice in responding to it, and you could become overwhelmed the next time stressful circumstances come your way. Remember that what we are going for is hormesis: building our capacity to respond to stressful circumstances (like the engine revving up) and then to quickly and efficiently downregulate (and return to an idle) afterward.

The **PRONEURO** approach provides you with a powerful toolkit for getting your body into a restorative state and maximizing the restoration that takes place while you are in that state—but it may take some work, emotionally and psychologically, to feel comfortable staying in that state and allowing yourself to rest. Building that sense of balance, and stepping out of the addiction to stress and overwork, is well worth focusing on. In fact, it is the most important thing you can do for the health of your brain.

CONCLUSION

"A word to the wise is sufficient."

—Proverb

Now that you've been introduced to the fantastical universe inside your skull—the human brain, with its intricate complexity, astounding ability to heal, and neurons as numerous as stars in the Milky Way—what will you do with this information?

My seventh-grade English teacher, Ms. Helen Curtis, was fond of quoting the proverb that opens this chapter. She impressed on me the idea that it's one thing to learn information, but implementing what you learn is another matter—and the mark of true wisdom. With this book, you have at your fingertips the toolkit for a healthy brain. Whether you use that toolkit is up to you.

Aside from my own and my mother's, I haven't included many stories in the book. Most of the evidence comes in the form of peer-reviewed research studies because I wanted you to have stronger evidence than simply "Someone I know said this helped them." This approach comes with the drawback of omitting some very compelling stories—so here in the conclusion, I want to share with you some success stories that capture the **PRONEURO** program's life-changing potential. These stories offer just a few examples of the concrete ways the approach detailed in this book can make a big difference in just a short time, both for people experiencing various sorts of brain damage and for their caregivers.

Andrés, a twenty-five-year-old master's degree student, had been struggling with persistent symptoms of long COVID since his acute infection three months earlier. After just one week of practicing the **PRONEURO** approach, Andrés said he noticed he had an easier time remembering addresses and phone numbers, that those types of information were "sticking" in a way he had not experienced in months. "This has helped me get back my clarity and my peace," he told us. "My verbal fluidity's back. My mental acuity's back. I don't have brain fog. I just feel better."

Scott, a thirty-year-old executive in finance, came to us in a state of desperation. He had been diagnosed with mold poisoning, Lyme disease, and long COVID—and was experiencing brain fog so severe he couldn't function. After less than one month of working with my team and the **PRONEURO** program, he reported higher energy levels and improved cognitive function, focus, motivation, and mood. "I saw an immediate improvement, starting the very first day," he told me. "Actually, I haven't had what I would call a bad day since starting the protocol."

The sixty-four-year-old woman you met in Chapter Nine, who was featured in our "Rapid Reversal of Cognitive Decline" research paper, also provided some enlightening quotes when we interviewed her. When she came to us, she said she was feeling frightened over her dementia diagnosis and the memory loss she was experiencing. She was taking medications for dementia but still perceived that her cognitive decline was worsening, and she viewed her diagnosis as a death sentence. After just one week, she told us she was starting to see changes that were giving her cause for hope. "I'm coming out of the fog," she told us. After four weeks, in addition to regaining her sense of smell and improving on cognitive measures as noted in Chapter Nine, the caregiver stress level of the woman's husband came down from a 6 to a 4 on the 10-point scale—an important metric for health and quality of life of both the patient and the caregiver.

If you've made it to the end of this book—as densely packed as it is with information—then you are clearly committed to doing something positive for your brain health (or that of someone you love). Don't just close the book and neglect to take action. Don't let yourself become overwhelmed with the many different lifestyle changes described here. Start with one small change. Build your ice cream sundae from the foundation up. And don't hesitate to reach out to my team for coaching if you would benefit from having support along the way.

If you've been reading this book as a caregiver of a parent with dementia, you might be wondering if the same fate awaits you. The answer is complicated: For Alzheimer's disease specifically, most of the associated genes are not deterministic (meaning that they do not directly cause the disease) but, rather, increase your risk. If a parent developed early-onset

Alzheimer's in their forties or fifties, they probably carried a deterministic gene, and in this case, your risk is significantly higher—but these genes are believed to account for less than ten percent of Alzheimer's cases worldwide, according to the U.S. National Institute on Aging. The more common APOE-ε4 allele increases an overall low level of Alzheimer's risk (having one copy of APOE-ε4 roughly doubles your risk and having two copies increases it roughly tenfold relative to the APOE-ε3 allele, which is neutral, and the APOE-ε2 allele, which plays a protective role) that is more easily influenced by the lifestyle changes represented in the **PRONEURO** program.

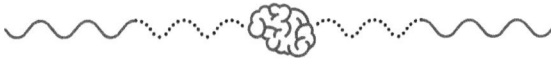

This book in many ways represents the culmination of my life's work thus far. You could say that I started working on it as far back as my undergraduate days when I studied writing. But the work began in earnest in 2019. After my mother's death, as my grief lifted and I began to refocus my life from the intense absorption of caregiving, I started pulling together the various research papers I'd published and talks I'd given in hopes of creating a "user's manual" for the **PRONEURO** approach that would explain all the science behind it. The effort picked up steam in late 2020 when I connected with Awaken Village Press and my eminently skilled coauthor.

As our work on the book has unfolded over the last two-plus years, it has become increasingly apparent that the approach presented in this book has relevance for a topic that has been at the top of all of our minds: COVID-19. A 2022 study found that women had an eighty-two percent increased risk and men a fifty percent increased risk of being diagnosed with dementia in the year after a COVID infection.[1077] Severe illness from SARS-CoV-2 has an uncanny amount of overlap with the symptoms that accompany Alzheimer's disease: elevated heart rate and blood pressure, reduced sensitivity of the autonomic nervous system, increased inflammation, reduced HRV, and cognitive impairment.[1078] For some people, the virus causes loss of sense of smell, which is also an early sign of

Alzheimer's and Parkinson's diseases. Research points to the virus's tendency to cause neuroinflammation—which we also see, of course, in TBI and Alzheimer's—and cognitive decline is a common outcome for both severe and mild COVID infections,[1079, 1080, 1081, 1082] again underscoring the relevance of all the information contained in this book. If we were previously facing an imminent wave of neurodegenerative conditions, now we are facing a tsunami. I take no pleasure in the fact that so many more people will soon desperately need the **PRONEURO** approach, but I am happy that we're in a position to provide them with hope for healing.

As a significant and growing portion of our population is suffering from post-viral illness, a number of studies have noted photobiomodulation's promise as a tool in helping people recover.[1083, 1084, 1085, 1086] As noted in the case studies cited earlier in this chapter, we are already using our method to help people suffering from long COVID, with encouraging results. We knew even before the pandemic that photobiomodulation could help reduce lung inflammation in people with chronic obstructive pulmonary disease and fibrosis of the lungs[1087]—so this treatment may prove valuable to people suffering from those conditions in the wake of COVID infection. Some have even suggested that photobiomodulation may have value in treating acute infections, based on findings from earlier SARS outbreaks[1088] and the intersection of the way photobiomodulation works (in a health-promoting sense) with the way the virus works (on the same dimensions in a health-diminishing sense).[1089, 1090, 1091, 1092, 1093, 1094, 1095, 1096, 1097] More research is needed to validate the hypotheses, but we have every reason to believe that photobiomodulation would have the power to inhibit viral replication, keep inflammation from spiraling out of control, and help the body heal due to its effects on mitochondrial function, nitric oxide, the balance of inflammation in the body, and entities that assist with cellular growth and repair. What's more, our newfound awareness of viruses' ability to cause long-lasting health implications may have opened a door for greater understanding of infections' role in triggering other chronic conditions—such as multiple sclerosis,[1098] fibromyalgia,[1099] and, yes, Alzheimer's.[1100] Since conditions such as myalgic encephalomyelitis/chronic fatigue syndrome and postural orthostatic tachycardia syndrome have unfortunately become more common in the wake of widespread COVID infection, the drive to alleviate suffering is leading to advances in research that reveal the role of dysautonomia in these conditions—and the role photobiomodulation and other treatments that help heal the nervous system can play in helping people recover. These fascinating links could be the subject of another entire book (and perhaps one day they will be)—but the overarching takeaway is that whatever helps the body heal will help tip the balance from neurodegeneration to neuroregeneration.

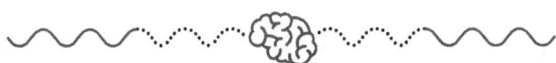

My mom loved to remind me that she had a master's degree. Even once Alzheimer's had robbed her of the ability to express herself through speech, she continued to express her love for education with simpler phrasing. One of the last things she said to me was "I love school!"

Mom's master's degree was in library science, and while I was in chiropractic college, she became the assistant librarian at Hobart and William Smith Colleges, where I initially started college before leaving for Montana. I inherited her love of libraries, or perhaps chose it as a way to feel connected to her. As the original chiropractic school, Palmer College had one of the greatest medical libraries in the world; during my studies, I spent much of my spare time (and my lunch money) in that library, making photocopies of articles at five cents per page. I wanted to make the most of my education, and this was a resource I'd been well trained by my mom to utilize. This obsession followed me to Italy; on my trips to the University of Verona Hospital, I delighted in the ability to access journal articles through their portal. I would also carve out a couple of hours to spend at the university library in Padua whenever I could. With journal articles now available on the internet, photocopies have been replaced by digital indexing tools that keep journal articles organized. (Oh, how times have changed! When I moved back to the U.S., I shipped back boxes of article printouts and then paid storage fees for those boxes for years.) All the same, I feel my mom's influence is well represented by the more than one thousand articles referenced in this book.

As you turn this last page, I hope you feel empowered to take positive action for your health. I hope you feel inspired to focus on increasing your capacity rather than avoiding challenges. I hope you understand that you don't need to go around avoiding stressful situations because your body is resilient. I hope you view your home as your hospital and your kitchen as your pharmacy. I hope you stop accepting brain fog as normal.

Remember that your body has an innate ability to heal. All you have to do is remove the interference.

Remember the triangle of disease and know that each side of the triangle—trauma, toxins, auto-suggestion—is not just a force that impacts your health negatively but an opportunity for healing. You can use your thoughts in a beneficial way. You can clear out the toxins and reduce your future intake. You can heal your trauma.

Remember, it's not just the years in our life we want to extend, it's the life in our years.

When you are tempted to say "I don't have time to take care of my health," remember that a more honest statement would be to say that it's not a priority right now. When are you going to make it a priority? As long as you are alive, you have time. How are you going to spend that time?

I've weathered quite a bit of adversity in my life: failed marriages, business partnerships that dissolved under unpleasant terms, ideas and intellectual property "borrowed" without permission or credit. I haven't dwelled on those obstacles much in the book because I'd rather focus on what I can teach you in terms of recovering and bouncing back. But if your life feels too stressful to implement what you've read, I want you to know that I've gone through times when the stress felt unbearable. I faced the fear of letting my family down. I felt the anguish of not knowing whether my greatest professional asset, my brain, would recover and heal from injury. Whatever "dark night of the soul" you encounter, know that I've experienced similar emotions. I've experienced misery, despair, and desperation—and the advice in this book is what helped me climb my way back to the light, step by painstaking step.

REFERENCES

1   Morris, Wooding, and Grant. "The answer is 17 years, what is the question: understanding time lags in translational research." *Journal of the Royal Society of Medicine*, 2011. https://www.ncbi.nlm.nih.gov/pmc/articles/PMC3241518/

2   Taylor. "Calorie restriction for long-term remission of type 2 diabetes." *Clinical Medicine*, 2019. https://www.ncbi.nlm.nih.gov/pmc/articles/PMC6399621/

3   DiDuro. "Improvement in hearing after chiropractic adjustment: a case series." *Chiropractic & Osteopathy*, 2006. https://www.ncbi.nlm.nih.gov/pmc/articles/PMC1395318/

4   Green and Johnson. "Fighting injustice: A historical review of the National Chiropractic Antitrust Committee." *Journal of Chiropractic Humanities*, 2019. https://www.ncbi.nlm.nih.gov/pmc/articles/PMC6911905/

5   Durieux, Wolff, and Dillin. "The cell non-autonomous nature of electron transport chain-mediated longevity." *Cell*, 2011. https://www.ncbi.nlm.nih.gov/pmc/articles/PMC3062502/

6   Chandel. "Mitochondria as signaling organelles." *BMC Biology*, 2014. https://www.ncbi.nlm.nih.gov/pmc/articles/PMC4035690/

7   Wang and Youle. "The role of mitochondria in apoptosis." *Annual Review of Genetics*, 2009. https://www.annualreviews.org/doi/10.1146/annurev-genet-102108-134850

8   Westermann. "Bioenergetic role of mitochondrial fusion and fission." *Biochimica et Biophysica Acta*, 2012. https://doi.org/10.1016/j.bbabio.2012.02.033

9   Cecchino, Seli, Alves da Motta, and García-Velasco. "The role of mitochondrial activity in female fertility and assisted reproductive technologies: overview and current insights." *Reproductive Biomedicine Online*, 2018. https://doi.org/10.1016/j.rbmo.2018.02.007

10   Benkhalifa, Ferreira, Chahine, Louanjli, Miron, Merviel, and Copin. "Mitochondria: participation to infertility as source of energy and cause of senescence." *International Journal of Biochemistry and Cell Biology*, 2014. https://doi.org/10.1016/j.biocel.2014.08.011

11   Espey, Kielwein, van der Ven, Steger, Allam, Paradowska-Dogan, and van der Ven. "Effects of pulsed-wave photobiomodulation therapy on human spermatozoa." *Lasers in Surgery and Medicine*, 2022. https://doi.org/10.1002/lsm.23399

12   https://www.painresearchforum.org/news/41532-painful-chemotherapy-induced-neuropathy-tk

13   Brannagan. "Current issues in peripheral neuropathy." *Journal of the Peripheral Nervous System*, 2012. https://onlinelibrary.wiley.com/doi/full/10.1111/j.1529-8027.2012.00387.x

14   Köhler, Freitas, Maes, de Andrade, Liu, Fernandes, Stubbs, Solmi, Veronese, Herrmann, Raison, Miller, Lanctôt, and Carvalho. "Peripheral cytokine and chemokine alterations in depression: a meta-analysis of 82 studies." *Acta Psychiatrica Scandinavica*, 2017. https://pubmed.ncbi.nlm.nih.gov/28122130/

15   Lee and Giuliani. "The role of inflammation in depression and fatigue." *Frontiers in Immunology*, 2019. https://www.ncbi.nlm.nih.gov/pmc/articles/PMC6658985/

16   Caldieraro, Salehpour, and Cassano. "Transcranial and systemic photobiomodulation for the enhancement of mitochondrial metabolism in depression." *Clinical Bioenergetics*, 2021. https://doi.org/10.1016/B978-0-12-819621-2.00028-0

17   Boudreau, Duchez, Cloutier, Soulet, Martin, Bollinger, Paré, Rousseau, Naika, Lévesque, Laflamme, Marcoux, Lambeau, Farndale, Pouliot, Hamzeh-Cognasse, Cognasse, Garraud, Nigrovic, Guderley, Lacrois, Thibault, Semple, Gelb, and Boilard. "Platelets release mitochondria serving as substrate for bactericidal group IIA-secreted phospholipase A_2 to promote inflammation." *Blood*, 2014. https://www.ncbi.nlm.nih.gov/pmc/articles/PMC4260364/

18   Knafl, Hughes, Dimeski, and Eley. "Rhabdomyolysis: Patterns, Circumstances, and Outcomes of Patients Presenting to the Emergency Department." *Ochsner Journal*, 2018. https://www.ncbi.nlm.nih.gov/pmc/articles/PMC6162117/

19   Mattson. "Hormesis defined." *Ageing Research Reviews*, 2009. https://www.ncbi.nlm.nih.gov/pmc/articles/PMC2248601/

20   Chandel, Maltepe, Goldwasser, Mathieu, Simon, and Schumacker. "Mitochondrial reactive oxygen species trigger hypoxia-induced transcription." *Proceedings of the National Academy of Sciences*, 1998. https://doi.org/10.1073%2Fpnas.95.20.11715

21   Gladyshev. "The free radical theory of aging is dead. Long live the damage theory!" *Antioxidants & Redox Signaling*, 2014. https://www.ncbi.nlm.nih.gov/pmc/articles/PMC3901353/

22   Picard and McEwen. "Psychological stress and mitochondria: a conceptual framework." *Psychosomatic Medicine*, 2018. https://www.ncbi.nlm.nih.gov/pmc/articles/PMC5901651/

23   Merry and Ristow. "Mitohormesis in exercise training." *Free Radical Biology and Medicine*, 2016. https://pubmed.ncbi.nlm.nih.gov/26654757/

24   Bárcena, Mayoral, and Quirós. "Mitohormesis, an antiaging paradigm. *International Review of Cellular and Molecular Biology*, 2018. https://pubmed.ncbi.nlm.nih.gov/30072093/

25   Bjelakovic, Nikolova, Gluud, Simonetti, and Gluud. "Mortality in randomized trials of antioxidant supplements for primary and secondary prevention: systematic review and meta-analysis." *Journal of the American Medical Association*, 2007. https://doi.org/10.1001/jama.297.8.842

26   Ristow and Schmeisser. "Extending life span by increasing oxidative stress." *Free Radical Biology and Medicine*, 2011. https://doi.org/10.1016/j.freeradbiomed.2011.05.010

27   Fiório, Silveira, Munin, de Lima, Fernandes, Mesquita-Ferrari, de Carvalho, Lopes-Martins, Aimbire, and de Carvalho. "Effect of incoherent LED radiation on third-degree burning wounds in rats." *Journal of Cosmetic and Laser Therapy*, 2011. https://doi.org/10.3109/14764172.2011.630082

28   Trajano, da Trajano, Dos Santos Silva, Venter, de Porto, de Fonseca, and Monte-Alto-Costa. "Low-level red laser improves healing of second-degree burn when applied during proliferative phase." *Lasers in Medical Science*, 2015. https://doi.org/10.1007/s10103-015-1729-2

29   Silveira, Ferreira, da Rocha, Pieri, Pedroso, De Souza, Nesi, and Pinho. "Effect of low-power laser and light-emitting diode on inflammatory response in burn wound healing." *Inflammation*, 2016. https://doi.org/10.1007/s10753-016-0371-x

30   Alsharnoubi, Shoukry, Fawzy, and Mohamed. "Evaluation of scars in children after treatment with low-level laser." *Lasers in Medical Science*, 2018. https://doi.org/10.1007/s10103-018-2572-z

31   Cotler, Chow, Hamblin, and Carroll. "The use of low level laser therapy (LLLT) for musculoskeletal pain." *MOJ Orthopedics & Rheumatology*, 2015. https://www.ncbi.nlm.nih.gov/pmc/articles/PMC4743666/

32   Mehrvar, Mostaghimi, Foomani, Abroe, Eells, Gopalakrishnan, and Ranji. "670 nm photo-
      biomodulation improves the mitochondrial redox state of diabetic wounds." *Quantitative
      Imaging in Medicine and Surgery*, 2021. https://doi.org/10.21037%2Fqims-20-522
33   Marković and Todorović. "Postoperative analgesia after lower third molar surgery: con-
      tribution of the use of long-acting local anesthetics, lower-power laser, and diclofenac."
      Oral Surgery, Oral Medicine, Oral Pathology, Oral Radiology, and Endodontics, 2006.
      https://doi.org/10.1016/j.tripleo.2006.02.024
34   Tanboga, Eren, Altinok, Peker, and Ertugral. "The effect of low level laser therapy on
      pain during dental tooth-cavity preparation in children." *European Archives of Paediatric
      Dentistry*, 2011. https://doi.org/10.1007/bf03262786
35   Chan, Armati, and Moorthy. "Pulsed ND:YAG laser induces pulpal analge-
      sia: a randomized clinical trial." *Journal of Dental Research*, 2012. https://doi.
      org/10.1177/0022034512447947
36   Peres e Serra and Ashmawi. "Influence of naloxone and methysergide on the anal-
      gesic effects of low-level laser in an experimental pain model." *Revista Brasileira de
      Anestesiologia*, 2010. https://doi.org/10.1016/s0034-7094(10)70037-4
37   Yan, Chow, and Armati. "Inhibitory effects of visible 650-nm and infrared 808-nm laser
      irradiation on somatosensory and compound muscle action potentials in rat sciatic
      nerve: implications for laser-induced analgesia." *Journal of the Peripheral Nervous System*,
      2011. https://doi.org/10.1111/j.1529-8027.2011.00337.x
38   Mosca, Ong, Albasha, Bass, and Arany. "Photobiomodulation therapy for wound
      care: a potent, noninvasive, photoceutical approach." *Advances in Skin & Wound
      Care*,   2019.   https://journals.lww.com/aswcjournal/Fulltext/2019/04000/
      Photobiomodulation_Therapy_for_Wound_Care__A.3.aspx
39   Keshri, Kumar, Sharma, Bora, Kumar, and Gupta. "Photobiomodulation effects of
      pulsed-NIR laser (810 nm) and LED (808 ±3 nm) with identical treatment regimen
      on burn wound healing: a quantitative label-free global proteomic approach." *Journal of
      Photochemistry and Photobiology*, 2021. https://www.sciencedirect.com/science/article/
      pii/S2666469021000099
40   Gavish, Zadik, and Raizman. "Supportive care of cancer patients with a self-applied
      photobiomodulation device: a case series." *Supportive Care in Cancer*, 2021. https://
      www.ncbi.nlm.nih.gov/pmc/articles/PMC7847302/
41   Gavish and Houreld. "Therapeutic efficacy of home-use photobiomodulation devices:
      a systematic literature review." *Photobiomodulation, Photomedicine, and Laser Surgery*,
      2019. https://doi.org/10.1089/photob.2018.4512
42   Salehpour and Hamblin. "Photobiomodulation for Parkinson's disease in animal
      models: a systematic review." *Biomolecules*, 2020. https://www.ncbi.nlm.nih.gov/pmc/
      articles/PMC7225948/
43   DiDuro. "Neuropathy patient satisfaction high with infrared LED care." Poster presen-
      tation, 10th Annual Conference of the North American Association for Laser Therapy,
      2010.
44   DiDuro and Burke. "A prospective study of changes in pain numeric rating scale with
      physiotherapy treatment for neuropathic pain." Poster presentation, PAINWeek, 2011.
45   DiDuro and Burke. "Pain relief and reduced viral load in HIV-associated sensory neu-
      ropathy using low level laser." Poster presentation, 28th Annual Meeting of the American
      Academy of Pain Medicine, 2012.
46   DiDuro and Marchese. "Clinical experience using NIR light therapy in subjects with
      type II diabetes complaining of neuropathy." Atlanta Pain Institute, 2016.

REFERENCES

47 DiDuro. "Regeneration of intraepidermal nerve fibers with infrared LED care in a 54-year-old female with Sjogren's syndrome: a case report." Poster presentation, 11th Annual Conference of the North American Association for Laser Therapy, 2011.

48 Jeziorska, Atkinson, Kass-Iliyya, Javed, Kobylecki, Gosal, Marshall, Silverdale, and Malik. "Increased intraepidermal nerve fiber degeneration and impaired regeneration relate to symptoms and deficits in Parkinson's disease." *Frontiers in Neurology*, 2019. https://www.ncbi.nlm.nih.gov/pmc/articles/PMC6383044/

49 Schatz. "The magic garden." *Annual Review of Biochemistry*, 2007. https://doi.org/10.1146/annurev.biochem.76.060806.091141

50 Salehpour and Hamblin. "Photobiomodulation for Parkinson's disease in animal models: a systematic review." *Biomolecules*, 2020. https://www.ncbi.nlm.nih.gov/pmc/articles/PMC7225948/

51 Hamblin. "Photobiomodulation for Alzheimer's disease: Has the light dawned?" *Photonics*, 2019. https://www.ncbi.nlm.nih.gov/pmc/articles/PMC6664299/

52 Amaroli, Pasquale, Zekiy, Utyuzh, Benedicenti, Signore, and Ravera. "Photobiomodulation and oxidative stress: 980nm diode laser light regulates mitochondrial activity and reactive oxygen species production." *Oxidative Medicine and Cellular Longevity*, 2021. https://doi.org/10.1155%2F2021%2F6626286

53 Hamblin. "Photobiomodulation for Alzheimer's disease: Has the light dawned?" *Photonics*, 2019. https://www.ncbi.nlm.nih.gov/pmc/articles/PMC6664299

54 Ramezani, Meshasteh-Riz, Ghadaksaz, Fazeli, Janzadeh, and Hamblin. "Mechanistic aspects of photobiomodulation therapy in the nervous system." *Lasers in Medical Science*, 2021. https://doi.org/10.1007/s10103-021-03277-2

55 Lunova, Smolková, Uzhytchak, Janoušková, Jirsa, Egorova, Kulikov, Kubinová, Dejneka, and Lunov. "Light-induced modulation of the mitochondrial respiratory chain activity: possibilities and limitations." *Cellular and Molecular Life Sciences*, 2020. https://doi.org/10.1007/s00018-019-03321-z

56 Blasco. "The epigenetic regulation of mammalian telomeres." *Nature Reviews Genetics*, 2007. https://doi.org/10.1038/nrg2047

57 Sibille, Witek-Janusek, Mathews, and Fillingim. "Telomeres and epigenetics: potential relevance to chronic pain." *Pain*, 2012. https://doi.org/10.1016/j.pain.2012.06.003

58 Liebert, Bicknell, and Adams. "Protein conformational modulation by photons: a mechanism for laser treatment effects." *Medical Hypotheses*, 2014. https://www.sciencedirect.com/science/article/pii/S0306987713005938

59 Chen, Arany, Huang, Tomkinson, Sharma, Kharkwal, Saleem, Mooney, Yull, Blackwell, and Hamblin. "Low-level laser therapy activates NF-kB via generation of reactive oxygen species in mouse embryonic fibroblasts." *PLoS One*, 2011. https://www.ncbi.nlm.nih.gov/pmc/articles/PMC3141042/

60 Wang, Tian, Soni, Gonzalez-Lima, and Liu. "Interplay between up-regulation of cytochrome-c-oxidase and hemoglobin oxygenation induced by near-infrared laser." *Scientific Reports*, 2016. https://pubmed.ncbi.nlm.nih.gov/27484673/

61 Salehpour, Mahmoudi, Kamari, Sadigh-Eteghad, Rasta, and Hamblin. "Brain photobiomodulation therapy: a narrative review." *Molecular Neurobiology*, 2018. https://www.ncbi.nlm.nih.gov/pmc/articles/PMC6041198/

62 Dache, Otandault, Tanos, Pastor, Meddeb, Sanchez, Arena, Lasorsa, Bennett, Grange, Messaoudi, Mazard, Prevostel, and Thierry. "Blood contains circulating cell-free respiratory competent mitochondria." *FASEB Journal: Official Publication of the Federation*

of American Societies for Experimental Biology, 2020. https://doi.org/10.1096/fj.201901917rr

63 Stephens, Grant, Frimel, Wanner, Yin, Willard, Erzurum, and Asosingh. "Characterization and origins of cell-free mitochondria in healthy murine and human blood." *Mitochondrion,* 2020. https://doi.org/10.1016/j.mito.2020.08.002

64 Salehpour and Hamblin. "Photobiomodulation for Parkinson's disease in animal models: a systematic review." *Biomolecules,* 2020. https://www.ncbi.nlm.nih.gov/pmc/articles/PMC7225948/

65 Machado, Micheletti, Vanderlei, Nakamura, Leal-Junior, Junior, and Pastre. "Effect of low-level laser therapy (LLLT) and light-emitting diodes (LEDT) applied during combined training on performance and post-exercise recovery: protocol for a randomized placebo-controlled trial." *Brazilian Journal of Physical Therapy,* 2017. https://doi.org/10.1016/j.bjpt.2017.05.010

66 Kumar, Kumar, Nordberg, Långström, and Darreh-Shori. "Proton pump inhibitors act with unprecedented potencies as inhibitors of the acetylcholine biosynthesizing enzyme—A plausible missing link for their association with incidence of dementia." *Alzheimer's & Dementia,* 2020. https://doi.org/10.1002/alz.12113

67 Ghebremariam, LePendu, Lee, Erlanson, Slaviero, Shah, Leiper, and Cooke. "An unexpected effect of proton pump inhibitors: elevation of the cardiovascular risk factor ADMA." *Circulation,* 2013. https://www.ncbi.nlm.nih.gov/pmc/articles/PMC3838201/

68 Yepuri, Sukhovershin, Nazari-Shafti, Petrascheck, Ghebre, and Cooke. "Proton pump inhibitors accelerate endothelial senescence." *Circulation Research,* 2016. https://www.ahajournals.org/doi/10.1161/CIRCRESAHA.116.308807

69 Gomm, von Holt, Thomé, Broich, Maier, Fink, Doblhammer, and Haenisch. "Association of proton pump inhibitors with risk of dementia: a pharmacoepidemiological claims data analysis." *JAMA Neurology,* 2016. https://jamanetwork.com/journals/jamaneurology/fullarticle/2487379

70 Hroudová, Fišar, Kitzlerová, Zvěová, and Raboch. "Mitochondrial respiration in blood platelets of depressive patients." *Mitochondrion,* 2013.

71 Bansal and Kuhad. "Mitochondrial dysfunction in depression." *Current Neuropharmacology,* 2016. https://www.ncbi.nlm.nih.gov/pmc/articles/PMC4981740/

72 Wang, Reddy, Nalawade, Pal, Gonzalez-Lima, and Liu. "Impact of heat on metabolic and hemodynamic changes in transcranial infrared laser stimulation measured by broadband near-infrared spectroscopy." *Neurophotonics,* 2018. https://pubmed.ncbi.nlm.nih.gov/28948191/

73 Salehpour, Mahmoudi, Kamari, Sadigh-Eteghad, Rasta, and Hamblin. "Brain photobiomodulation therapy: a narrative review." *Molecular Neurobiology,* 2018. https://www.ncbi.nlm.nih.gov/pmc/articles/PMC6041198/

74 Rojas, Lee, John, and Gonzalez-Lima. "Neuroprotective effects of near-infrared light in an *in vivo* model of mitochondrial optic neuropathy." *Journal of Neuroscience,* 2008. https://doi.org/10.1523/jneurosci.3457-08.2008

75 Salehpour, Cassano, Rouhi, Hamblin, De Taboada, Farajdokht, and Mahmoudi. "Penetration profiles of visible and near-infrared lasers and light-emitting diode light through the head tissues in animal and human species: a review of literature." *Photobiomodulation, Photomedicine, and Laser Surgery,* 2019. https://doi.org/10.1089/photob.2019.4676

REFERENCES

[76] Hamblin. "Mechanisms and applications of the anti-inflammatory effects of photo-biomodulation." *AIMS Biophysics*, 2017. https://www.ncbi.nlm.nih.gov/pmc/articles/PMC5523874/

[77] Sousa, Rodrigues, de Souza Santos, Mesquita-Ferrari, Nunes, de Fátima Teixeira da Silva, Bussadori, and Fernandes. "Differential expression of inflammatory and anti-inflammatory mediators by M1 and M2 macrophages after photobiomodulation with red or infrared lasers." *Lasers in Medical Science*, 2020. https://doi.org/10.1007/s10103-019-02817-1

[78] Salehpour, Mahmoudi, Kamari, Sadigh-Eteghad, Rasta, and Hamblin. "Brain photobiomodulation therapy: a narrative review." *Molecular Neurobiology*, 2018. https://doi.org/10.1007/s12035-017-0852-4

[79] Liebert, Krause, Goonetilleke, Bicknell, and Kiat. "A role for photobiomodulation in the prevention of myocardial ischemic reperfusion injury: a systematic review and potential molecular mechanisms." *Scientific Reports*, 2017. https://www.nature.com/articles/srep42386

[80] Gavish, Rubinstein, Bulut, Berlatzky, Beeri, Gilon, Gavish, Harlev, Reissman, and Gertz. "Low-level laser irradiation inhibits abdominal aortic aneurysm progression in apolipoprotein E-deficient mice." *Cardiovascular Research*, 2009. https://academic.oup.com/cardiovascres/article/83/4/785/371679

[81] Gavish, Beeri, Gilon, Rubinstein, Berlatzky, Bulut Reissman, Gavish, and Gertz. "Arrest of progression of pre-induced abdominal aortic aneurysm in apolipoprotein E-deficient mice by low level laser phototherapy." *Lasers in Surgery and Medicine*, 2014. https://doi.org/10.1002/lsm.22306

[82] Tatmatsu-Rocha, Tim, Avo, Bernardes-Filho, Brassolatti, Kido, Hamblin, and Parizotto. "Mitochondrial dynamics (fission and fusion) and collagen production in a rat model of diabetic wound healing treated by photobiomodulation: comparison of 904 nm laser and 850 nm light-emitting diode (LED)." *Journal of Photochemistry and Photobiology B: Biology*, 2018. https://www.ncbi.nlm.nih.gov/pmc/articles/PMC6131055/

[83] Correia Rocha, Perez-Reyes, and Chacur. "Effect of photobiomodulation on mitochondrial dynamics in peripheral nervous system in streptozotocin-induced type 1 diabetes in rats." *Photochemical & Photobiological Sciences*, 2021. https://doi.org/10.1007/s43630-021-00018-w

[84] Rosso, Buchaim, Kawano, Furlanette, Pomini, and Buchaim. "Photobiomodulation therapy (PBMT) in peripheral nerve regeneration: a systematic review." *Bioengineering*, 2018. https://doi.org/10.3390/bioengineering5020044

[85] Martignago, Assis, Deusdara de Alexandria, Tatmatsu-Rocha, Parizotto, and Tim. "Effects of photobiomodulation therapy in the integration of skin graft in rats." *Lasers in Medical Science*, 2020. https://link.springer.com/article/10.1007/s10103-019-02909-y

[86] Cassano, Petrie, Mischoulon, Cusin, Katnani, Yeung, de Taboada, Archibald, Bui, Baer, Chang, Chen, Pedrelli, Fisher, Farabaugh, Hamblin, Alpert, Fava, and Iosifescu. "Transcranial photobiomodulation for the treatment of major depressive disorder." *Photomedicine and Laser Surgery*, 2018. https://www.ncbi.nlm.nih.gov/pmc/articles/PMC7864111/

[87] Askalsky and Iosifescu. "Transcranial photobiomodulation for the management of depression: current perspectives." *Neuropsychiatric Disease and Treatment*, 2019. https://doi.org/10.2147/ndt.s188906

[88] Cassano, Petrie, Hamblin, Henderson, and Iosifescu. "Review of transcranial photobiomodulation for major depressive disorder: targeting brain metabolism, inflammation,

oxidative stress, and neurogenesis." *Neurophotonics*, 2016. https://www.ncbi.nlm.nih.gov/pmc/articles/PMC4777909/

[89] Salehpour and Rasta. "The potential of transcranial photobiomodulation therapy for treatment of major depressive disorder." *Reviews in the Neurosciences*, 2017. https://doi.org/10.1515/revneuro-2016-0087

[90] Schiffer, Johnston, Ravichandran, Polcari, Teicher, Webb, and Hamblin. "Psychological benefits 2 and 4 weeks after a single treatment with near infrared light to the forehead: a pilot study of 10 patients with major depression and anxiety." *Behavioral and Brain Functions*, 2009. https://doi.org/10.1186/1744-9081-5-46

[91] Marks. "Photobiomodulation, depression, anxiety, and cognition." *Journal of Aging Research and Healthcare*, 2021. https://doi.org/10.14302/issn.2474-7785.jarh-21-3935

[92] Chang, Ren, Wang, Li, Wang, and Chu. "Transcranial low-level laser therapy for depression and Alzheimer's disease." *Neuropsychiatry*, 2018. https://www.jneuropsychiatry.org/peer-review/transcranial-lowlevel-laser-therapy-for-depression-and-alzheimers-disease-12428.html

[93] Cassano and Caldieraro. "Photobiomodulation." *The Massachusetts General Hospital Guide to Depression, Springer International Publishing*, 2018. https://link.springer.com/chapter/10.1007/978-3-319-97241-1_18

[94] Disner, Beevers, and Gonzalez-Lima. "Transcranial laser stimulation as neuroenhancement for attention bias modification in adults with elevated depression symptoms." *Brain Stimulation*, 2016. https://www.ncbi.nlm.nih.gov/pmc/articles/PMC5007141/

[95] Salehpour, Rasta, Mohaddes, Sadigh-Eteghad, and Salarirad. "A comparison between antidepressant effects of transcranial near-infrared laser and Citalopram in a rat model of depression." *Clinical and Translational Neurophotonics*, 2017. https://doi.org/10.1117/12.2251598

[96] Eshaghi, Sadigh-Eteghad, Mohaddes, and Rasta. "Transcranial photobiomodulation prevents anxiety and depression via changing serotonin and nitric oxide levels in brain of depression model mice: a study of three different doses of 810 nm laser." *Lasers in Surgery and Medicine*, 2019. https://onlinelibrary.wiley.com/doi/10.1002/lsm.23082

[97] Ceranoglu, Hoskova, Cassano, Biederman, and Joshi. "Efficacy of transcranial near-infrared light treatment in ASD: interim analysis of an open-label proof of concept study of a novel approach." *Journal of the American Academy of Child and Adolescent Psychiatry*, 2018. https://doi.org/10.1016/j.jaac.2019.09.009

[98] Leisman, Machado, Machado, and Chinchilla-Acosta. "Effects of low-level laser therapy in autism spectrum disorder." *Advances in Experimental Medicine and Biology*, 2018. https://doi.org/10.1007/5584_2018_234

[99] Ceranoglu, Cassano, Hoskova, Green, Dallenbach, DiSalvo, Biederman, and Joshi. "Transcranial photobiomodulation in adults with high-functioning autism spectrum disorder: positive findings from a proof-of-concept study." *Photobiomodulation, Photomedicine, and Laser Surgery*, 2022. https://doi.org/10.1089/photob.2020.4986

[100] Pallanti, Di Ponzio, Grassi, Vannini, and Cauli. "Transcranial photobiomodulation for the treatment of children with autism spectrum disorder (ASD): a retrospective study." *Children*, 2022. https://www.ncbi.nlm.nih.gov/pmc/articles/PMC9139753/

[101] Naviaux, Zolkipli, Wang, Nakayama, Naviaux, Le, Schuchbauer, Rogac, Tang, Dugan, and Powell. "Antipurinergic therapy corrects the autism-like features in the poly(IC) mouse model." *PLoS One*, 2013. https://journals.plos.org/plosone/article?id=10.1371/journal.pone.0057380

REFERENCES

102   Naviaux, Schuchbauer, Li, Wang, Risbrough, Powell, and Naviaux. "Reversal of autism-like behaviors and metabolism in adult mice with single-dose antipurinergic therapy." *Translational Psychiatry*, 2014. https://www.nature.com/articles/tp201433

103   Hopkins, McLoda, Seegmiller, and Baxter. "Low-level laser therapy facilitates superficial wound healing in humans: a triple-blind, sham-controlled study." *Journal of Athletic Training*, 2004. https://www.ncbi.nlm.nih.gov/pmc/articles/PMC522143/

104   Wickenheisser, Zywot, Rabjohns, Lee, Lawrence, and Tarrant. "Laser light therapy in inflammatory, musculoskeletal, and autoimmune disease." *Current Allergy and Asthma Reports*, 2020. https://doi.org/10.1007/s11882-019-0869-z

105   Cassano, Dording, Thomas, Foster, Yeung, Uchida, Hamblin, Bui, Fava, Mischoulon, and Iosifescu. "Effects of transcranial photobiomodulation with near-infrared light on sexual dysfunction." *Lasers in Surgery and Medicine*, 2019. https://doi.org/10.1002/lsm.23011

106   Caldieraro and Cassano. "Transcranial photobiomodulation for major depressive and anxiety disorders and for posttraumatic stress disorder." *Photobiomodulation in the Brain: Low-Level Laser (Light) Therapy in Neurology and Neuroscience*, 2019. https://doi.org/10.1016/B978-0-12-815305-5.00035-X

107   Maiello, Losiewicz, Bui, Spera, Hamblin, Marques, and Cassano. "Transcranial photobiomodulation with near-infrared light for generalized anxiety disorder: a pilot study." *Photobiomodulation, Photomedicine, and Laser Surgery*, 2019. https://doi.org/10.1089/photob.2019.4677

108   Kerppers, Gonçalves dos Santos, Ribeiro Cordeiro, da Silva Pereira, Barbosa, Pezzini, Ferreira Cunha, Fonseca, Bragnholo, Salgado, and Kerppers. "Study of transcranial photobiomodulation at 945-nm wavelength: anxiety and depression." *Lasers in Medical Science*, 2020. https://doi.org/10.1007/s10103-020-02983-7

109   O'Donnell, Barrett, Fink, Garcia-Pittman, and Gonzalez-Lima. "Transcranial infrared laser stimulation improves cognition in older bipolar patients: proof of concept study." *Journal of Geriatric Psychiatry and Neurology*, 2021. https://doi.org/10.1177/0891988720988906

110   Mannu, Saccaro, Spera, and Cassano. "Transcranial photobiomodulation to augment lithium in bipolar I disorder." *Photobiomodulation, Photomedicine, and Laser Surgery*, 2019. https://doi.org/10.1089/photob.2019.4674

111   Barolet and Boucher. "LED photoprevention: reduced MED response following multiple LED exposures." *Lasers in Surgery and Medicine*, 2008. https://doi.org/10.1002/lsm.20615

112   Dirican, Andacoglu, Johnson, McGuire, Mager, and Soran. "The short-term effects of low-level laser therapy in the management of breast-cancer-related lymphedema." *Supportive Care in Cancer*, 2011.

113   Smoot, Chiavola-Larson, Lee, Manibusan, and Allen. "Effect of low-level laser therapy on pain and swelling in women with breast cancer-related lymphedema: a systematic review and meta-analysis." *Journal of Cancer Survivorship*, 2014. https://doi.org/10.1007/s00520-010-0888-8

114   Li, Xia, Liu, Nicoli, Constantinides, D'Ambrosia, Lazzeri, Tremp, Zhang, and Zhang. "Far infrared ray (FIR) therapy: an effective and oncological safe treatment modality for breast cancer related lymphedema." *Journal of Photochemistry and Photobiology B*, 2017. https://doi.org/10.1016/j.jphotobiol.2017.05.011

115   Schiffer, Reichmann, Flynn, Hamblin, and McCormack. "A novel treatment of opioid cravings with an effect size of .73 for unilateral transcranial photobiomodulation over

sham." *Frontiers in Psychiatry*, 2020. https://www.frontiersin.org/articles/10.3389/fpsyt.2020.00827/full

[116] Schiffer, Khan, Bolger, Flynn, Seltzer, and Teicher. "An effective and safe novel treatment of opioid use disorder: unilateral transcranial photobiomodulation." *Frontiers in Psychiatry*, 2021. https://www.ncbi.nlm.nih.gov/pmc/articles/PMC8382852/

[117] Ohshiro. "Personal overview of the application of LLLT in severely infertile Japanese females." *Laser Therapy*, 2012. https://www.ncbi.nlm.nih.gov/pmc/articles/PMC3944482/

[118] Iwahata, Endoh, and Hirai. "Treatment of female infertility incorporating low-reactive laser therapy (LLLT): an initial report." *Laser Therapy*, 2006. https://doi.org/10.5978/ISLSM.15.37

[119] Taniguchi, Ohshiro, Ohshiro, and Sasaki. "Analysis of the curative effect of GaAlAs diode laser therapy in female infertility." *Laser Therapy*, 2010. https://doi.org/10.5978/ISLSM.19.257

[120] Fujii, Ohshiro, Ohshiro, Sasaki, and Taniguchi. "Proximal priority treatment using the neck irradiator for adjunctive treatment of female infertility." *Laser Therapy*, 2007. https://doi.org/10.5978/ISLSM.16.133

[121] Yazdi, Bakhshi, Alipoor, Akhoond, Borhani, Farrahi, Panah, and Gilani. "Effect of 830-nm diode laser irradiation on human sperm motility." *Lasers in Medical Science*, 2014. https://doi.org/10.1007/s10103-013-1276-7

[122] Gabel, Carroll, and Harrison. "Sperm motility is enhanced by low level laser and light emitting diode photobiomodulation with a dose-dependent response and differential effects in fresh and frozen samples." *Laser Therapy*, 2018. https://doi.org/10.5978/islsm.18-or-13

[123] Frangez, Frangez, Verdenik, Jansa, and Klun. "Photobiomodulation with light-emitting diodes improves sperm motility in men with asthenozoospermia." *Lasers in Medical Science*, 2015. https://doi.org/10.1007/s10103-014-1653-x

[124] Safian, Novin, Karimi, Kazemi, Zare, Ghoreishi, and Bayat. "Photobiomodulation with 810 nm wavelengths improves human sperm's motility and viability *in vitro*." *Photobiomodulation, Photomedicine, and Laser Surgery*, 2020. https://doi.org/10.1089/photob.2019.4773

[125] Moskvin and Apolikhin. "Effectiveness of low level laser therapy for treating male infertility." *Biomedicine*, 2018. https://www.ncbi.nlm.nih.gov/pmc/articles/PMC5992952/

[126] Preece, Chow, Gomez-Godinez, Gustafson, Esener, Ravida, Durrant, and Berns. "Red light improves spermatozoa motility and does not induce oxidative DNA damage." *Scientific Reports*, 2017. https://www.ncbi.nlm.nih.gov/pmc/articles/PMC5397839/

[127] Zupin, Pascolo, Luppi, Ottaviani, Crovella, and Ricci. "Photobiomodulation therapy for male infertility." *Lasers in Medical Science*, 2020. https://doi.org/10.1007/s10103-020-03042-x

[128] Zaizar, Papini, Gonzalez-Lima, and Telch. "Singular and combined effects of transcranial infrared laser stimulation and exposure therapy on pathological fear: a randomized clinical trial." *Psychological Medicine*, 2021. https://doi.org/10.1017/s0033291721002270

[129] Zhu, Xiao, Hua, Yang, Hu, Zhu, and Zhong. "Near infrared (NIR) light therapy of eye diseases: a review." *International Journal of Medical Sciences*, 2021. https://www.ncbi.nlm.nih.gov/pmc/articles/PMC7738953/

[130] Salehpour, Gholipour-Khalili, Farajdokht, Kamari, Walski, Hamblin, DiDuro, and Cassano. "Therapeutic potential of intranasal photobiomodulation therapy for neurological and neuropsychiatric disorders: a narrative review." *Reviews in the Neurosciences*, 2020.

REFERENCES

https://pubmed.ncbi.nlm.nih.gov/31812948/

[131] Ferraresi, Huang, and Hamblin. "Photobiomodulation in human muscle tissue: an advantage in sports performance?" *Journal of Biophotonics*, 2016. https://doi.org/10.1002/jbio.201600176

[132] Pinto, Guimarães, Souza, Leonardo, Neves, Lima, Lima, and Lopes-Martins. "Sensorymotor and cardiorespiratory sensory rehabilitation associated with transcranial photobiomodulation in patients with central nervous system injury: trial protocol for a single-center, randomized, double-blind, and controlled clinical trial." *Medicine*, 2019. https://doi.org/10.1097/md.0000000000015851

[133] Pires de Sousa, Ferraresi, Kawakubo, Kaippert, Yoshimura, and Hamblin. "Transcranial low-level laser therapy (810 nm) temporarily inhibits peripheral nociception: photoneuromodulation of glutamate receptors, prostatic acid phosphatase, and adenosine triphosphate." *Neurophotonics*, 2016. https://www.spiedigitallibrary.org/journals/neurophotonics/volume-3/issue-01/015003/Transcranial-low-level-laser-therapy-810nm-temporarily-inhibits-peripheral-nociception/10.1117/1.NPh.3.1.015003.full?SSO=1

[134] Pires de Sousa, Kawakubo, Ferraresi, Kaippert, Yoshimura, and Hamblin. "Pain management using photobiomodulation: mechanisms, location, and repeatability quantified by pain threshold and neural biomarkers in mice." *Journal of Biophotonics*, 2018. https://doi.org/10.1002/jbio.201700370

[135] Chow, Johnson, Lopes-Martins, and Bjordal. "Efficacy of low-level laser therapy in the management of neck pain: a systematic review and meta-analysis of randomised placebo or active-treatment controlled trials." *Lancet*, 2009. https://doi.org/10.1016/s0140-6736(09)61522-1

[136] De Oliveira, Antonio, Silva, de Carvalho, Feliciano, Yoshizaki, Vieira, de Melo, Leal-Junior, Labat, Bocalini, Silva Junior, Tucci, and Serra. "Protective effects of photobiomodulation against resistance exercise-induced muscle damage and inflammation in rats." *Journal of Sports Sciences*, 2018. https://doi.org/10.1080/02640414.2018.1457419

[137] Hersant, SidAhmed-Mezi, Bosc, and Meningaud. "Current indications of low-level laser therapy in plastic surgery: a review." *Photomedicine and Laser Surgery*, 2015. https://doi.org/10.1089/pho.2014.3822

[138] Cotler, Chow, Hamblin, and Carroll. "The use of low level laser therapy (LLLT) for musculoskeletal pain." *MedCrave Online Journal of Orthopedics & Rheumatology*, 2015. https://www.ncbi.nlm.nih.gov/pmc/articles/PMC4743666/

[139] Dos Anjos, Salvador, de Souza, de Souza da Fonseca, de Paoli, and Gameiro. "Modulation of immune response to induced arthritis by low-level laser therapy." *Journal of Biophotonics*, 2018. https://doi.org/10.1002/jbio.201800120

[140] Brusaca, Barbieri, Beltrame, Milan-Mattos, Catai, and Oliveira. "Cardiac autonomic responses to different tasks in office workers with access to a sit-stand table: a study in a real work setting." *Ergonomics*, 2021. https://doi.org/10.1080/00140139.2020.1830184

[141] Brugnero, Zarbo, Tarvainen, Marchettini, Adorni, and Compare. "Heart rate variability during acute psychosocial stress: a randomized cross-over trial of verbal and non-verbal laboratory stressors." *International Journal of Psychophysiology*, 2018. https://doi.org/10.1016/j.ijpsycho.2018.02.016

[142] Brosschot, Verkuil, and Thayer. "Generalized unsafety theory of stress: unsafe environments and conditions, and the default stress response." *International Journal of*

Environmental Research and Public Health, 2018. https://www.ncbi.nlm.nih.gov/pmc/articles/PMC5877009/

[143] La Rovere, Bigger, Marcus, Mortara, and Schwartz. "Baroreflex sensitivity and heart-rate variability in prediction of total cardiac mortality after myocardial infarction." *Lancet*, 1998. https://doi.org/10.1016/s0140-6736(97)11144-8

[144] Ernst. "Heart-rate variability: more than heart beats?" *Frontiers in Public Health*, 2017. https://doi.org/10.3389/fpubh.2017.00240

[145] Arab, Martins Dias, de Almeida Barbosa, de Carvalho, Valenti, Crocetta, Ferreira, de Abreu, and Ferreira. "Heart rate variability measure in breast cancer patients and survivors: a systematic review." *Psychoneuroendocrinology*, 2016. https://doi.org/10.1016/j.psyneuen.2016.02.018

[146] Zhou, Ma, Zhang, Zhou, Wang, Wang, and Fu. "Heart rate variability in the prediction of survival in patients with cancer: a systematic review and meta-analysis." *Journal of Psychosomatic Research*, 2016. https://doi.org/10.1016/j.jpsychores.2016.08.004

[147] Giese-Davis, Wilhelm, Tamagawa, Palesh, Neri, Taylor, Kraemer, and Spiegel. "Higher vagal activity as related to survival in patients with advanced breast cancer: an analysis of autonomic dysregulation." *Psychosomatic Medicine*, 2015. https://doi.org/10.1097/psy.0000000000000167

[148] Masel, Huber, Schur, Kierner, Nemecek, and Watzke. "Predicting discharge of palliative care inpatients by measuring their heart rate variability." *Annals of Palliative Medicine*, 2014. https://doi.org/10.3978/j.issn.2224-5820.2014.08.01

[149] Chiang, Koo, Kuo, and Fu. "Association between cardiovascular autonomic functions and time to death in patients with terminal hepatocellular carcinoma." *Journal of Pain and Symptom Management*, 2010.

[150] Elias, Goodell, and Dore. "Hypertension and cognitive functioning: a perspective in historical context." *Hypertension*, 2012. https://doi.org/10.1016/j.jpainsymman.2009.09.014

[151] Buratti, Cruciani, Pulcini, Rocchi, Totaro, Lattanzi, Viticchi, Falsetti, and Silvestrini. "Lacunar stroke and heart rate variability during sleep." *Sleep Medicine*, 2020. https://www.sciencedirect.com/science/article/abs/pii/S1389945720301660?via%3Dihub

[152] Boissoneault, Letzen, Robinson, and Staud. "Cerebral blood flow and heart rate variability predict fatigue severity in patients with chronic fatigue syndrome." *Brain Imaging and Behavior*, 2019. https://doi.org/10.1007/s11682-018-9897-x

[153] Lombardi, Mäkikallio, Myerburg, and Huikuri. "Sudden cardiac death: role of heart rate variability to identify patients at risk." *Cardiovascular Research*, 2001. https://academic.oup.com/cardiovascres/article/50/2/210/273315

[154] Kamaleswaran, Akbilgic, Hallman, West, Davis, and Shah. "Applying artificial intelligence to identify physiomarkers predicting severe sepsis in the PICU." *Pediatric Critical Care Medicine*, 2018. https://doi.org/10.1097/pcc.0000000000001666

[155] Reed, Robertson, and Addison. "Heart rate variability measurements and the prediction of ventricular arrhythmias." *QJM: An International Journal of Medicine*, 2005. https://doi.org/10.1093/qjmed/hci018

[156] Kong, Hoyos, Phillips, McKinnon, Lin, Duffy, Mowszowski, LaMonica, Grunstein, Naismith, and Gordon. "Altered heart rate variability during sleep in mild cognitive impairment." *Sleep*, 2021. https://doi.org/10.1093/sleep/zsaa232

[157] Viljoen and Claassen. "Allostatic load and heart rate variability as health risk indicators." *African Health Sciences*, 2017. https://doi.org/10.4314/ahs.v17i2.17

[158] Kidwell and Ellenbroek. "Heart and soul: heart rate variability and major depression." *Behavioural Pharmacology*, 2018. https://www.researchgate.net/publication/324139627_Heart_and_soul_Heart_rate_variability_and_major_depression

159 Kemp, Koenig, and Thayer. "From psychological moments to mortality: a multidisciplinary synthesis on heart rate variability spanning the continuum of time." *Neuroscience & Biobehavioral Reviews*, 2017. https://doi.org/10.1016/j.neubiorev.2017.09.006

160 Allen, Jennings, Gianaros, Thayer, and Manuck. "Resting high-frequency heart rate variability is related to resting brain perfusion." *Psychophysiology*, 2014. https://doi.org/10.1111/psyp.12321

161 Shi, Yang, Zhao, Su, Mao, Zhang, and Liu. "Differences of heart rate variability between happiness and sadness emotion states: a pilot study." *Journal of Medical and Biological Engineering*, 2017. https://link.springer.com/article/10.1007/s40846-017-0238-0

162 Blood, Wu, Chaplin, Hommer, Vazquez, Rutherford, Mayes, and Crowley. "The variable heart: high frequency and very low frequency correlates of depressive symptoms in children and adolescents." *Journal of Affective Disorders*, 2015. https://www.ncbi.nlm.nih.gov/pmc/articles/PMC4565756/

163 Williams, Cash, Rankin, Bernardi, Koenig, and Thayer. "Resting heart rate variability predicts self-reported difficulties in emotion regulation: a focus on different facets of emotion regulation." *Frontiers in Psychology*, 2015. https://www.ncbi.nlm.nih.gov/pmc/articles/PMC4354240/

164 An, Nolty, Amano, Rizzo, Buckwalter, and Rensberger. "Heart rate variability as an index of resilience." *Military Medicine*, 2020. https://academic.oup.com/milmed/article/185/3-4/363/5586497

165 Wei, Han, Zhang, Hannak, Dai, and Liu. "Affective emotion increases heart rate variability and activates left dorsolateral prefrontal cortex in post-traumatic growth." *Scientific Reports*, 2017. https://www.nature.com/articles/s41598-017-16890-5

166 Telles, Singh, Joshi, and Balkrishna. "Post-traumatic stress symptoms and heart rate variability in Bihar flood survivors following yoga: a randomized controlled study." *BMC Psychiatry*, 2010. https://www.ncbi.nlm.nih.gov/pmc/articles/PMC2836997/

167 Makovac, Carnevali, Hernandez-Medina, Sgoifo, Petrocchi, and Ottaviani. "Safe in my heart: resting heart rate variability longitudinally predicts emotion regulation, worry, and sense of safeness during COVID-19 lockdown." *Stress*, 2022. https://www.medrxiv.org/content/10.1101/2021.06.17.21259071v1

168 Kemp, Quintana, Kuhnert, Griffiths, Hickie, and Guastella. "Oxytocin increases heart rate variability in humans at rest: implications for social approach-related motivation and capacity for social engagement." *PLoS One*, 2012. https://doi.org/10.1371/journal.pone.0044014

169 An, Nolty, Amano, Rizzo, Buckwalter, and Rensberger. "Heart rate variability as an index of resilience." *Military Medicine*, 2020. https://academic.oup.com/milmed/article/185/3-4/363/5586497

170 Benjamin, Valstad, Elvsåshagen, Jönsson, Moberget, Winterton, Haram, Høegh, Lagerberg, Steen, Larsen, Andreassen, Westlye, and Quintana. "Heart rate variability is associated with disease severity in psychosis spectrum disorders." *Progress in Neuro-Psychopharmacology and Biological Psychiatry*, 2020.

171 Carnevali, Koenig, Sgoifo, and Ottaviani. "Autonomic and brain morphological predictors of stress resilience." *Frontiers in Neuroscience*, 2018. https://doi.org/10.1016/j.pnpbp.2020.110108

172 Ge, Yuan, Li, and Zhang. "Posttraumatic stress disorder and alterations in resting heart rate variability: a systematic review and meta-analysis." *Psychiatry Investigation*, 2020. https://doi.org/10.30773/pi.2019.0112

173 He, Wang, Zhang, Wang, Dong, and Yang. "Admission heart rate variability is associated with poststroke depression in patients with acute mild-moderate ischemic stroke." *Frontiers in Psychiatry*, 2020. https://doi.org/10.3389/fpsyt.2020.00696

174 van der Kooy, van Hout, van Marwijk, de Haan, Stehouwer, and Beekman. "Differences in heart rate variability between depressed and non-depressed elderly." *International Journal of Geriatric Psychiatry*, 2006. https://pubmed.ncbi.nlm.nih.gov/16416460/

175 Beaumont, Burton, Lemon, Bennett, Lloyd, and Vollmer-Conna. "Reduced cardiac vagal modulation impacts on cognitive performance in chronic fatigue syndrome." *PLoS One*, 2012. https://www.ncbi.nlm.nih.gov/pmc/articles/PMC3498107/

176 Pignotti and Steinberg. "Heart rate variability as an outcome measure for thought field therapy in clinical practice." *Journal of Clinical Psychology*, 2001. https://www.marksteinberg.com/pdf/HRV.pdf

177 Park, Oh, Noh, Kim, and Kim. "Heart rate variability as a marker of distress and recovery: the effect of brief supportive expressive group therapy with mindfulness in cancer patients." *Integrative Cancer Therapies*, 2018. https://journals.sagepub.com/doi/pdf/10.1177/1534735418756192

178 Kircanski, Williams, and Gotlib. "Heart rate variability as a biomarker of anxious depression response to antidepressant medication." *Depression & Anxiety*, 2018. https://doi.org/10.1002/da.22843

179 Borrione, Brunoni, Sampaio-Junior, Aparicio, Kemp, Benseñor, Lotufo, and Fraguas. "Associations between symptoms of depression and heart rate variability: an exploratory study." *Psychiatry Research*, 2018. https://doi.org/10.1016/j.psychres.2017.09.028

180 Shu, Yu, Chen, Hua, Li, Jin, and Xu. "Wearable emotion recognition using heart rate data from a smart bracelet." *Sensors*, 2020. https://doi.org/10.3390/s20030718

181 Brown, Brosschot, Versluis, Thayer, and Verkuil. "Assessing new methods to optimally detect episodes of non-metabolic heart rate variability reduction as an indicator of psychological stress in everyday life: a thorough evaluation of six methods." *Frontiers in Neuroscience*, 2020. https://doi.org/10.3389/fnins.2020.564123

182 Alabdulgader. "The human heart rate variability: neurobiology of psychophysiological well-being and planetary resonance." *General Internal Medicine and Clinical Innovations*, 2017. https://www.researchgate.net/publication/318614079 The Human Heart Rate Variability Neurobiology of Psychophysiological well being and Planetary Resonance

183 Wu, Chen, Chang, Wu, Chang, Chu, and Jiang. "Study of autonomic nervous activity of night shift workers treated with laser acupuncture." *Photomedicine and Laser Surgery*, 2009. https://doi.org/10.1089/pho.2007.2235

184 Choi, Kim, Kim, Kim, and Choi. "Reactivity of heart rate variability after exposure to colored lights in healthy adults with symptoms of anxiety and depression." *International Journal of Psychophysiology*, 2011. https://doi.org/10.1016/j.ijpsycho.2010.09.011

185 Momota, Takano, Kani, Matsumoto, Motegi, Aota, Yamamura, Omori, Tomioka, and Azuma. "Frequency analysis of heart rate variability: a useful assessment tool of linearly polarized near-infrared irradiation to stellate ganglion area for burning mouth syndrome." *Pain Medicine*, 2013. https://doi.org/10.1111/pme.12008

186 Liao, Rau, Liou, Tsao, and Lin. "Effects of linearly polarized near-infrared irradiation near the stellate ganglion region on pain and heart rate variability in patients with neuropathic pain." *Pain Medicine*, 2017. https://doi.org/10.1093/pm/pnw145

187 Wu. "Photobiomodulation therapy (PBMT) as a complementary medicine for women to adjust their autonomic nervous systems and induce specific brain waves: a case

report." *OBM Integrative and Complementary Medicine*, 2019. https://www.research-gate.net/publication/334610827_Photobiomodulation_Therapy_PBMT_as_a_Complementary_Medicine_for_Women_to_Adjust_Their_Autonomic_Nervous_Systems_and_Induce_Specific_Brain_Waves_-_A_Case_Report

188 Machado, Machado, Chinchilla, Machado, and Foyaca-Sibat. "Assessing the autonomic effect of vagal nerve stimulation with low level lasers by heart rate variability." *Internet Journal of Neurology*, 2019. https://ispub.com/doi/10.5580/IJN.54164

189 Chen, Liu, Ali, and Huizinga. "Effects of sacral photobiomodulation on the autonomic nervous system in patients with colonic dysmotility." *Journal of the Canadian Association of Gastroenterology*, 2021. https://doi.org/10.1093/jcag/gwab002.233

190 Di Bello, Ottaviani, and Petrocchi. "Compassion is not a benzo: distinctive associations of heart rate variability with its empathic and action components." *Frontiers in Neuroscience*, 2021. https://doi.org/10.3389/fnins.2021.617443

191 Zhang, Liao, Wang, Yuan, Zhao, Han, Tang, and Zhao. "Effects of joy and sorrow on pulse-graph parameters in healthy female college students based on emotion-evoked experiments." *Explore*, 2020. https://doi.org/10.1016/j.explore.2020.09.011

192 Ross and Mason. "The effects of preferred natural stimuli on humans' affective states, physiological stress, and mental health, and the potential implications for well-being in captive animals." *Neuroscience & Behavioral Reviews*, 2017. https://doi.org/10.1016/j.neubiorev.2017.09.012

193 Völker and Kistemann. "The impact of blue space on human health and well-being—salutogenetic health effects of inland surface waters: a review." *International Journal of Hygiene and Environmental Health*, 2011. https://doi.org/10.1016/j.ijheh.2011.05.001

194 De Vries, Ten Have, van Dorsselaer, van Wezep, Hermans, and de Graaf. "Local availability of green and blue space and prevalence of common mental disorders in the Netherlands." *British Journal of Psychiatry Open*, 2016. https://www.ncbi.nlm.nih.gov/pmc/articles/PMC5609776/

195 Lanki, Siponen, Ojala, Korpela, Pennanen, Tiittanen, Tsunetsugu, Kagawa, and Tyrväinen. "Acute effects of visits to urban green environments on cardiovascular physiology in women: a field experiment." *Environmental Research*, 2017. https://doi.org/10.1016/j.envres.2017.07.039

196 He, Litscher, Wang, Jing, Shi, Shang, and Zhu. "Intravenous laser blood irradiation, interstitial laser acupuncture, and electroacupuncture in an animal experimental setting: Preliminary results from heart rate variability and electrocorticographic recordings." *Evidence-Based Complementary and Alternative Medicine*, 2013. https://doi.org/10.1155/2013/169249

197 Yang, Litscher, Sun, and Sun. "The application of laser acupuncture in animal experiments: A narrative review of biological aspects." *Evidence-Based Complementary and Alternative Medicine*, 2021 https://doi.org/10.1155/2021/6646237

198 Wu, Chen, Chang, Wu, Chang, Chu, and Jiang. "Study of autonomic nervous activity of night shift workers treated with laser acupuncture." *Photomedicine and Laser Surgery*, 2009. https://doi.org/10.1089/pho.2007.2235

199 Wheat and Larkin. "Biofeedback of heart rate variability and related physiology: a critical review." *Applied Psychophysiology and Biofeedback*, 2010. https://pubmed.ncbi.nlm.nih.gov/20443135/

200 Wells, Outhred, Heathers, Quintana, and Kemp. "Matter over mind: a randomised controlled trial of single-session biofeedback training on performance anxiety and heart rate variability in musicians." *PLos One*, 2012. https://doi.org/10.1371/journal.pone.0046597

201   Azulay, Smart, Mott, and Cicerone. "A pilot study examining the effect of mindful-ness-based stress reduction on symptoms of chronic mild traumatic brain injury/post-concussive syndrome." *Journal of Head Trauma Rehabilitation*, 2013. https://doi.org/10.1097/htr.0b013e318250ebda

202   Lin, Fan, Lu, Lin, Chu, Kuo, Lee, and Lu. "Randomized controlled trial of heart rate variability biofeedback in cardiac autonomic and hostility among patients with coro-nary artery disease." *Behaviour Research and Therapy*, 2015. https://doi.org/10.1016/j.brat.2015.05.001

203   Breach. "Heart rate variability biofeedback in the treatment of major depression." Doctoral dissertation, 2012. https://rucore.libraries.rutgers.edu/rutgers-lib/39081/PDF/

204   Pinter, Szatmari, Horvath, Penzlin, Barlinn, Siepmann, and Siepmann. "Cardiac dysau-tonomia in depression: heart rate variability biofeedback as a potential add-on therapy." *Neuropsychiatric Disease and Treatment*, 2019. https://www.ncbi.nlm.nih.gov/pmc/articles/PMC6529729/

205   Pizzoli, Marzorati, Gatti, Monzani, Mazzocco, and Pravettoni. "A meta-analysis on heart rate variability biofeedback and depressive symptoms." *Scientific Reports*, 2021. https://www.ncbi.nlm.nih.gov/pmc/articles/PMC7988005/

206   Blase, van Dijke, Cluitmans, and Vermetten. "Efficacy of HRV-biofeedback as additional treatment of depression and PTSD." *Tijdschrift voor psychiatrie*, 2016. https://pubmed.ncbi.nlm.nih.gov/27075221/

207   Gevensleben, Holl, Albrecht, Schlamp, Kratz, Studer, Rothenberger, Moll, and Heinrich. "Neurofeedback training in children with ADHD: 6-month follow-up of a randomised controlled trial." *European Child & Adolescent Psychiatry*, 2010. https://doi.org/10.1007/s00787-010-0109-5

208   Tsui-Caldwell and Steffen. "Adding HRV biofeedback to psychotherapy increases heart rate variability and improves the treatment of major depressive disorder." International Journal of Psychophysiology, 2018. https://www.ncbi.nlm.nih.gov/pubmed/29307738

209   Blanck, Stoffel, Bents, Ditzen, and Mander. "Heart rate variability in individual psy-chotherapy." *Journal of Nervous and Mental Disease*, 2019. https://doi.org/10.1097/NMD.0000000000000994

210   Kudo, Shinohara, and Kodama. "Heart rate variability biofeedback intervention for reduction of psychological stress during the early postpartum period." *Applied Psychophysiology and Biofeedback*, 2014. https://www.ncbi.nlm.nih.gov/pmc/articles/PMC4220117/

211   Lehrer and Gevirtz. "Heart rate variability biofeedback: How and why does it work?" *Frontiers in Psychology*, 2014. https://www.ncbi.nlm.nih.gov/pmc/articles/PMC4104929/

212   McCraty, Atkinson, Lipsenthal, and Arguelles. "New hope for correctional officers: an innovative program for reducing stress and health risks." *Applied Psychophysiology and Biofeedback*, 2009. https://doi.org/10.1007/s10484-009-9087-0

213   Mather and Thayer. "How heart rate variability affects emotion regulation brain net-works." *Current Opinion in Behavioral Sciences*, 2018. https://www.ncbi.nlm.nih.gov/pmc/articles/PMC5761738/

214   Brosschot, Verkuil, and Thayer. "Generalized unsafety theory of stress: unsafe envi-ronments and conditions, and the default stress response." *International Journal of Environmental Research and Public Health*, 2018. https://www.ncbi.nlm.nih.gov/pmc/articles/PMC5877009/

REFERENCES

215 Cacioppo, Cacioppo, Capitanio, and Cole. "The neuroendocrinology of social isolation." *Annual Review of Psychology*, 2015. https://doi.org/10.1146%2Fannurev-psych-010814-015240

216 Momota, Takano, Kani, Matsumoto, Motegi, Aota, Yamamura, Omori, Tomioka, and Azuma. "Frequency analysis of heart rate variability: a useful assessment tool of linearly polarized near infrared irradiation to stellate ganglion area for burning mouth syndrome." *Pain Medicine*, 2013. https://doi.org/10.1111/pme.12008

217 Liao, Rau, Liou, Tsauo, and Lin. "Effects of linearly polarized near-infrared irradiation near the stellate ganglion region on pain and heart rate variability in patients with neuropathic pain." *Pain Medicine*, 2017. https://doi.org/10.1093/pm/pnw145

218 Valencia, Brown, Mair, Smith, and Gurovich. "Heart rate variability response to experimental pain procedure." *Journal of Pain*, 2017. https://doi.org/10.1016/j.jpain.2017.02.230

219 Chalmers, Quintana, Abbott, and Kemp. "Anxiety disorders are associated with reduced heart rate variability: a meta-analysis." *Frontiers in Psychiatry*, 2014. https://doi.org/10.3389/fpsyt.2014.00080

220 Nugent, Bain, Thayer. Sollers, and Drevets. "Heart rate variability during motor and cognitive tasks in females with major depressive disorder." *Psychiatry Research*, 2011. https://doi.org/10.1016/j.pscychresns.2010.08.013

221 Alvares, Quintana, Hickie, and Guastella. "Autonomic nervous system dysfunction in psychiatric disorders and the impact of psychotropic medications: a systematic review and meta-analysis." *Journal of Psychiatry & Neuroscience*, 2016. https://doi.org/10.1503/jpn.140217

222 Schiffer, Johnston, Ravichandran, Polcari, Teicher, Webb, and Hamblin. "Psychological benefits 2 and 4 weeks after a single treatment with near infrared light to the forehead: a pilot study of 10 patients with major depression and anxiety." *Behavioral and Brain Functions*, 2009. https://doi.org/10.1186/1744-9081-5-46

223 Cassano, Cusin, Mischoulon, Hamblin, De Taboada, Pisoni, Chang, Yeung, Ionescu, Petrie, Nierenberg, Fava, and Iosifescu. "Near-infrared transcranial radiation for major depressive disorder: proof of concept study." *Psychiatry Journal*, 2015. https://doi.org/10.1155/2015/352979

224 Tsai and Wang. "Effect of laser stimulation of acupoint Taichong (LR3) on blood pressure and heart rate variability. *Internet Journal of Alternative Medicine*, 2014. https://www.academia.edu/en/76562795/Effect_of_Laser_Stimulation_of_Acupoint_Taichong_LR3_on_Blood_Pressure_and_Heart_Rate_Variability

225 Chen, Liu, Ali, and Huizinga. "Effects of sacral photobiomodulation on the autonomic nervous system in patients with colonic dysmotility." *Journal of the Canadian Association of Gastroenterology*, 2021. http://dx.doi.org/10.1093/jcag/gwab002.233

226 Jang, Hwang, Padhye, and Meininger. "Effects of cognitive behavioral therapy on heart rate variability in young females with constipation-predominant irritable bowel syndrome: a parallel group trial." *Journal of Neurogastroenterology and Motility*, 2017. http://www.jnmjournal.org/journal/view.html?doi=10.5056/jnm17017

227 Hamblin. "Mechanisms and applications of the anti-inflammatory effects of photobiomodulation." *AIMS Biophysics*, 2017. https://doi.org/10.3934/biophy.2017.3.337

228 Neves, Gonçalves, Cavalli, Vieira, Laurindo, Simões, Coelho, Santos, Marcolino, Cola, and Dutra. "Photobiomodulation therapy improves acute inflammatory response in mice: the role of cannabinoid receptors/ATP-sensitive K+ channel/P38-MAPK

signaling pathway." *Molecular Neurobiology*, 2018. https://pubmed.ncbi.nlm.nih.gov/28980210/

229 Rojas and Gonzalez-Lima. "Neurological and psychological applications of transcranial lasers and LEDs." *Biochemical Pharmacology*, 2013. https://doi.org/10.1016/j.bcp.2013.06.012

230 Salehpour, Gholipour-Khalili, Farajdokht, Kamari, Walski, Hamblin, DiDuro, and Cassano. "Therapeutic potential of intranasal photobiomodulation therapy for neurological and neuropsychiatric disorders: a narrative review." *Reviews in the Neurosciences*, 2020. https://doi.org/10.1515/revneuro-2019-0063

231 Nawashiro, Sato, Kawauchi, Takeuchi, Nagatani, Yoshihara, and Shinmoto. "Blood-oxygen-level-dependent (BOLD) functional magnetic resonance imaging (fMRI) during transcranial near-infrared laser irradiation." *Brain Stimulation*, 2017. https://doi.org/10.1016/j.brs.2017.08.010

232 Chaney. "Brain injury in American football: 130 years of knowledge and denial." ChaneysBlog.com, 2016. https://doi.org/10.1227/01.neu.0000053210.76063.e4

233 For more on this topic, you may want to check out his TED talk, "Growing Evidence of Brain Plasticity": https://www.ted.com/talks/michael_merzenich_growing_evidence_of_brain_plasticity

234 McInnes, Friesen, MacKenzie, Westwood, and Boe. "Mild traumatic brain injury (mTBI) and chronic cognitive impairment: a scoping review." *PLoS One*, 2017. https://doi.org/10.1371/journal.pone.0174847

235 Siegel. *Second Impact*, 2019.

236 Yuan and Wang. "Emotional lability as a unique presenting sign of suspected chronic traumatic encephalopathy." *Case Reports in Neurological Medicine*, 2018. https://www.hindawi.com/journals/crinm/2018/2621416/

237 Rodrigues, Lasmar, and Caramelli. "Effects of soccer heading on brain structure and function." *Frontiers in Neurology*, 2016. https://www.ncbi.nlm.nih.gov/pmc/articles/PMC4800441/

238 Paniccia, Taha, Keightley, Thomas, Verweel, Murphy, Wilson, and Reed. "Autonomic function following concussion in youth athletes: an exploration of heart rate variability using 24-hour recording methodology." *Journal of Visualized Experiments*, 2018. https://www.ncbi.nlm.nih.gov/pmc/articles/PMC6235273/

239 Sicard, Lortie, Moore, and Ellemberg. "Cognitive testing and exercise to assess the readiness to return to play after a concussion." *Translational Journal of the American College of Sports Medicine*, 2020. https://journals.lww.com/acsm-tj/Fulltext/2020/07150/Cognitive_Testing_and_Exercise_to_Assess_the.6.aspx

240 Zhou and Greenwald. "Update on insomnia after mild traumatic brain injury." *Brain Sciences*, 2018. https://www.ncbi.nlm.nih.gov/pmc/articles/PMC6315624/

241 For more on the impact of TBI, see:
Belanger, Kretzmer, Vanderploeg, and French. "Symptom complaints following combat-related traumatic brain injury: relationship to traumatic brain injury severity and posttraumatic stress disorder." *Journal of the International Neuropsychological Society*, 2010. https://www.cambridge.org/core/journals/journal-of-the-international-neuropsychological-society/article/abs/symptom-complaints-following-combatrelated-traumatic-brain-injury-relationship-to-traumatic-brain-injury-severity-and-posttraumatic-stress-disorder/BEC6C8887C6481D4FA419D7351E78359
Bivona, D'Ippolito, Giustini, Vignally, Longo, Taggi, and Formisano. "Return to driving after severe traumatic brain injury: increased risk of traffic accidents and personal

responsibility." *Journal of Head Trauma Rehabilitation*, 2012. https://pubmed.ncbi.nlm.nih.gov/21829135/

Blechert, Michael, Grossman, Lajtman, and Wilhelm. "Autonomic and respiratory characteristics of posttraumatic stress disorder and panic disorder." *Psychosomatic Medicine*, 2007. https://journals.lww.com/psychosomaticmedicine/Abstract/2007/11000/Autonomic_and_Respiratory_Characteristics_of.20.aspx

Fisk, Schneider, and Novack. "Driving following traumatic brain injury: prevalence, exposure, advice and evaluations." *Brain Injury*, 1998. https://pubmed.ncbi.nlm.nih.gov/9724839/

Jarrahi, Braun, Ahluwalia, Gupta, Wilson, Munie, Ahluwalia, Vender, Vale, Dhandapani, and Vaibhav. "Revisiting traumatic brain injury: from molecular mechanisms to therapeutic interventions." *Biomedicines*, 2020. https://doi.org/10.3390/biomedicines8100389

Jonsson and Andersson. "Mild traumatic brain injury: a description of how children and youths between 16 and 18 years of age perform leisure activities after 1 year." *Developmental Neurorehabilitation*, 2013. https://pubmed.ncbi.nlm.nih.gov/23030702/

King, Law, King, Hurley, Hanna, Kertoy, and Rosenbaum. "Measuring children's participation in recreation and leisure activities: construct validation of the CAPE and PAC." *Child: Care, Health and Development*, 2007. https://www.researchgate.net/publication/6618097_Measuring_children's_participation_in_recreation_and_leisure_activities_Construct_validation_of_the_CAPE_and_PAC

Leddy, Kozlowski, Fung, Pendergast, and Willer. "Regulatory and autoregulatory physiological dysfunction as a primary characteristic of post-concussion syndrome: implications for treatment. *Neurorehabilitation*, 2007. https://www.researchgate.net/publication/5928182_Regulatory_and_autoregulatory_physiological_dysfunction_as_a_primary_characteristic_of_post_concussion_syndrome_Implications_for_treatment]

Macpherson, Fridman, Scolnik, Corallo, and Guttmann. "A population-based study of paediatric emergency department and office visits for concussions from 2003 to 2010." *Paediatrics & Child Health*, 2014. https://www.ncbi.nlm.nih.gov/pmc/articles/PMC4276389/

McCrory, Meeuwisse, Aubry, Cantu, Dvorak, Echemendia, Engebretsen, Johnston, Kutcher, Raftery, Sills, Benson, Davis, Ellenbogen, Guskiewicz, Herring, Iverson, Jordan, Kissick, McCrea, McIntosh, Maddocks, Makdissi, Purcell, Putukian, Schneider, Tator, and Turner. "Consensus statement on concussion in sport." *Physical Therapy in Sport*, 2013. https://doi.org/10.1016/j.ptsp.2013.03.002

Milleville-Pennel, Pothier, Hoc, and Mathé. "Consequences of cognitive impairments following traumatic brain injury: Pilot study on visual exploration while driving." *Brain Injury*, 2010. https://pubmed.ncbi.nlm.nih.gov/20235770/

Preece, Horswill, and Geffen. "Driving after concussion: the acute effect of mild traumatic brain injury on drivers' hazard perception." *Neuropsychology*, 2010. https://pubmed.ncbi.nlm.nih.gov/20604623/

Ingebrigtsen, Waterloo, Marup-Jensen, Attner, and Romner. "Quantification of post-concussion symptoms 3 months after minor head injury in 100 consecutive patients." *Journal of Neurology*, 1998. https://pubmed.ncbi.nlm.nih.gov/9758300/

Zemek, Farion, Sampson, and McGahern. "Prognosticators of persistent symptoms following pediatric concussion: a systematic review." *JAMA Pediatrics*, 2013. https://jamanetwork.com/journals/jamapediatrics/fullarticle/1548768

[242] Weber. "Altered calcium signaling following traumatic brain injury." *Frontiers in Pharmacology*, 2012. https://www.ncbi.nlm.nih.gov/pmc/articles/PMC3324969/

[243] Jorge, Robinson, Moser, Tateno, Crespo-Facorro, and Arndt. "Major depression following traumatic brain injury." *Archives of General Psychiatry*, 2004. https://jamanetwork.com/journals/jamapsychiatry/fullarticle/481944

[244] Fann, Burlington, Leonetti, Jaffe, Katon, and Thompson. "Psychiatric illness following traumatic brain injury in an adult health maintenance organization population." *Archives of General Psychiatry*, 2004. https://doi.org/10.1001/archpsyc.61.1.53

[245] Henderson, van Lierop, McLean, Uszler, Thornton, Siow, Pavel, Cardaci, and Cohen. "Functional neuroimaging in psychiatry—aiding in diagnosis and guiding treatment: what the American Psychiatric Association does not know." *Frontiers in Psychiatry*, 2020. https://doi.org/10.3389/fpsyt.2020.00276

[246] Dams-O'Connor, Cantor, Brown, Dijkers, Spielman, and Gordon. "Screening for traumatic brain injury: Findings and public health implications." *Journal of Head Trauma Rehabilitation*, 2014. https://doi.org/10.1097/htr.0000000000000099

[247] Mayer and Quinn. "Neuroimaging biomarkers of new-onset psychiatric disorders following traumatic brain injury." *Biological Psychiatry*, 2021. https://doi.org/10.1016/j.biopsych.2021.06.005

[248] Corsellis, Bruton, and Freeman-Browne. "The aftermath of boxing." *Psychological Medicine*, 1973. https://doi.org/10.1017/s0033291700049588

[249] Antonius, Mathew, Picano, Hinds, Cogswell, Olympia, Brooks, DiGiacomo, Baker, Willer, and Leddy. "Behavioral health symptoms associated with chronic traumatic encephalopathy: a critical review of the literature and recommendations for treatment and research." *Journal of Neuropsychiatry and Clinical Neurosciences*, 2014. https://neuro.psychiatryonline.org/doi/10.1176/appi.neuropsych.13090201?url_ver=Z39.88-2003&rfr_id=ori%3Arid%3Acrossref.org&rfr_dat=cr_pub++0pubmed&

[250] Johnson, Stewart, and Smith. "Axonal pathology in traumatic brain injury." *Experimental Neurology*, 2013. https://www.ncbi.nlm.nih.gov/pmc/articles/PMC3979341/

[251] Thompson, Thompson, Reid-Chung, and Thompson. "Managing traumatic brain injury: Appropriate assessment and a rationale for using neurofeedback and biofeedback to enhance recovery in postconcussion syndrome. *Biofeedback*, 2013. https://meridian.allenpress.com/biofeedback/article-abstract/41/4/158/113318/Managing-Traumatic-Brain-Injury-Appropriate

[252] Hiebert, Shen, Thimmesch, and Pierce. "Traumatic brain injury and mitochondrial dysfunction." *American Journal of the Medical Sciences*, 2015. https://doi.org/10.1097/maj.0000000000000506

[253] Lamade, Anthonymuthu, Hier, Gao, Kagan, and Bayir. "Mitochondrial damage and lipid signaling in traumatic brain injury." *Experimental Neurology*, 2020. https://www.ncbi.nlm.nih.gov/pmc/articles/PMC7237325/

[254] Zinchenko, Navolokin, Shirokov, Khlebtsov, Dubrovsky, Saranceva, Abdurashitov, Khorovodov, Terskov, Mamedova, Klimova, Agranovich, Martinov, Tuchin, Semyachkina-Glushkovskaya, and Kurts. "Pilot study of transcranial photobiomodulation of lymphatic clearance of beta-amyloid from the mouse brain: breakthrough strategies for non-pharmacologic therapy of Alzheimer's disease." *Biomedical Optics Express*, 2019. https://www.ncbi.nlm.nih.gov/pmc/articles/PMC6701516/

[255] Zinchenko, Klimova, Mamedova, Agranovich, Blokhina, Antonova, Terskov, Shirokov, Navolokin, Morgun, Osipova, Boytsova, Yu, Zhu, Kurths, and Semyachkina-Glushkovskaya. "Photostimulation of extravasation of beta-amyloid through the model of

blood-brain barrier." *Electronics*, 2020. https://www.mdpi.com/2079-9292/9/6/1056/htm

256   Petraglia, Plog, Dayawansa, Chen, Dashnaw, Czerniecka, Walker, Viterise, Hyrien, Iliff, Deane, Nedergaard, and Huang. "The spectrum of neurobehavioral sequelae after repetitive mild traumatic brain injury: a novel mouse model of chronic traumatic encephalopathy." *Journal of Neurotrauma*, 2014. https://www.ncbi.nlm.nih.gov/pmc/articles/PMC4082360/

257   Francis, Fisher, Rushby, and McDonald. "Reduced heart rate variability in chronic severe traumatic brain injury: association with impaired emotional and social functioning, and potential for treatment using biofeedback." *Neuropsychological Rehabilitation*, 2016. https://pubmed.ncbi.nlm.nih.gov/25627984/

258   Su, Kuo, Kuo, Lai, and Chen. "Sympathetic and parasympathetic activities evaluated by heart-rate variability in head injury of various severities." *Clinical Neurophysiology*, 2005. https://doi.org/10.1016/j.clinph.2005.01.010

259   Lagos, Thompson, and Vaschillo. "A preliminary study: heart rate variability biofeedback for treatment of postconcussion syndrome." *Biofeedback*, 2013. http://dx.doi.org/10.5298/1081-5937-41.3.02

260   Reid-Chung, Thompson, and Thompson. "Heart rate variability and traumatic brain injury: clinical applications." *Biofeedback*, 2015. http://dx.doi.org/10.5298/1081-5937-43.1.02

261   Abaji, Curnier, Moore, and Ellemberg. "Persisting effects of concussion on heart rate variability during physical exertion." *Journal of Neurotrauma*, 2016. http://dx.doi.org/10.1089/neu.2015.3989

262   Bishop, Dech, Guzik, and Neary. "Heart rate variability and implication for sport concussion." *Clinical Physiology and Functional Imaging*, 2018. https://doi.org/10.1111/cpf.12487

263   Huang, Frantz, Moralez, Sabo, Davis, Davis, Bell, and Purkayastha. "Reduced resting and increased elevation of heart rate variability with cognitive task performance in concussed athletes." *Journal of Head Trauma Rehabilitation*, 2019. https://doi.org/10.1097/htr.0000000000000409

264   Sung, Lee, Chiang, Chiu, Chu, Ou, Tsai, Liao, Lin, Lin, Chen, Li, and Wang. "Early dysautonomia detected by heart rate variability predicts late depression in female patients following mild traumatic brain injury." *Psychophysiology*, 2015. https://onlinelibrary.wiley.com/doi/abs/10.1111/psyp.12575

265   Khalid, Yang, McGuire, Robson, Foreman, Ngwenya, and Lorenz. "Autonomic dysfunction following traumatic brain injury: translational insights." *Neurosurgical Focus*, 2019. https://thejns.org/focus/view/journals/neurosurg-focus/47/5/article-pE8.xml

266   Faden, Wu, Stoica, and Loane. "Progressive inflammation-mediated neurodegeneration after traumatic brain or spinal cord injury." *British Journal of Pharmacology*, 2016. https://www.ncbi.nlm.nih.gov/pmc/articles/PMC4742301/

267   Lim and Baumann. "Sleep-wake disorders in patients with traumatic brain injury." Uptodate.com, 2019. https://www.uptodate.com/contents/sleep-wake-disorders-in-patients-with-traumatic-brain-injury

268   Leng, Byers, Barnes, Peltz, Li, and Yaffe. "Traumatic brain injury and incidence risk of sleep disorders in nearly 200,000 U.S. veterans." *Neurology*, 2021. https://www.ncbi.nlm.nih.gov/pmc/articles/PMC8055309/

269   Chao, Mohlenhoff, Weiner, and Neylan. "Associations between subjective sleep quality and brain volume in Gulf War veterans." *Sleep*, 2014. https://www.ncbi.nlm.nih.gov/pmc/articles/PMC3920309/

270 Mantua, Henry, Garskovas, and Spencer. "Mild traumatic brain injury chronically impairs sleep- and wake-dependent emotional processing." *Sleep*, 2017. https://doi.org/10.1093/sleep/zsx062

271 Salehpour, Farajdokht, Erfani, Sadigh-Eteghad, Shotorbani, Hamblin, Karimi, Rasta, and Mahmoudi. "Transcranial near-infrared photobiomodulation attenuates memory impairment and hippocampal oxidative stress in sleep-deprived mice." *Brain Research*, 2018. https://www.ncbi.nlm.nih.gov/pmc/articles/PMC5801165/

272 Zhang, Zhou, Hamblin, and Wu. "Low-level laser therapy effectively prevents secondary brain injury induced by immediate early responsive gene X-1 deficiency." *Journal of Cerebral Blood Flow & Metabolism*, 2014. https://www.ncbi.nlm.nih.gov/pmc/articles/PMC4126101/

273 Thunshelle and Hamblin. "Transcranial low-level laser (light) therapy for brain injury." *Photomedicine and Laser Surgery*, 2016. https://www.ncbi.nlm.nih.gov/pmc/articles/PMC5180077/

274 Naeser, Zafonte, Krengel, Martin, Frazier, Hamblin, Knight, Meehan, and Baker. "Significant improvements in cognitive performance post-transcranial red/near-infrared light-emitting diode treatments in chronic, mild traumatic brain injury: open-protocol study." *Journal of Neurotrauma*, 2014. https://www.ncbi.nlm.nih.gov/pmc/articles/PMC4043367/

275 Naeser, Saltmarche, Krengel, Hamblin, and Knight. "Transcranial LED therapy for cognitive dysfunction in chronic, mild traumatic brain injury: two case reports." *Proceedings of SPIE - The International Society for Optical Engineering*, 2010. https://www.researchgate.net/publication/229011472_Transcranial_LED_therapy_for_cognitive_dysfunction_in_chronic_mild_traumatic_brain_injury_Two_case_reports

276 Stephan, Banas, Bennett, and Tunceroglu. "Efficacy of super-pulsed 905 nm low level laser therapy (LLLT) in the management of traumatic brain injury (TBI): a case study." *World Journal of Neuroscience*, 2012. https://www.scirp.org/html/8-1390063_24793.htm

277 Chao, Barlow, Karimpoor, and Lim. "Changes in brain function and structure after self-administered home photobiomodulation treatment in a concussion case." *Frontiers in Neurology*, 2020. https://doi.org/10.3389%2Ffneur.2020.00952

278 Henderson and Morries. "Multi-watt near-infrared phototherapy for the treatment of comorbid depression: an open-label single-arm study." *Frontiers in Psychiatry*, 2017. https://www.ncbi.nlm.nih.gov/pmc/articles/PMC5627142/

279 Morries, Cassano, and Henderson. "Treatments for traumatic brain injury with emphasis on transcranial near-infrared laser phototherapy." *Neuropsychiatric Disease and Treatment*, 2015. https://www.ncbi.nlm.nih.gov/pmc/articles/PMC4550182/

280 Bogdanova, Gilbert, Baird, and Naeser. "LED home treatment program for chronic TBI and PTSD: clinical program evaluation." *Archives of Physical Medicine and Rehabilitation*, 2019. http://dx.doi.org/10.1016/j.apmr.2019.10.077

281 Poiani, Zaninotto, Carneiro, Zangaro, Salgado, Parreira, de Andrade, Teixeira, and Paiva. "Photobiomodulation using low-level laser therapy (LLLT) for patients with chronic traumatic brain injury: a randomized controlled trial study protocol." *Trials*, 2018. https://www.ncbi.nlm.nih.gov/pmc/articles/PMC5759360/

282 Xuan, Vatansever, Huang, Wu, Xuan, Dai, Ando, Xu, Huang, and Hamblin. "Transcranial low-level laser therapy improves neurological performance in traumatic brain injury in mice: effect of treatment repetition regimen." *PLOS One*, 2013. https://journals.plos.org/plosone/article?id=10.1371/journal.pone.0053454

REFERENCES

283 Wu, Xuan, Ando, Xu, Huang, Huang, Dai, Dhital, Sharma, Whalen, and Hamblin. "Low-level laser therapy for closed-head traumatic brain injury in mice: effect of different wavelengths." *Lasers in Surgery and Medicine*, 2012. https://pubmed.ncbi.nlm.nih.gov/22275301/

284 Ando, Xuan, Xu, Dai, Sharma, Kharkwal, Huang, Wu, Whalen, Sato, Obara, and Hamblin. "Comparison of therapeutic effects between pulsed and continuous wave 810-nm wavelength laser irradiation for traumatic brain injury in mice." *PLoS One*, 2011. https://doi.org/10.1371/journal.pone.0026212

285 Quirk, Torbey, Buchmann, Verma, and Whelan. "Near-infrared photobiomodulation in an animal model of traumatic brain injury: improvements at the behavioral and biochemical levels." *Photomedicine and Laser Surgery*, 2012. https://doi.org/10.1089/pho.2012.3261

286 Mocciaro, Grant, Esenaliev, Petrov, Petrov, Sell, Hausser, Guptarak, Bishop, Parsley, Bolding, Johnson, Lidstone, Prough, and Micci. "Non-invasive transcranial nano-pulsed laser therapy ameliorates cognitive function and prevents aberrant migration of neural progenitor cells in the hippocampus of rats subjected to traumatic brain injury." *Journal of Neurotrauma*, 2020. https://doi.org/10.1089/neu.2019.6534

287 Dong, Zhang, Hamblin, and Wu. "Low-level light in combination with metabolic modulators for effective therapy of injured brain." *Journal of Cerebral Blood Flow & Metabolism*, 2015. https://www.ncbi.nlm.nih.gov/pmc/articles/PMC4640344/

288 Oron, Oron, Streeter, De Taboada, Alexandrovich, Trembovler, and Shohami. "Near infrared transcranial laser therapy applied at various modes to mice following traumatic brain injury significantly reduces long-term neurological deficits." *Journal of Neurotrauma*, 2012. https://doi.org/10.1089/neu.2011.2062

289 Figueiro Longo, Tan, Chan, Welt, Avesta, Ratai, Mercaldo, Yendiki, Namati, Chico-Calero, Parry, Drake, Anderson, Rauch, Diaz-Arrastia, Lev, Lee, Hamblin, Vakoc, and Gupta. "Effect of transcranial low-level light therapy vs. sham therapy among patients with moderate traumatic brain injury: a randomized clinical trial." *JAMA Network Open*, 2020. https://www.ncbi.nlm.nih.gov/pmc/articles/PMC7490644/

290 Cherry, Tripodis, Alvarez, Huber, Kiernan, Daneshvar, Mez, Montenigro, Solomon, Alosco, Stern, McKee, and Stein. "Microglial neuroinflammation contributes to tau accumulation in chronic traumatic encephalopathy." *Acta Neuropathologica Communications*, 2016. https://doi.org/10.1186/s40478-016-0382-8

291 Gabel, Petrie, Mischoulon, Hamblin, Yeung, Sangermano, and Cassano. "Case control series for the effect of photobiomodulation in patients with low back pain and concurrent depression." *Laser Therapy*, 2018. https://www.ncbi.nlm.nih.gov/pmc/articles/PMC7034249/

292 Bourassa. "The effects of photobiostimulation in brain injury: a new consideration for clinical practice." Working paper, 2017. http://dx.doi.org/10.13140/RG.2.2.11591.91045

293 Bourassa. "Transcranial low level laser therapy (tLLLT) in the chiropractic management of mild traumatic brain injury." Working paper, 2017. https://www.researchgate.net/publication/316145447_Transcranial_Low_Level_Laser_Therapy_tLLLT_in_the_Chiropractic_Management_of_Mild_Traumatic_Brain_Injury

294 Carneiro, Poiani, Zaninnoto, Osorio, Oliveira, Paiva, and Zângaro. "Transcranial photobiomodulation therapy in the cognitive rehabilitation of patients with cranioencephalic trauma." *Photobiomodulation, Photomedicine, and Laser Surgery*, 2019. https://www.ncbi.nlm.nih.gov/pmc/articles/PMC6818475/

295 Naeser, Martin, Ho, Krengel, Bogdanova, Knight, Yee, Zafonte, Frazier, Hamblin, and Koo. "Transcranial, red/near-infrared light-emitting diode therapy to improve cognition in chronic traumatic brain injury." *Photomedicine and Laser Surgery*, 2016. https://doi.org/10.1089/pho.2015.4037

296 Naeser, Martin, Ho, Krengel, Bogdanova, Knight, Fedoruk, Hamblin, and Koo. "Transcranial, red/near-infrared light-emitting diode therapy for chronic traumatic brain injury and post-stroke aphasia: clinical studies." *Photobiomodulation in the Brain*, 2019. http://dx.doi.org/10.1089/pho.2015.4037

297 Yang, Youngblood, Wu, and Zhang. "Mitochondria as a target for neuroprotection: role of methylene blue and photobiomodulation." *Translational Neurodegeneration*, 2020. https://doi.org/10.1186/s40035-020-00197-z

298 Goldin and Bogdanova. "Novel neurorehabilitation interventions for cognition in ABI." *Brain Injury Professional*, 2014. https://www.researchgate.net/publication/349752584_Novel_Neurorehabilitation_Interventions_for_Cognition_in_ABI

299 Hashmi, Huang, Osmani, Sharma, Naeser, and Hamblin. "Role of low-level laser therapy in neurorehabilitation." *Physical Medicine and Rehabilitation*, 2010. https://www.ncbi.nlm.nih.gov/pmc/articles/PMC3065857/

300 Dos Santos, Paiva, and Teixeira. "Transcranial light-emitting diode therapy for neuropsychological improvement after traumatic brain injury: a new perspective for diffuse axonal lesion management." *Medical Devices: Evidence and Research*, 2018. https://www.ncbi.nlm.nih.gov/pmc/articles/PMC5927185/

301 Henderson and Morries. "Near-infrared photonic energy penetration: Can infrared phototherapy effectively reach the human brain?" *Neuropsychiatric Disease and Treatment*, 2015. https://doi.org/10.2147/ndt.s78182

302 Naviaux. "Metabolic features of the cell danger response." *Mitochondrion*, 2014. https://www.sciencedirect.com/science/article/pii/S1567724913002390

303 Yang, Dong, Wu, Li, Guo, Yang, Zong, Hamblin, Liu, and Zhang. "Photobiomodulation preconditioning prevents cognitive impairment in a neonatal rat model of hypoxia-ischemia." *Journal of Biophotonics*, 2019. https://doi.org/10.1002/jbio.201800359

304 Yu, Liu, Zhao, Li, McCarthy, Tedford, Lo, and Wang. "Near infrared radiation rescues mitochondrial dysfunction in cortical neurons after oxygen-glucose deprivation." *Metabolic Brain Disease*, 2014. https://doi.org/10.1007/s11011-014-9515-6

305 Wang, Dong, Lu, Zhang, Brann, and Zhang. "Photobiomodulation for global cerebral ischemia: targeting mitochondrial dynamics and functions." *Molecular Neurobiology*, 2019. https://www.ncbi.nlm.nih.gov/pmc/articles/PMC6310117/

306 Kumar, Bukowski, Wider, Reynolds, Calo, Lepore, Tousignant, Jones, Przyklenk, and Sanderson. "Mitochondrial dynamics following global cerebral ischemia." *Molecular and Cellular Neuroscience*, 2016. https://doi.org/10.1016/j.mcn.2016.08.010

307 Sanderson, Wider, Lee, Reynolds, Liu, Lepore, Tousignant, Bukowski, Johnston, Fite, Raghunayakula, Kamholz, Grossman, Przyklenk, and Hüttemann. "Inhibitory modulation of cytochrome c oxidase activity with specific near-infrared light wavelengths attenuates brain ischemia/reperfusion injury." *Scientific Reports*, 2018. https://www.nature.com/articles/s41598-018-21869-x

308 Tucker, Lu, Dong, Yang, Li, Zhao, and Zhang. "Photobiomodulation therapy attenuates hypoxic-ischemic injury in a neonatal rat model." *Journal of Molecular Neuroscience*, 2018. https://www.ncbi.nlm.nih.gov/pmc/articles/PMC6109412/

309 Scuteri, Miloso, Foudah, Orciani, Cavaletti, and Tredici. "Mesenchymal stem cells neuronal differentiation ability: a real perspective for nervous system repair?" *Current Stem Cell Research & Therapy*, 2011. https://doi.org/10.2174/157488811795495486

REFERENCES

310   Arany. "Special issue on stem cells and photobiomodulation therapy." *Photomedicine and Laser Surgery*, 2016. https://doi.org/10.1089/pho.2016.4216

311   Rojas and Gonzalez-Lima. "Low-level light therapy of the eye and brain." *Eye and Brain*, 2011. https://www.ncbi.nlm.nih.gov/pmc/articles/PMC5436183/

312   Abrahamse. "Regenerative medicine, stem cells, and low-level laser therapy: future directives." *Photomedicine and Laser Surgery*, 2012. https://doi.org/10.1089/pho.2012.9881

313   Tuby, Maltz, and Oron. "Induction of autologous mesenchymal stem cells in the bone marrow by low-level laser therapy has profound beneficial effects on the infarcted rat heart." *Lasers in Surgery and Medicine*, 2011. https://pubmed.ncbi.nlm.nih.gov/21674545/

314   Oron, Tuby, Maltz, Sagi-Assif, Abu-Hamed, Yaakobi, Doenyas-Barak, and Efrati. "Autologous bone marrow stem cells stimulation reverses post-ischemic-reperfusion kidney injury in rats." *American Journal of Nephrology*, 2014. https://www.karger.com/Article/Abstract/368721

315   Blatt, Elbaz-Greener, Tuby, Maltz, Siman-Tov, Ben-Aharon, Copel, Eisenberg, Efrati, Jonas, Vered, Tal, Goitein, and Oron. "Low-level laser therapy to the bone marrow reduces scarring and improves heart function post-acute myocardial infarction in the pig." *Photomedicine and Laser Surgery*, 2016. https://doi.org/10.1089/pho.2015.3988

316   Kouhkheil, Fridoni, Piryaei, Taheri, Chirani, Anarkooli, Nejatbakhsh, Shafikhani, Schuger, Reddy, Ghoreishi, Jalalifirouzkouhi, Chien, and Bayat. "The effect of combined pulsed wave low-level laser therapy and mesenchymal stem cell-conditioned medium on the healing of an infected wound with methicillin-resistant *Staphyloccus aureus* in diabetic rats." *Journal of Cellular Biochemistry*, 2018. https://pubmed.ncbi.nlm.nih.gov/29574990/

317   Fallahnezhad, Piryaei, Tabeie, Nazarian, Darbandi, Amini, Mostafavinia, Ghoreishi, Jalalifirouzkouhi, and Bayat. "Low-level laser therapy with helium-neon laser improved variability of osteoporotic bone marrow-derived mesenchymal stem cells from ovariectomy-induced osteoporotic rats." *Journal of Biomedical Optics*, 2016. https://www.researchgate.net/publication/308758331

318   Xuan, Huang, Vatansever, Agrawal, and Hamblin. "Transcranial low-level laser therapy increases memory, learning, neuroprogenitor cells, BDNF and synaptogenesis in mice with traumatic brain injury." *Proceedings of the Society of Photo-optical Instrumentation Engineers*, 2015. https://www.researchgate.net/publication/281765834

319   Xuan, Agrawal, Huang, Gupta, and Hamblin. "Low-level laser therapy for traumatic brain injury in mice increases brain derived neurotrophic factor (BDNF) and synaptogenesis." *Journal of Biophotonics*, 2015. https://pubmed.ncbi.nlm.nih.gov/25196192/

320   Xuan, Vatansever, Huang, and Hamblin. "Transcranial low-level laser therapy enhances learning, memory, and neuroprogenitor cells after traumatic brain injury in mice." *Journal of Biomedical Optics*, 2014. http://ncbi.nlm.nih.gov/pmc/articles/PMC4189010/

321   AlGhamdi, Kumar, and Moussa. "Low-level laser therapy: a useful technique for enhancing the proliferation of various cultured cells." *Lasers in Medical Science*, 2011. https://pubmed.ncbi.nlm.nih.gov/21274733/

322   Hamajima, Hiratsuka, Kiyama-Kishikawa, Tagawa, Kawahara, Ohta, Sasahara, and Abiko. "Effect of low-level laser irradiation on osteoglycin gene expression in osteoblasts." *Lasers in Medical Science*, 2003 https://doi.org/10.1007/s10103-003-0255-9 .

323   Ginani, Soares, Barreto, and Barboza. "Effect of low-level laser therapy on mesenchymal stem cell proliferation: a systematic review." *Lasers in Medical Science*, 2015. https://doi.org/10.1007/s10103-015-1730-9

[324] Amaroli, Agas, Laus, Cuteri, Hanna, Sabbieti, and Benedicenti. "The effects of photo-biomodulation of 808 nm diode laser therapy at higher fluence on the *in vitro* osteogenic differentiation of bone marrow stromal cells." *Frontiers in Physiology*, 2018. https://doi.org/10.3389/fphys.2018.00123

[325] Tuby, Maltz, and Oron. "Implantation of low-level laser irradiated mesenchymal stem cells into the infarcted rat heart is associated with reduction in infarct size and enhanced angiogenesis." *Photomedicine and Laser Surgery*, 2009. https://doi.org/10.1089/pho.2008.2272

[326] Tuby, Maltz, and Oron. "Induction of autologous mesenchymal stem cells in the bone marrow by low-level laser therapy has profound beneficial effects on the infarcted rat heart." *Lasers in Surgery and Medicine*, 2011. https://doi.org/10.1002/lsm.21063

[327] Yoon, Hong, Lee, and Ahn. "Photobiomodulation with a 660-nanometer light-emitting diode promotes cell proliferation in astrocyte culture." *Cells*, 2021. https://www.ncbi.nlm.nih.gov/pmc/articles/PMC8307591/

[328] Min, Byun, Chan, Heo, Kim, Choi, and Pak. "Effect of low-level laser therapy on human adipose-derived stem cells: *in vitro* and *in vivo* studies." *Aesthetic Plastic Surgery*, 2015. https://doi.org/10.1007/s00266-015-0524-6

[329] Guermonprez, Declercq, Decaux, and Grimaud. "Safety and efficacy of a novel home-use device for light-potentiated (LED) skin treatment." *Journal of Biophotonics*, 2020. https://doi.org/10.1002/jbio.202000230

[330] Chang and Lee. "Photobiomodulation with a wavelength > 800 nm induces morpholog-ical changes in stem cells within otic organoids and scala media of the cochlea." *Lasers in Medical Science*, 2021. https://link.springer.com/article/10.1007/s10103-021-03268-3

[331] Wang, Huang, Wang, Lyu, and Hamblin. "Photobiomodulation (blue and green light) encourages osteoblastic differentiation of human adipose-derived stem cells: role of intracellular calcium and light-gated ion channels." *Scientific Reports*, 2016. https://www.ncbi.nlm.nih.gov/pmc/articles/PMC5030629/

[332] Grassia, Vitale, d'Apuzzo, Paiusco, Caccianiga, and Perillo. "Analysis of changes induced in human periodontal ligament, dental pulp, bone marrow and adipose stem cells by low level laser therapy: a review and new perspectives." *Biomedical Journal of Scientific & Technical Research*, 2018. http://dx.doi.org/10.26717/BJSTR.2018.04.0001039

[333] Dompe, Moncrieff, Matys, Grzech-Leśniak, Kocherova, Bryja, Bruska, Dominiak, Mozdziak, Skiba, Shibli, Volponi, Kempisty, and Dyszkiewicz-Konwińska. "Photobiomodulation—underlying mechanism and clinical applications." *Journal of Clinical Medicine*, 2020. https://doi.org/10.3390/jcm9061724

[334] El Gammal, Zaher, and El-Badri. "Effect of low-level laser-treated mesenchymal stem cells on myocardial infarction." *Lasers in Medical Science*, 2017. https://pubmed.ncbi.nlm.nih.gov/28681086/

[335] Liebert, Chow, Bicknell, and Varigos. "Neuroprotective effects against POCD by pho-tobiomodulation: Evidence from assembly/disassembly of the cytoskeleton." *Journal of Experimental Neuroscience*, 2016. https://www.ncbi.nlm.nih.gov/pmc/articles/PMC4737522/

[336] Yang, Tucker, Dong, Wu, Lu, Li, Zhang, Liu, and Zhang. "Photobiomodulation therapy promotes neurogenesis by improving post-stroke local microenvironment and stimu-lating neuroprogenitor cells." *Experimental Neurology*, 2018. https://www.ncbi.nlm.nih.gov/pmc/articles/PMC5723531/

[337] Lapchak, Wei, and Zivin. "Transcranial infrared laser therapy improves clinical rating scores after embolic strokes in rabbits." *Stroke*, 2004. https://doi.org/10.1161/01.str.0000131808.69640.b7

[338] Oron, Oron, Chen, Eilam, Zhang, Sadeh, Lampl, Streeter, De Taboada, and Chopp. "Low-level laser therapy applied transcranially to rats after induction of stroke significantly reduces long-term neurological deficits." *Stroke*, 2006. https://doi.org/10.1161/01.str.0000242775.14642.b8

[339] De Taboada, Ilic, Leichliter-Martha, Oron, Oron, and Streeter. "Transcranial application of low-energy laser irradiation improves neurological deficits in rats following acute stroke." *Lasers in Surgery and Medicine*, 2006. https://doi.org/10.1002/lsm.20256

[340] Gavish, Perez, Reissman, and Gertz. "Irradiation with 780 nm diode laser attenuates inflammatory cytokines but upregulates nitric oxide in lipopolysaccharide-stimulated macrophages: implications for the prevention of aneurysm progression." *Lasers in Surgery and Medicine*, 2008. https://doi.org/10.1002/lsm.20635

[341] Hesse, Werner, and Byhahn. "Transcranial low-level laser therapy may improve alertness and awareness in traumatic brain injured subjects with severe disorders of consciousness: a case series." *International Archives of Medicine*, 2015. http://imed.pub/ojs/index.php/iam/article/view/1232

[342] Lampl, Zivin, Fisher, Lew, Welin, Dahlof, Borenstein, Andersson, Perez, Caparo, Ilic, and Oron. "Infrared laser therapy for ischemic stroke: a new treatment strategy—results of the NeuroThera Effectiveness and Safety Trial-1 (NEST-1)." *Stroke*, 2007. https://doi.org/10.1161/strokeaha.106.478230

[343] Zivin, Albers, Bornstein, Chippendale, Dahlof, Devlin, Fisher, Hacke, Holt, Ilic, Kasner, Lew, Nash, Perez, Rymer, Schellinger, Schneider, Schwab, Veltkamp, Walker, and Streeter. "Effectiveness and safety of transcranial laser therapy for acute ischemic stroke." *Stroke*, 2009. https://doi.org/10.1161/strokeaha.109.547547

[344] Stemer, Huisa, and Zivin. "The evolution of transcranial laser therapy for acute ischemic stroke, including a pooled analysis of NEST-1 and NEST-2." *Current Cardiology Reports*, 2010. https://doi.org/10.1007/s11886-009-0071-3

[345] Naeser, Ho, Martin, Hamblin, and Koo. "Increased functional connectivity within intrinsic neural networks in chronic stroke following treatment with red/near-infrared transcranial photobiomodulation: case series with improved naming in aphasia." *Photobiomodulation, Photomedicine, and Laser Surgery*, 2020. https://doi.org/10.1089/photob.2019.4630

[346] Maksimovich. "Transcatheter intracerebral laser photobiomodulation therapy for treatment of the consequences of ischemic stroke with distal atherosclerotic lesion." *OBM Integrative and Complementary Medicine*, 2021. https://www.lidsen.com/journals/icm/icm-06-04-036

[347] Zhou and Greenwald. "Update on insomnia after mild traumatic brain injury." *Brain Sciences*, 2018. https://www.ncbi.nlm.nih.gov/pmc/articles/PMC6315624/

[348] Knorr, Akay, and Mellman. "Heart rate variability during sleep and the development of PTSD following traumatic injury." Proceedings of the 25th Annual Conference of the IEEE EMBS, 2003. https://ieeexplore.ieee.org/document/1279649

[349] Pyne, Constans, Wiederhold, Gibson, Kimbrell, Kramer, Pitcock, Han, Williams, Chartrand, Gevirtz, Spira, Wiederhold, McCraty, and McCune. "Heart rate variability: pre-deployment predictor of post-deployment PTSD symptoms." *Biological Psychology*, 2016. https://doi.org/10.1016/j.biopsycho.2016.10.008

350 Li, Dong, Yang, Tucker, Zong, Brann, Hamblin, Vazdarjanova, and Zhang. "Photobiomodulation prevents PTSD-like memory impairments in rats." *Molecular Psychiatry*, 2021. https://www.nature.com/articles/s41380-021-01088-z

351 Hoge, McGurk, Thomas, Cox, Engel, and Castro. "Mild traumatic brain injury in U.S. soldiers returning from Iraq." *New England Journal of Medicine*, 2008. https://www.nejm.org/doi/10.1056/NEJMoa072972?url_ver=Z39.88-2003&rfr_id=ori%3Arid%3Acrossref.org&rfr_dat=cr_pub++0www.ncbi.nlm.nih.gov

352 Bogdanova and Verfaellie. "Cognitive sequelae of blast-induced traumatic brain injury: recovery and rehabilitation." *Neuropsychology Review*, 2012. https://www.ncbi.nlm.nih.gov/pmc/articles/PMC4372457/

353 Morries, Cassano, and Henderson. "Treatments for traumatic brain injury with emphasis on transcranial near-infrared laser phototherapy." *Neuropsychiatric Disease and Treatment*, 2015. https://pubmed.ncbi.nlm.nih.gov/26347062/

354 Naeser, Saltmarche, Krengel, Hamblin, and Knight. "Improved cognitive function after transcranial light-emitting diode treatments in chronic traumatic brain injury: two case reports." *Photomedicine and Laser Surgery*, 2011. https://doi.org/10.1089/pho.2010.2814

355 Hipskind, Grover, Fort, Helffenstein, Burke, Quint, Bussiere, Stone, and Hurtado. "Pulsed transcranial red/near-infrared light therapy using light-emitting diodes improves cerebral blood flow and cognitive function in veterans with chronic traumatic brain injury: a case series." *Photobiomodulation, Photomedicine, and Laser Surgery*, 2019. https://doi.org/10.1089/photob.2018.4489

356 Chao. "Improvements in Gulf War Illness symptoms after near-infrared transcranial and intranasal photobiomodulation: two case reports." *Military Medicine*, 2019. https://pubmed.ncbi.nlm.nih.gov/30916762/

357 Martin, Chao, Krengel, Ho, Yee, Lew, Knight, Hamblin, and Naeser. "Transcranial photobiomodulation to improve cognition in Gulf War Illness." *Frontiers in Neurology*, 2021. https://www.ncbi.nlm.nih.gov/pmc/articles/PMC7859640/#B1

358 Hamblin. "Photobiomodulation for traumatic brain injury and stroke." *Journal of Neuroscience Research*, 2017. https://www.ncbi.nlm.nih.gov/pmc/articles/PMC5803455/

359 Hamblin. "Shining light on the head: photobiomodulation for brain disorders." *BBA Clinical*, 2016. https://pubmed.ncbi.nlm.nih.gov/27752476/

360 Azulay, Smart, Mott, and Cicerone. "A pilot study examining the effect of mindfulness-based stress reduction on symptoms of chronic mild traumatic brain injury/post-concussive syndrome." *Journal of Head Trauma Rehabilitation*, 2013. https://pubmed.ncbi.nlm.nih.gov/22688212/

361 Bonn. "The effectiveness of neurofeedback and heart rate variability biofeedback for individuals with long-term post-concussive symptoms." University of Western Ontario Electronic Thesis and Dissertation Repository, 2018. https://ir.lib.uwo.ca/cgi/viewcontent.cgi?article=7698&context=etd

362 Lagos, Thompson, and Vaschillo. "A preliminary study: heart rate variability biofeedback for treatment of postconcussion syndrome." *Biofeedback*, 2013. https://doi.org/10.5298/1081-5937-41.3.02

363 Conder and Conder. "Heart rate variability interventions for concussion and rehabilitation." *Frontiers in Psychology*, 2014. https://doi.org/10.3389/fpsyg.2014.00890

364 Wong-Riley, Liang, Eells, Chance, Salzman, Buchmann, Kane, and Whelan. "Photobiomodulation directly benefits primary neurons functionally inactivated by

toxins: role of cytochrome c oxidase." *Journal of Biological Chemistry*, 2005. https://doi.org/10.1074/jbc.m409650200

365 Jenkins, Andrewes, Nicholas, Drummond, Moffat, Phal, and Desmond. "Emotional reactivity following surgery to the prefrontal cortex." *Journal of Neuropsychology*, 2018. https://doi.org/10.1111/jnp.12110

366 Gillie and Thayer. "Individual differences in resting heart rate variability and cognitive control in post-traumatic stress disorder." *Frontiers in Psychology*, 2014. https://doi.org/10.3389/fpsyg.2014.00758

367 Tian, Yennu, Smith-Osborne, Gonzalez-Lima, North, and Liu. "Prefrontal responses to digit span memory phases in patients with post-traumatic stress disorder: a functional near infrared spectroscopy study." *NeuroImage Clinical*, 2014. https://www.ncbi.nlm.nih.gov/pmc/articles/PMC4055895/

368 Thayer, Hansen, Saus-Rose, and Johnsen. "Heart rate variability, prefrontal neural function, and cognitive performance: the neurovisceral integration perspective on self-regulation, adaptation, and health." *Annals of Behavioral Medicine*, 2009. https://academic.oup.com/abm/article/37/2/141/4565855

369 Maier and Hare. "Higher heart-rate variability is associated with ventromedial prefrontal cortex activity and increased resistance to temptation in dietary self-control challenges." *Journal of Neuroscience*, 2017. https://doi.org/10.1523/jneurosci.2815-16.2016

370 Mäkinen, Mäntysaari, Pääkönen, Jokelainen, Palinkas, Hassi, Leppäluoto, Tahvanainen, and Rintamäki. "Autonomic nervous function during whole-body cold exposure before and after cold acclimation." *Aviation, Space, and Environmental Medicine*, 2008. https://pubmed.ncbi.nlm.nih.gov/18785356/

371 Šrámek, Šimečková, Janský, Šavlíková, and Vybíral. "Human physiological responses to immersion in water of different temperatures." *European Journal of Applied Physiology*, 2000. https://link.springer.com/article/10.1007/s004210050065

372 Kinoshita, Nagata, Baba, Kohmoto, and Iwagaki. "Cold-water face immersion per se elicits cardiac parasympathetic activity." *Circulation Journal*, 2006. https://www.ncbi.nlm.nih.gov/pubmed/16723802

373 Laukkanen, Kunutsor, Kauhanen, and Laukkanen. "Sauna bathing is inversely associated with dementia and Alzheimer's disease in middle-aged Finnish men." *Age and Ageing*, 2016. https://academic.oup.com/ageing/article/46/2/245/2654230

374 Kunutsor, Khan, Zaccardi, Laukkanen, Willeit, and Laukkanen. "Sauna bathing reduces the risk of stroke in Finnish men and women: a prospective cohort study." *Neurology*, 2018. https://pubmed.ncbi.nlm.nih.gov/29720543/

375 Kunutsor, Laukkanen, and Laukkanen. "Longitudinal associations of sauna bathing with inflammation and oxidative stress: the KIHD prospective cohort study." *Annals of Medicine*, 2018. https://www.tandfonline.com/doi/pdf/10.1080/07853890.2018.1489143

376 Kunbootsri, Janyacharoen, Arrayawichanon, Chainansamit, Kanpittaya, Auvichayapat, and Sawanyawisuth. "The effect of six weeks of sauna treatment on autonomic nervous system, peak nasal inspiratory flow, and lung functions of allergic rhinitis Thai patients." *Asian Pacific Journal of Allergy and Immunology*, 2013. https://doi.org/10.12932/ap0262.31.2.2013

377 Laukkanen, Lipponen, Kunutsor, Zaccardi, Araújo, Mäkikallio, Khan, Willeit, Lee, Poikonen, Tarvainen, and Laukkanen. "Recovery from sauna bathing favorably modulates cardiac autonomic nervous system." *Complementary Therapies in Medicine*, 2019. https://doi.org/10.1016/j.ctim.2019.06.011

378 Gutsaeva, Carraway, Suliman, Demchenko, Shitara, Yonekawa, and Piantadosi. "Transient hypoxia stimulates mitochondrial biogenesis in brain subcortex by a neuronal nitric oxide synthase-dependent mechanism." *Journal of Neuroscience*, 2008. https://pubmed.ncbi.nlm.nih.gov/18305236/

379 Putz, Martos, Németh, Körei, Vági, Kempler, and Kempler. "Is there an association between diabetic neuropathy and low vitamin D levels?" *Current Diabetes Reports*, 2014. https://doi.org/10.1007/s11892-014-0537-6

380 Anjum, Jaffery, Fayyaz, Samoo, and Anjum. "The role of vitamin D in brain health: a mini literature review." *Cureus*, 2018. https://doi.org/10.7759/cureus.2960

381 Frei, Haile, Mutsch, and Rohrmann. "Relationship of serum vitamin D concentrations and allostatic load as a measure of cumulative biological risk among the U.S. population: a cross-sectional study." *PLoS One*, 2015. https://doi.org/10.1371/journal.pone.0139217

382 McIntosh, Faden, Yamakami, and Vink. "Magnesium deficiency exacerbates and pretreatment improves outcome following traumatic brain injury in rats: 31P magnetic resonance spectroscopy and behavioral studies." *Journal of Neurotrauma*, 1988. https://doi.org/10.1089/neu.1988.5.17

383 Pivovarova, Stanika, Kazanina, Villanueva, and Andrews. "The interactive roles of zinc and calcium in mitochondrial dysfunction and neurodegeneration." *Journal of Neurochemistry*, 2014. https://www.ncbi.nlm.nih.gov/pmc/articles/PMC3946206/

384 Yang, Wang, Huang, He, Xu, Luo, and Huang. "Zinc enhances the cellular energy supply to improve cell motility and restore impaired energetic metabolism in a toxic environment induced by OTA." *Scientific Reports*, 2017. https://www.nature.com/articles/s41598-017-14868-x

385 Chipuk. "Think we understand the role of DRP1 in mitochondrial biology? Zinc again!" *Molecular Cell*, 2019. https://doi.org/10.1016/j.molcel.2018.12.024

386 Steiner, Mathersul, MacMillan, Camfield, Klupp, Seto, Huang, Hohenberg, and Chang. "A systematic review of intervention studies examining nutritional and herbal therapies for mild cognitive impairment and dementia using neuroimaging methods: study characteristics and intervention efficacy." *Evidence-Based Complementary and Alternative Medicine*, 2017. https://www.hindawi.com/journals/ecam/2017/6083629/

387 Filler, Lyon, Bennett, McCain, Elswick, Lukkahatai, and Saligan. "Association of mitochondrial dysfunction and fatigue: a review of the literature." *BBA Clinical*, 2014. https://www.ncbi.nlm.nih.gov/pmc/articles/PMC4136529/

388 Hagen, Liu, Lykkesfeldt, Wehr, Ingersoll, Vinarsky, Bartholomew, and Ames. "Feeding acetyl-L-carnitine and lipoic acid to old rats significantly improves metabolic function while decreasing oxidative stress." *Proceedings of the National Academy of Sciences of the United States of America*, 2002. https://pubmed.ncbi.nlm.nih.gov/11854487/

389 Chowanadisai, Bauerly, Tchaparian, Wong, Cortopassi, and Rucker. "Pyrroloquinoline quinone stimulates mitochondrial biogenesis through cAMP response element-binding phosphorylation and increased PGC-1α expression." *Journal of Biological Chemistry*, 2010. https://www.ncbi.nlm.nih.gov/pmc/articles/PMC2804159/

390 Saihara, Kamikubo, Ikemoto, Uchida, and Akagawa. "Pyrroloquinoline quinone, a redox-active o-quinone, stimulates mitochondrial biogenesis by activating the SIR1/PGC-1α signaling pathway." *Biochemistry*, 2017. https://pubmed.ncbi.nlm.nih.gov/29185343

391 Hwang and Willoughby. "Mechanisms behind pyrroloquinoline quinone supplementation on skeletal muscle mitochondrial biogenesis: possible synergistic effects with exer-

cise." *Journal of the American College of Nutrition*, 2018. https://pubmed.ncbi.nlm.nih.gov/29714638/

392 Hwang, Machek, Cardaci, Wilburn, Kim, Suezaki, and Willoughby. "Effects of pyrroloquinoline quinone (PQQ) supplementation on aerobic exercise performance and indices of mitochondrial biogenesis in untrained men." *Journal of the American College of Nutrition*, 2019. https://www.tandfonline.com/doi/abs/10.1080/07315724.2019.1705203

393 Andreux, Blanco-Bose, Ryu, Burdet, Ibberson, Aebischer, Auwerx, Singh, and Rinsch. "The mitophagy activator urolithin A is safe and induces a molecular signature of improved mitochondrial and cellular health in humans." *Nature Metabolism*, 2019. https://www.nature.com/articles/s42255-019-0073-4

394 Braidy, Essa, Poljak, Selvaraju, Al-Adawi, Manivasagm, Thenmozhi, Ooi, Sachdev, and Guillemin. "Consumption of pomegranates improves synaptic function in a transgenic mice model of Alzheimer's disease." *Oncotarget*, 2016. https://doi.org/10.18632/oncotarget.10905

395 Sastre, Millán, Asunción, Plá, Juan, Pallardó, O'Connor, Martin, Droy-Lefaix, and Viña. "Ginkgo biloba extract (EGb 761) prevents mitochondrial aging by protecting against oxidative stress." *Free Radical Biology & Medicine*, 1998. https://doi.org/10.1016/s0891-5849(97)00228-1

396 Sastre, Lloret, Borrás, Pereda, García-Sala, Droy-Lefaix, Pallardó, and Viña. "Ginkgo biloba extract EGb 761 protects against mitochondrial aging in the brain and in the liver." *Cellular and Molecular Biology*, 2002. https://pubmed.ncbi.nlm.nih.gov/12396080/

397 Wu, Li, Zu, Du, and Wang. "Ginkgo biloba extract improves coronary artery circulation in patients with coronary artery disease: contribution of plasma nitric oxide and endothelin-1." *Phytotherapy Research*, 2008. https://pubmed.ncbi.nlm.nih.gov/18446847/

398 Darbinyan, Kteyan, Panossian, Gabrielian, Wikman, and Wagner. "Rhodiola rosea in stress-induced fatigue: a double-blind crossover study of a standardized extract SHR-5 with a repeated low-dose regimen on the mental performance of healthy physicians during night duty." *Phytomedicine*, 2000. https://pubmed.ncbi.nlm.nih.gov/11081987/

399 Shevtsov, Zholus, Shervarly, Vol'skij, Korovin, Khristich, Roslyakova, and Wikman. "A randomized trial of two different doses of a SHR-5 Rhodiola rosea extract versus placebo and control of capacity for mental work." *Phytomedicine*, 2003. https://pubmed.ncbi.nlm.nih.gov/12725561/

400 De Bock, Eijnde, Ramaekers, and Hespel. "Acute Rhodiola rosea intake can improve endurance exercise performance." *International Journal of Sport Nutrition and Exercise Metabolism*, 2004. https://pubmed.ncbi.nlm.nih.gov/15256690/

401 Trewin, Hopkins, and Pyne. "Relationship between world-ranking and Olympic performance of swimmers." *Journal of Sports Sciences*, 2007. https://www.tandfonline.com/doi/abs/10.1080/02640410310001641610

402 Duncan and Clarke. "The effect of acute *Rhodiola rosea* ingestion on exercise heart rate, substrate utilisation, mood state, and perceptions of exertion, arousal, and pleasure/displeasure in active men." *Journal of Sports Medicine*, 2014. https://www.ncbi.nlm.nih.gov/pmc/articles/PMC4590898/

403 Noreen, Buckley, Lewis, Brandauer, and Stuempfle. "The effects of an acute dose of Rhodiola rosea on endurance exercise performance." *Journal of Strength and Conditioning Research*, 2013. https://pubmed.ncbi.nlm.nih.gov/23443221/

404 Liu, Li, Simoneau, Jafari, and Zi. "Rhodiola rosea extracts and salidroside decrease the growth of bladder cancer cell lines via inhibition of the mTOR pathway and induc-

tion of autophagy. *Molecular Carcinogenesis*, 2012. https://pubmed.ncbi.nlm.nih.gov/21520297/

[405] Fan, Wang, Wang, and Zhu. "Salidroside induces apoptosis and autophagy in human colorectal cancer cells through inhibition of PI3K/Akt/mTOR pathway." *Oncology Reports*, 2016. https://pubmed.ncbi.nlm.nih.gov/27748934/

[406] Tu, Roberts, Shetty, and Schneider. "Rhodiola crenulata induces death and inhibits growth of breast cancer cell lines." *Journal of Medicinal Food*, 2008. https://pubmed.ncbi.nlm.nih.gov/18800886/

[407] Liu, Peng, Hu, Zhao, He, Li, and Zhong. "Effects of overexpression of ANXA10 gene on proliferation and apoptosis of hepatocellular carcinoma cell line HepG2." *Journal of Huazhong University of Science and Technology*, 2012. https://pubmed.ncbi.nlm.nih.gov/23073794/

[408] Liu, Zhao, and Luo. "Anti-aging implications of *Astragalus membranaceus* (Huangqi): a well-known Chinese tonic." *Aging and Disease*, 2017. https://www.ncbi.nlm.nih.gov/pmc/articles/PMC5758356/

[409] Tsoukalas, Fragkiadaki, Docea, Alegakis, Sarandi, Thanasoula, Spandidos, Tsatsakis, Razgonova, and Calina. "Discovery of potent telomerase activators: unfolding new therapeutic and anti-aging perspectives." *Molecular Medicine Reports*, 2019. https://www.ncbi.nlm.nih.gov/pmc/articles/PMC6755196/

[410] Auddy, Hazra, Mitra, Abedon, and Ghosal. "A standardized *Withania somnifera* extract significantly reduces stress-related parameters in chronically stressed humans: a double-blind, randomized, placebo-controlled study." *Journal of the American Nutraceutical Association*, 2008. https://blog.priceplow.com/wp-content/uploads/2014/08/withania_review.pdf

[411] Chandrasekhar, Kapoor, and Anishetty. "A prospective, randomized, double-blind, placebo-controlled study of safety and efficacy of a high-concentration, full-spectrum extract of ashwagandha root in reducing stress and anxiety in adults." *Indian Journal of Psychological Medicine*, 2012. https://pubmed.ncbi.nlm.nih.gov/23439798/

[412] Noshahr, Shahraki, Ahmadvand, Nourabadi, and Nakhaei. "Protective effects of Withania somnifera root on inflammatory markers and insulin resistance in fructose-fed rats." *Reports of Biochemistry & Molecular Biology*, 2015. https://pubmed.ncbi.nlm.nih.gov/26989739/

[413] Orrù, Casu, Tambaro, Marchese, Casu, and Ruiu. "Withania somnífera (L.) Dunal root extract alleviates formalin-induced nociception in mice: involvement of the opioidergic system." *Behavioural Pharmacology*, 2016. https://pubmed.ncbi.nlm.nih.gov/26397759/

[414] Vyas and Singh. "Molecular targets and mechanisms of cancer prevention and treatment by withaferin A, a naturally occurring steroidal lactone." *AAPS Journal*, 2014. https://pubmed.ncbi.nlm.nih.gov/24046237/

[415] Nishikawa, Okuzaki, Fukushima, Mukai, Ohno, Ozaki, Yabuta, and Nojima. "Withaferin A induces cell death selectively in androgen-independent prostate cancer cells but not in normal fibroblast cells." *PLoS One*, 2015. https://pubmed.ncbi.nlm.nih.gov/26230090/

[416] Bhat, Damle, Vaishnav, Albers, Joshi, and Banerjee. "In vivo enhancement of natural killer cell activity through tea fortified with Ayurvedic herbs." *Phytotherapy Research*, 2010. https://pubmed.ncbi.nlm.nih.gov/19504465/

[417] Mikolai, Erlandsen, Murison, Brown, Gregory, Raman-Caplan, and Zwickey. "In vivo effects of Ashwagandha (Withania somnifera) extract on the activation of lymphocytes." *Journal of Alternative and Complementary Medicine*, 2009. https://pubmed.ncbi.nlm.nih.gov/19388865/

REFERENCES

418   Valerio, D'Antona, and Nisoli. "Branched-chain amino acids, mitochondrial biogenesis, and healthspan: an evolutionary perspective." *Aging*, 2011. https://www.ncbi.nlm.nih.gov/pmc/articles/PMC3156598/

419   Shay, Moreau, Smith, Smith, and Hagen. "Alpha-lipoic acid as a dietary supplement: molecular mechanisms and therapeutic potential." *Biochimica et Biophysica Acta*, 2009. https://pubmed.ncbi.nlm.nih.gov/19664690/

420   Dajas, Abin-Carriquiry, Arredondo, Blasina, Echeverry, Martínez, Rivera, and Vaamonde. "Quercetin in brain diseases: potential and limits." *Neurochemistry International*, 2015. https://www.sciencedirect.com/science/article/abs/pii/S019701861530005X#:~:text=Besides%20its%20activities%20at%20neurons,insults%2C%20potentiating%20the%20protective%20capacity

421   Oliveira, Nabavi, Braidy, Setzer, Ahmed, and Nabavi. "Quercetin and the mitochondria: a mechanistic view." *Biotechnology Advances*, 2016. https://doi.org/10.1016/j.biotechadv.2015.12.014

422   Samuni, Goldstein, Dean, and Berk. "The chemistry and biological activities of N-acetylcysteine." *Biochimica et Biophysica Acta*, 2013. https://www.sciencedirect.com/science/article/abs/pii/S030441651300144X

423   Dean, Giorlando, and Berk. "N-acetylcysteine in psychiatry: current therapeutic evidence and potential mechanisms of action." *Journal of Psychiatry and Neuroscience*, 2011. https://www.ncbi.nlm.nih.gov/pmc/articles/PMC3044191/

424   Pomportes, Davranche, Brisswalter, Hays, and Brisswalter. "Heart rate variability and cognitive function following a multivitamin and mineral supplementation with added guarana (*Paullinia cupana*)." *Nutrients*, 2014. https://www.ncbi.nlm.nih.gov/pmc/articles/PMC4303833/

425   Supakul, Pintana, Apaijai, Chattipakorn, Shinlapawittayatorn, and Chattipakorn. "Protective effects of garlic extract on cardiac function, heart rate variability, and cardiac mitochondria in obese insulin-resistant rats." *European Journal of Nutrition*, 2014. https://doi.org/10.1007/s00394-013-0595-6

426   Sabarwal, Agarwal, and Singh. "Fisetin inhibits cellular proliferation and induces mitochondria-dependent apoptosis in human gastric cancer cells." *Molecular Carcinogenesis*, 2017. https://pubmed.ncbi.nlm.nih.gov/27254419/

427   Wang, Hu, Lin, Yang, Hsieh, Chien, and Yang. "Fisetin induces apoptosis through mitochondrial apoptosis pathway in human uveal melanoma cells." *Environmental Toxicology*, 2018. https://pubmed.ncbi.nlm.nih.gov/29383865/

428   Begley, Hill, and Gahan. "Bile salt hydrolase activity in probiotics." *Applied and Environmental Microbiology*, 2006. https://pubmed.ncbi.nlm.nih.gov/16517616/

429   Kumar, Nagpal, Kumar, Hemalatha, Verma, Kumar, Chakraborty, Singh, Marotta, Jain, and Yadav. "Cholesterol-lowering probiotics as potential biotherapeutics for metabolic diseases." *Experimental Diabetes Research*, 2012. https://pubmed.ncbi.nlm.nih.gov/22611376/

430   Agerholm-Larsen, Bell, Grunwald, and Astrup. "The effect of probiotic milk product on plasma cholesterol: a meta-analysis of short-term intervention studies." *European Journal of Clinical Nutrition*, 2000. https://pubmed.ncbi.nlm.nih.gov/11114681/

431   Kiessling, Schneider, and Jahreis. "Long-term consumption of fermented dairy products over six months increases HDL cholesterol." *European Journal of Clinical Nutrition*, 2002. https://pubmed.ncbi.nlm.nih.gov/12209372/

[432] Khalesi, Sun, Buys, and Jayasinghe. "Effect of probiotics on blood pressure: a systematic review and meta-analysis of randomized, controlled trials." *Hypertension*, 2014. https://pubmed.ncbi.nlm.nih.gov/25047574/

[433] Chi, Cao, Zhang, Su, Yang, Li, Li, She, Wang, Gao, Ma, Zheng, Li, and Cui. "Environmental noise stress disturbs commensal microbiota homeostasis and induces oxi-inflammation and AD-like neuropathology through epithelial barrier disruption in the EOAD mouse model." *Journal of Neuroinflammation*, 2021. https://doi.org/10.1186/s12974-020-02053-3

[434] Akbari, Asemi, Kakhaki, Bahmani, Kouchaki, Tamtaji, Hamidi, and Salami. "Effect of probiotic supplementation on cognitive function and metabolic status in Alzheimer's disease: a randomized, double-blind and controlled trial." *Frontiers in Aging Neuroscience*, 2016. https://doi.org/10.3389/fnagi.2016.00256

[435] Jiang, Li, Huang, Liu, and Zhao. "The gut microbiota and Alzheimer's disease." *Journal of Alzheimer's Disease*, 2017. https://doi.org/10.3233/jad-161141

[436] Kowalski and Mulak. "Brain-gut-microbiota axis in Alzheimer's disease." *Journal of Neurogastroenterology and Motility*, 2019. https://www.ncbi.nlm.nih.gov/pmc/articles/PMC6326209/

[437] Meyer, Lulla, Debroy, Shikany, Yaffe, Meirelles, and Launer. "Association of the gut microbiota with cognitive function in midlife." *JAMA Network Open*, 2022. https://jamanetwork.com/journals/jamanetworkopen/fullarticle/2788843

[438] Forsythe, Bienenstock, and Kunze. "Vagal pathways for microbiome-brain-gut axis communication." *Advances in Experimental Medicine and Biology*, 2014. https://www.ncbi.nlm.nih.gov/pubmed/24997031

[439] Zhu, Grandhi, Patterson, and Nicholson. "A review of traumatic brain injury and the gut microbiome: insights into novel mechanisms of secondary brain injury and promising targets for neuroprotection. *Brain Sciences*, 2018. https://www.ncbi.nlm.nih.gov/pmc/articles/PMC6025245/

[440] Rice, Pandya, and Shear. "Gut microbiota as a therapeutic target to ameliorate the biochemical, neuroanatomical, and behavioral effects of traumatic brain injuries." *Frontiers in Neurology*, 2019. https://www.ncbi.nlm.nih.gov/pmc/articles/PMC6706789/

[441] Saleh, Peyssonnaux, Singh, and Edeas. "Mitochondria and microbiota dysfunction in COVID-19 pathogenesis." *Mitochondrion*, 2020. https://doi.org/10.1016/j.mito.2020.06.008

[442] Bicknell, Liebert, Johnstone, and Kiat. "Photobiomodulation of the microbiome: implications for metabolic and inflammatory diseases." *Lasers in Medical Science*, 2019. https://doi.org/10.1007/s10103-018-2594-6

[443] Bicknell, Liebert, McLachlan, and Kiat. "Microbiome changes in humans with Parkinson's disease after photobiomodulation therapy: a retrospective study." *Journal of Personalized Medicine*, 2022. https://doi.org/10.3390/jpm12010049

[444] Shil and Chichger. "Artificial sweeteners negatively regulate pathogenic characteristics of two model gut bacteria, E. coli and E. faecalis." *International Journal of Molecular Sciences*, 2021. https://www.mdpi.com/1422-0067/22/10/5228

[445] Ruiz-Ojeda, Plaza-Díaz, Sáez-Lara, and Gil. "Effects of sweeteners on the gut microbiota: a review of experimental studies and clinical trials." *Advances in Nutrition*, 2019. https://www.ncbi.nlm.nih.gov/pmc/articles/PMC6363527/

[446] Lutsey, Steffen, and Stevens. "Dietary intake and the development of metabolic syndrome: the Atherosclerosis Risk in Communities study." *Circulation*, 2008. https://pubmed.ncbi.nlm.nih.gov/18212291/

447 Fowler, Williams, Resendez, Hunt, Hazuda, and Stern. "Fueling the obesity epidemic? Artificially sweetened beverage use and long-term weight gain." *Obesity*, 2008. https://pubmed.ncbi.nlm.nih.gov/18535548/

448 Stellman and Garfinkel. "Artificial sweetener use and one-year weight change among women." *Preventive Medicine*, 1986. https://pubmed.ncbi.nlm.nih.gov/3714671/

449 Bianchi, Herrera, and Laura. "Effect of nutrition on neurodegenerative diseases. A systematic review." *Nutritional Neuroscience*, 2019. https://doi.org/10.1080/10284 15x.2019.1681088

450 Keys, Menotti, Karvonen, Aravanis, Blackburn, Buzina, Djordjevic, Dontas, Fidanza, and Keys. "The diet and 15-year death rate in the seven countries study." *American Journal of Epidemiology*, 1986. https://doi.org/10.1093/oxfordjournals.aje.a114480

451 Wu and Sun. "Adherence to Mediterranean diet and risk of developing cognitive disorders: an updated systematic review and meta-analysis of prospective cohort studies." *Scientific Reports*, 2017. https://doi.org/10.1038/srep41317

452 Anastasiou, Yannakoulia, Kosmidis, Dardiotis, Hadjigeorgiou, Sakka, Arampatzi, Bougea, Labropoulos, and Scarmeas. "Mediterranean diet and cognitive health: initial results from the Hellenic Longitudinal Investigation of Ageing and Diet." *PLoS One*, 2017. https://journals.plos.org/plosone/article?id=10.1371/journal.pone.0182048

453 Samadi, Moradi, Moradinazar, Mostafai, and Pasdar. "Dietary pattern in relation to the risk of Alzheimer's disease: a systematic review." *Neurological Sciences*, 2019. https://doi.org/10.1007/s10072-019-03976-3

454 Rusek, Pluta, Ulamek-Koziol, and Czuczwar. "Ketogenic diet in Alzheimer's disease." *International Journal of Molecular Sciences*, 2019. https://www.ncbi.nlm.nih.gov/pmc/articles/PMC6720297/

455 Wang, Hou, Lu, Jia, Qiu, Wang, Zhang, and Jiang. "Ketogenic diet attenuates neuronal injury via autophagy and mitochondrial pathways in pentylenetetrazol-kindled seizures." *Brain Research*, 2018. https://pubmed.ncbi.nlm.nih.gov/29056525/

456 Ruskin, Murphy, Slade, and Masino. "Ketogenic diet improves behaviors in a maternal immune activation model of autism spectrum disorder." *PLoS One*, 2017. https://www.ncbi.nlm.nih.gov/pmc/articles/PMC5293204/

457 Bourassa. "The use of transcranial low level laser therapy for the management of mild traumatic brain injury." *Chiropractic Economics*, 2017. https://www.chiroeco.com/mild-traumatic-brain-injury/

458 Pinto, Bonucci, Maggi, Corsi, and Businaro. "Anti-oxidant and anti-inflammatory activity of ketogenic diet: new perspectives for neuroprotection in Alzheimer's disease." *Antioxidants*, 2018. https://www.ncbi.nlm.nih.gov/pmc/articles/PMC5981249/

459 Dupuis, Curatolo, Benoist, and Auvin. "Ketogenic diet exhibits anti-inflammatory properties." *Epilepsia*, 2015. https://www.ilae.org/files/dmfile/Dupuis 2015 Epilepsia.pdf

460 Lange, Lange, Makulska-Gertruda, Nakamura, Reissmann, Kanaya, and Hauser. "Ketogenic diets and Alzheimer's disease." *Food Science and Human Wellness*, 2017. https://doi.org/10.1016/j.fshw.2016.10.003

461 Horner, Berger, and Gibas. "Nutritional ketosis and photobiomodulation remediate mitochondria warding off Alzheimer's disease in a diabetic ApoE4+ patient with mild cognitive impairment: a case report." *Photodiagnosis and Photodynamic Therapy*, 2020. https://doi.org/10.1016/j.pdpdt.2020.101777

462 Lin, Zhang, Gao, and Watts. "Caloric restriction increases ketone bodies metabolism and preserves blood flow in aging brain." *Neurobiology of Aging*, 2015. https://doi.org/10.1016/j.neurobiolaging.2015.03.012

463 Pinto, Bonucci, Maggi, Corsi, and Businaro. "Anti-oxidant and anti-inflammatory activity of ketogenic diet: new perspectives for neuroprotection in Alzheimer's disease." *Antioxidants*, 2018. https://www.ncbi.nlm.nih.gov/pmc/articles/PMC5981249/

464 Schulz, Zarse, Voigt, Urban, Birringer, and Ristow. "Glucose restriction extends *Caenorhabditis elegans* lifespan by inducing mitochondrial respiration and increasing oxidative stress." *Cell Metabolism*, 2007. https://www.sciencedirect.com/science/article/pii/S1550413107002562

465 Klaus and Ost. "Mitochondrial uncoupling and longevity – A role for mitokines?" *Experimental Gerontology*, 2020. https://doi.org/10.1016/j.exger.2019.110796

466 Lee, Duan, Long, Ingram, and Mattson. "Dietary restriction increases the number of newly generated neural cells and induces BDNF expression in the dentate gyrus of rats." *Journal of Molecular Neuroscience*, 2000. https://doi.org/10.1385/jmn:15:2:99

467 Brownlow, Benner, Joly-Amado, Azam, D'Agostino, Gordon, and Morgan. "Calorie restriction, but not ketogenic diet, improves cognition in mouse models of Alzheimer's pathology." *Alzheimer's & Dementia*, 2013. https://doi.org/10.1016/j.jalz.2013.05.240

468 Wang, Yang, Liao, Li, Zhang, Santos, Kord-Varkaneh, and Abshirini. "Effects of intermittent fasting diets on plasma concentrations of inflammatory biomarkers: a systematic review and meta-analysis of randomized controlled trials." *Nutrition*, 2020. https://doi.org/10.1016/j.nut.2020.110974

469 Mattson, Moehl, Ghena, Schmaedick, and Cheng. "Intermittent metabolic switching, neuroplasticity, and brain health." *Nature Reviews Neuroscience*, 2018. https://www.ncbi.nlm.nih.gov/pmc/articles/PMC5913738/

470 Andika, Yoon, Kim, and Jeong. "Intermittent fasting alleviates cognitive impairments and hippocampal neuronal loss but enhances astrocytosis in mice with subcortical vascular dementia." *Journal of Nutrition*, 2021. https://doi.org/10.1093/jn/nxaa384

471 Dias, Murphy, Stangl, Ahmet, Morisse, Nix, Aimone, Aimone, Kuro-O, Gage, and Thuret. "Intermittent fasting enhances long-term memory consolidation, adult hippocampal neurogenesis, and expression of longevity gene Klotho." *Molecular Psychiatry*, 2021. https://www.nature.com/articles/s41380-021-01102-4

472 Goodrick, Ingram, Reynolds, Freeman, and Cider. "Effects of intermittent feeding upon growth and life span in rats." *Gerontology*, 1982. https://doi.org/10.1159/000212538

473 Sogawa and Kubo. "Influence of short-term repeated fasting on the longevity of female (NZB x NZW)F1 mice." *Mechanisms of Ageing and Development*, 2000. https://doi.org/10.1016/s0047-6374(00)00109-3

474 Baik, Rajeev, Fann, Jo, and Arumugam. "Intermittent fasting increases adult hippocampal neurogenesis." *Brain and Behavior*, 2020. https://www.ncbi.nlm.nih.gov/pmc/articles/PMC6955834/

475 Zhu, Yan, Gius, and Vassilopoulos. "Metabolic regulation of sirtuins upon fasting and the implication for cancer." *Current Opinion in Oncology*, 2013. https://www.ncbi.nlm.nih.gov/pmc/articles/PMC5525320/

476 Rudman, Feller, Nagraj, Gergans, Lalitha, Goldberg, Schlenker, Cohn, Rudman, and Mattson. "Effects of human growth hormone in men over 60 years old." *New England Journal of Medicine*, 1990. https://www.ncbi.nlm.nih.gov/pmc/articles/PMC7856758/

477 Mager, Wan, Brown, Cheng, Wareski, Abernethy, and Mattson. "Caloric restriction and intermittent fasting alter spectral measures of heart rate and blood pressure variability in rats." *FASEB Journal: Official Publication of the Federation of American Societies for Experimental Biology*, 2006. https://faseb.onlinelibrary.wiley.com/doi/epdf/10.1096/fj.05-5263com

[478] Shin, Kang, Kim, and Park. "Intermittent fasting protects against the deterioration of cognitive function, energy metabolism, and dyslipidemia in Alzheimer's disease-induced estrogen-deficient rats." *Experimental Biology and Medicine*, 2018. https://www.ncbi.nlm.nih.gov/pmc/articles/PMC6022926/

[479] Varady, Cienfuegos, Ezpeleta, and Gabel. "Cardiometabolic benefits of intermittent fasting." *Annual Review of Nutrition*, 2021. https://doi.org/10.1146/annurev-nutr-052020-041327

[480] Yang, Liu, Liu, Pan, Li, Tian, Sun, Yang, Zhao, An, Yang, Gao, and Xing. "Effect of epidemic intermittent fasting on cardiometabolic risk factors: a systematic review and meta-analysis of randomized controlled trials." *Frontiers in Nutrition*, 2021. https://www.ncbi.nlm.nih.gov/pmc/articles/PMC8558421/

[481] Albosta and Bakke. "Intermittent fasting: Is there a role in the treatment of diabetes? A review of the literature and guide for primary care physicians." *Clinical Diabetes and Endocrinology*, 2021. https://www.ncbi.nlm.nih.gov/pmc/articles/PMC7856758/

[482] Cignarella, Cantoni, Ghezzi, Salter, Dorsett, Chen, Phillips, Weinstock, Fontana, Cross, Zhou, and Piccio. "Intermittent fasting confers protection in CNS autoimmunity by altering the gut microbiota." *Cell Metabolism*, 2018. https://www.ncbi.nlm.nih.gov/pmc/articles/PMC6460288/

[483] Bagherniya, Butler, Barreto, and Sahebkar. "The effect of fasting or calorie restriction on autophagy induction: a review of the literature." *Ageing Research Reviews*, 2018. https://doi.org/10.1016/j.arr.2018.08.004

[484] Chung and Chung. "The effects of calorie restriction on autophagy: role on aging intervention." *Nutrients*, 2019. https://www.ncbi.nlm.nih.gov/pmc/articles/PMC6950580/

[485] Longo and Mattson. "Fasting: molecular mechanisms and clinical applications." *Cell Metabolism*, 2015. https://www.ncbi.nlm.nih.gov/pmc/articles/PMC3946160/

[486] Martin, Mattson, and Maudsley. "Caloric restriction and intermittent fasting: two potential diets for successful brain aging." *Ageing Research Reviews*, 2006. https://www.ncbi.nlm.nih.gov/pmc/articles/PMC2622429/

[487] Zhu, Yan, Gius, and Vassilopoulos. "Metabolic regulation of Sirtuins upon fasting and the implication for cancer." *Current Opinion in Oncology*, 2013. https://pubmed.ncbi.nlm.nih.gov/24048020/

[488] Kim and Lemasters. "Mitochondrial degradation by autophagy (mitophagy) in GFP-LC3 transgenic hepatocytes during nutrient deprivation." *American Journal of Physiology: Cell Physiology*, 2011. https://pubmed.ncbi.nlm.nih.gov/21106691/

[489] Alirezaei, Kemball, Flynn, Wood, Whitton, and Kiosses. "Short-term fasting induces profound neuronal autophagy." *Autophagy*, 2010. https://www.ncbi.nlm.nih.gov/pmc/articles/PMC3106288/

[490] Heilbronn, Smith, Martin, Anton, and Ravussin. "Alternate-day fasting in nonobese subjects: effects on body weight, body composition, and energy metabolism." *American Journal of Clinical Nutrition*, 2005. https://doi.org/10.1093/ajcn/81.1.69

[491] Rudman, Feller, Nagraj, Gergans, Lalitha, Goldberg, Schlenker, Cohn, Rudman, and Mattson. "Effects of human growth hormone in men over 60 years old." *New England Journal of Medicine*, 1990. https://www.nejm.org/doi/full/10.1056/NEJM199007053230101

[492] Blackman, Sorkin, Münzer, Bellantoni, Busby-Whitehead, Stevens, Jayme, O'Connor, Christmas, Tobin, Stewart, Cottrell, St. Clair, Pabst, and Harman. "Growth hormone and sex steroid administration in healthy aged women and men: a randomized con-

trolled trial." *Journal of the American Medical Association*, 2002. https://jamanetwork.com/journals/jama/fullarticle/1108358

[493] Hartman, Veldhuis, Johnson, Lee, Alberti, Samojlik, and Thorner. "Augmented growth hormone (GH) secretory burst frequency and amplitude mediate enhanced GH secretion during a two-day fast in normal men." *Journal of Clinical Endocrinology and Metabolism*, 1992. https://pubmed.ncbi.nlm.nih.gov/1548337/

[494] Ho, Veldhuis, Johnson, Furlanetto, Evans, Alberti, and Thorner. "Fasting enhances growth hormone secretion and amplifies the complex rhythms of growth hormone secretion in man." *Journal of Clinical Investigation*, 1988. https://www.ncbi.nlm.nih.gov/pmc/articles/PMC329619/

[495] Barnosky, Hoddy, Unterman, and Varady. "Intermittent fasting vs daily calorie restriction for type 2 diabetes prevention: a review of human findings." *Translational Research*, 2014. https://www.sciencedirect.com/science/article/abs/pii/S193152441400200X

[496] Lewis and Bailes. "Neuroprotection for the warrior: dietary supplementation with omega-3 fatty acids." *Military Medicine*, 2011. https://doi.org/10.7205/MILMED-D-10-00466

[497] Raatz and Bibus. *Fish and Fish Oil in Health and Disease Prevention*. Elsevier, 2016. https://doi.org/10.1016/C2014-0-02727-X

[498] Scrimgeour and Condlin. "Nutritional treatment for traumatic brain injury." *Journal of Neurotrauma*, 2014. https://doi.org/10.1089/neu.2013.3234

[499] Breit, Kupferberg, Rogler, and Hasler. "Vagus nerve as modulator of the brain-gut axis in psychiatric and inflammatory disorders." *Frontiers in Psychiatry*, 2018. https://www.frontiersin.org/article/10.3389/fpsyt.2018.00044

[500] Holt-Lunstad, Smith, Baker, Harris, and Stephenson. "Loneliness and Social Isolation as Risk Factors for Mortality: A Meta-Analytic Review." *Perspectives on Psychological Science*, 2015. https://doi.org/10.1177/1745691614568352

[501] Baumgarten, Hanley, Infante-Rivard, Battista, Becker, and Gauthier. "Health of family members caring for elderly persons with dementia: a longitudinal study." *Annals of Internal Medicine*, 1994. https://doi.org/10.7326/0003-4819-120-2-199401150-00005

[502] Pinquart and Sörensen. "Differences between caregivers and noncaregivers in psychological health and physical health: a meta-analysis." *Psychology and Aging*, 2003. https://www.researchgate.net/publication/10691251

[503] Allen, Curran, Duggan, Cryan, Chorcoráin, Dinan, Molloy, Kearney, and Clarke. "A systematic review of the psychological burden of informal caregiving for patients with dementia: focus on cognitive and biological markers of chronic stress." *Neuroscience & Biobehavioral Reviews*, 2017. https://doi.org/10.1016/j.neubiorev.2016.12.006

[504] Ma, Dorstyn, Ward, and Prentice. "Alzheimer's disease and caregiving: a meta-analytic review comparing the mental health of primary carers to controls." *Aging & Mental Health*, 2017. https://doi.org/10.1080/13607863.2017.1370689

[505] Kim. "Relationships between caregiving stress, depression, and self-esteem in family caregivers of adults with a disability." *Occupational Therapy International*, 2017. https://www.ncbi.nlm.nih.gov/pmc/articles/PMC5664279/

[506] Hawken, Turner-Cobb, and Barnett. "Coping and adjustment in caregivers: a systematic review." *Health Psychology Open*, 2018. https://journals.sagepub.com/doi/pdf/10.1177/2055102918810659

[507] Fonareva and Oken. "Physiological and functional consequences of caregiving for relatives with dementia." *International Psychogeriatrics*, 2014. https://doi.org/10.1017/S1041610214000039

REFERENCES

508 Alzheimer's Association 2022 *Alzheimer's Disease Facts and Figures*. https://www.alz.org/alzheimers-dementia/facts-figures

509 Chiu, Lee, Wang, Chang, Li, Hsu, and Lee. "Family caregivers' sleep disturbance and its associations with multilevel stressors when caring for patients with dementia." *Aging & Mental Health*, 2014. https://doi.org/10.1080/13607863.2013.837141

510 Gao, Chapagain, and Scullin. "Sleep duration and sleep quality in caregivers of patients with dementia: a systematic review and meta-analysis." *JAMA Network Open*, 2019. https://jamanetwork.com/journals/jamanetworkopen/fullarticle/2748661

511 de Vugt, Jolles, van Osch, Stevens, Aalten, Lousberg, and Verhey. "Cognitive functioning in spousal caregivers of dementia patients: findings from the prospective MAASBED study." *Age and Ageing*, 2006. https://doi.org/10.1093/ageing/afj044

512 Vitaliano, Zhang, Young, Caswell, Scanlan, and Echeverria. "Depressed mood mediates decline in cognitive processing speed in caregivers." *Gerontologist*, 2009. https://doi.org/10.1093/geront/gnp004

513 Oken, Fonareva, and Wahbeh. "Stress-related cognitive dysfunction in dementia caregivers." *Journal of Geriatric Psychiatry and Neurology*, 2011. https://www.ncbi.nlm.nih.gov/pmc/articles/PMC3340013/

514 Corrêa, Vedovelli, Giacobbo, de Souza, Ferrari, de Lima Argimon, Walz, Kapczinski, and Bromberg. "Psychophysiological correlates of cognitive deficits in family caregivers of patients with Alzheimer disease." *Neuroscience*, 2015. https://doi.org/10.1016/j.neuroscience.2014.11.052

515 Dassel, Carr, and Vitaliano. "Does caring for a spouse with dementia accelerate cognitive decline? Findings from the Health and Retirement Study." *Gerontologist*, 2017. https://doi.org/10.1093/geront/gnv148

516 Schulz, O'Brien, Bookwala, and Fleissner. "Psychiatric and physical morbidity effects of dementia caregiving: prevalence, correlates, and causes." *Gerontologist*, 1995. https://doi.org/10.1093/geront/35.6.771

517 Dassel and Carr. "Does dementia caregiving accelerate frailty? Findings from the Health and Retirement Study." *Gerontologist*, 2016. https://doi.org/10.1093/geront/gnu078

518 Norton, Smith, Ostbye, Tschanz, Corcoran, Schwartz, Piercy, Rabins, Steffens, Skoog, Breitner, and Welsh-Bohmer. "Increased risk of dementia when spouse has dementia? The Cache County Study." *Journal of the American Geriatrics Society*, 2010. https://www.ncbi.nlm.nih.gov/pmc/articles/PMC2945313/

519 Roepke, Mausbach, Patterson, von Känel, Ancoli-Israel, Harmell, Dimsdale, Aschbacher, Mills, Ziegler, Allison, and Grant. "Effects of Alzheimer caregiving on allostatic load." *Journal of Health Psychology*, 2011. https://www.ncbi.nlm.nih.gov/pmc/articles/PMC3161622/

520 Karg, Graessel, Randzio, and Pendergrass. "Dementia as a predictor of care-related quality of life in informal caregivers: a cross-sectional study to investigate differences in health-related outcomes between dementia and non-dementia caregivers." *BMC Geriatrics*, 2018. https://link.springer.com/article/10.1186/s12877-018-0885-1

521 DiDuro. "Care for the caregivers: a novel, home-based therapy to boost caregiver resiliency." medium.com, 2023. https://drjoe-69223.medium.com/care-for-the-caregiver-a-novel-home-based-therapy-to-boost-caregiver-resiliency-e0bfa66b8d91

522 Salehpour, Hamblin, and DiDuro. "Rapid reversal of cognitive decline, olfactory dysfunction, and quality of life using multi-modality photobiomodulation therapy: case report." *Photobiomodulation, Photomedicine, and Laser Surgery*, 2019. https://doi.org/10.1089/photob.2018.4569

523 Alzheimer's Association 2022 *Alzheimer's Disease Facts and Figures*. https://www.alz.org/alzheimers-dementia/facts-figures

524 GBD 2019 Dementia Forecasting Collaborators. "Estimation of the global prevalence of dementia in 2019 and forecasted prevalence in 2050: an analysis for the Global Burden of Disease Study 2019." *The Lancet Public Health*, 2022. https://www.thelancet.com/journals/lanpub/article/PIIS2468-2667(21)00249-8/fulltext#seccestitle10

525 Alzheimer's Research & Prevention Foundation website, 2022. https://alzheimersprevention.org/

526 Alzheimer's Association 2022 *Alzheimer's Disease Facts and Figures*. https://www.alz.org/alzheimers-dementia/facts-figures

527 Liu, Hlavka, Hillestad, and Mattke. "Assessing the preparedness of the U.S. health care system infrastructure for an Alzheimer's treatment." RAND Corporation, 2017. https://www.rand.org/pubs/research_reports/RR2272.html

528 Hlavka, Mattke, and Liu. "Assessing the preparedness of the health care system infrastructure in six European countries for an Alzheimer's treatment." *Rand Health Quarterly*, 2019. https://www.ncbi.nlm.nih.gov/pmc/articles/PMC6557037/

529 Deb, Thornton, Sambamoorthi, and Innes. "Direct and indirect cost of managing Alzheimer's disease and related dementias in the United States." *Expert Review of Pharmacoeconomics & Outcomes Research*, 2017. https://www.ncbi.nlm.nih.gov/pmc/articles/PMC5494694/

530 Jessen, Munk, Lundgaard, and Nedergaard. "The glymphatic system: a beginner's guide." *Neurochemical Research*, 2015. https://link.springer.com/article/10.1007/s11064-015-1581-6

531 Xin, Tan, Cao, Yu, and Tan. "Clearance of amyloid beta and tau in Alzheimer's disease: from mechanisms to therapy." *Neurotoxicity Research*, 2018. https://link.springer.com/article/10.1007/s12640-018-9895-1

532 Lananna, McKee, King, Del-Aguila, Dimitry, Farias, Nadarajah, Xiong, Guo, Cammack, Elias, Zhang, Cruchaga, and Musiek. "*Chi3l1*/YKL-40 is controlled by the astrocyte circadian clock and regulates neuroinflammation and Alzheimer's disease pathogenesis." *Science Translational Medicine*, 2020. https://www.science.org/doi/10.1126/scitranslmed.aax3519

533 Mogensen, Delle, and Nedergaard. "The glymphatic system (en)during inflammation." *International Journal of Molecular Sciences*, 2021. https://www.researchgate.net/publication/353240231

534 Xie, Kang, Xu, Chen, Liao, Thiyagarajan, O'Donnell, Christensen, Iliff, Takano, Deane, and Nedergaard. "Sleep drives metabolite clearance from the adult brain." *Science*, 2013. https://www.ncbi.nlm.nih.gov/pmc/articles/PMC3880190/

535 Fultz, Bonmassar, Setsompop, Stickgold, Rosen, Polimeni, and Lewis. "Coupled electrophysiological, hemodynamic, and cerebrospinal fluid oscillations in human sleep." *Science*, 2019. https://science.sciencemag.org/content/366/6465/628/tab-article-info

536 Han, Chen, Belkin-Rosen, Gu, Luo, Buxton, and Liu. "Reduced coupling between cerebrospinal fluid flow and global brain activity is linked to Alzheimer's disease-related pathology." *PLOS Biology*, 2021. https://journals.plos.org/plosbiology/article?id=10.1371/journal.pbio.3001233

537 Chylinski, Van Egroo, Narbutas, Muto, Bahri, Berthomier, Salmon, Bastin, Phillips, Collette, Maquet, Carrier, Lina, and Vandewalle. "Timely coupling of sleep spindles and slow waves linked to early amyloid-ß burden and predicts memory decline." *eLife*, 2022. https://www.ncbi.nlm.nih.gov/pmc/articles/PMC9177143/

REFERENCES

538   Ju, Lucey, and Holtzman. "Sleep and Alzheimer disease pathology: a bidirectional relationship." *Nature Reviews: Neurology*, 2014. https://www.ncbi.nlm.nih.gov/pmc/articles/PMC3979317/

539   Louveau, da Mesquita, and Kipnis. "Lymphatics in neurological disorders? A neuro-lympho-vascular component of multiple sclerosis and Alzheimer's disease?" *Neuron*, 2016. https://pubmed.ncbi.nlm.nih.gov/27608759/

540   de la Torre. "The Mobius circle of Alzheimer research." *Biochemistry and Molecular Biology*, 2013.

541   da Mesquita, Louveau, Vaccari, Smirnov, Cornelison, Kingsmore, Contarino, Onengut-Gumuscu, Farber, Raper, Viar, Powell, Baker, Dabhi, Bai, Cao, Hu, Rich, Munson, Lopes, Overall, Acton, and Kipnis. "Functional aspects of meningeal lymphatics in ageing and Alzheimer's disease." *Nature*, 2018. https://pubmed.ncbi.nlm.nih.gov/30046111/

542   Zou, Pu, Feng, Lu, Zheng, Du, Xiao, and Hu. "Blocking meningeal lymphatic drainage aggravates Parkinson's disease-like pathology in mice overexpressing mutated α-synuclein." *Translational Neurodegeneration*, 2019. https://translationalneurodegeneration.biomedcentral.com/articles/10.1186/s40035-019-0147-y

543   Iliff, Chen, Plog, Zeppenfeld, Soltero, Yang, Singh, Deane, and Nedergaard. "Impairment of glymphatic pathway function promotes tau pathology after traumatic brain injury." *Journal of Neuroscience*, 2014. https://www.ncbi.nlm.nih.gov/pmc/articles/PMC4252540/

544   Nedergaard and Goldman. "Glymphatic failure as a final common pathway to dementia." *Science*, 2020. https://www.ncbi.nlm.nih.gov/pmc/articles/PMC8186542/

545   Piantino, Lim, Newgard, and Iliff. "Linking traumatic brain injury, sleep disruption and post-traumatic headache: a potential role for glymphatic pathway dysfunction." *Current Pain and Headache Reports*, 2019. https://pubmed.ncbi.nlm.nih.gov/31359173/

546   Semyachkina-Glushkovskaya, Postnov, Lavrova, Fedosov, Borisova, Nikolenko, Penzel, Kurths, and Tuchin. "Biophotonic strategies of measurement and stimulation of the cranial and the extracranial lymphatic drainage function." *IEEE Journal of Selected Topics in Quantum Electronics*, 2021. https://ieeexplore.ieee.org/document/9298844

547   Zhao, Liu, Wei, Li, Liu, Ma, Shang, Jiang, Huo, Wang, and Qu. "Chronic sleep restriction induces Aß accumulation by disrupting the balance of Aß production and clearance in rats." *Neurochemical Research*, 2019. https://link.springer.com/article/10.1007/s11064-019-02719-2

548   Qiu, Zhong, Liu, Zhang, Li, and Le. "Chronic sleep deprivation exacerbates learning memory disability and Alzheimer's disease-like pathologies in AßPP(swe)/PS1(ΔE9) mice." *Journal of Alzheimer's Disease*, 2016. https://pubmed.ncbi.nlm.nih.gov/26757041/

549   Ju, McLeland, Toedebusch, Xiong, Fagan, Duntley, Morris, and Holtzman. "Sleep quality and preclinical Alzheimer disease." *JAMA Neurology*, 2013. https://jamanetwork.com/journals/jamaneurology/fullarticle/1663363

550   Robbins, Weaver, Barger, Wang, Quan, and Czeisler. "Sleep difficulties, incident dementia and all-cause mortality among older adults across 8 years: Findings from the National Health and Aging Trends Study." *Journal of Sleep Research*, 2021. https://onlinelibrary.wiley.com/doi/10.1111/jsr.13395

551   Sabia, Fayosse, Dumurgier, van Hees, Paquet, Sommerlad, Kivimäki, Dugravot, and Singh-Manoux. "Association of sleep duration in middle and old age with incidence of dementia." *Nature Communications*, 2021. https://www.nature.com/articles/s41467-021-22354-2

552   Abulafia, Duarte-Abritta, Villarreal, Ladrón-de-Guevara, Garcia, Sequeyra, Sevlever, Fiorentini, Bär, Gustafson, Vigo, and Guinjoan. "Relationship between cognitive and sleep-wake variables in asymptomatic offspring of patients with late-onset Alzheimer's disease." *Frontiers in Aging Neuroscience*, 2017. https://www.ncbi.nlm.nih.gov/pmc/articles/PMC5380732/

553   Reddy and van der Werf. "The sleeping brain: harnessing the power of the glymphatic system through lifestyle choices." *Brain Science*, 2020. https://www.ncbi.nlm.nih.gov/pmc/articles/PMC7698404/

554   Shokri-Kojori, Wang, Wiers, Demiral, Guo, Kim, Lindgren, Ramirez, Zehra, Freeman, Miller, Manza, Srivastava, Santi, Tomasi, Benveniste, and Volkow. "ß-amyloid accumulation in the human brain after one night of sleep deprivation." *Proceedings of the National Academy of Science*, 2018. https://www.pnas.org/doi/10.1073/pnas.1721694115

555   Ahmadian, Hejazi, Mahmoudi, and Talebi. "Tau pathology of Alzheimer disease: possible role of sleep deprivation." *Basic and Clinical Neuroscience*, 2018. https://bcn.iums.ac.ir/article-1-1039-en.html

556   Holth, Fritschi, Wang, Pedersen, Cirrito, Mahan, Finn, Manis, Geerling, Fuller, Lucey, and Holtzman. "The sleep-wake cycle regulates brain interstitial fluid tau in mice and CSF tau in humans." *Science*, 2019. https://www.ncbi.nlm.nih.gov/pmc/articles/PMC6410369/

557   Sprecher, Koscik, Carlsson, Zetterberg, Blennow, Okonkwo, Sager, Asthana, Johnson, Benca, and Bendlin. "Poor sleep is associated with CSF biomarkers of amyloid pathology in cognitively normal adults." *Neurology*, 2017. https://www.ncbi.nlm.nih.gov/pmc/articles/PMC5539733/

558   Ju, Ooms, Sutphen, Macauley, Zangrilli, Jerome, Fagan, Mignot, Zempel, Claassen, and Holtzman. "Slow wave sleep disruption increases cerebrospinal fluid amyloid-ß levels." *Brain*, 2017. https://academic.oup.com/brain/article/140/8/2104/3933862

559   Martucci, Conte, Ostan, Chiarello, Miele, Franceschi, Salvioli, Santoro, and Provini. "Both objective and paradoxical insomnia elicit a stress response involving mitokine production." *Aging*, 2020. https://www.ncbi.nlm.nih.gov/pmc/articles/PMC7346035/

560   Winer, Mander, Helfrich, Maass, Harrison, Baker, Knight, Jagust, and Walker. "Sleep as a potential biomarker of tau and ß-amyloid burden in the human brain." *Journal of Neuroscience*, 2019. https://www.ncbi.nlm.nih.gov/pmc/articles/PMC6687908/

561   Kresge, Khan, Wagener, Liu, Terry, Nair, Cambronero, Gifford, Osborn, Hohman, Pechman, Bell, Wang, Carr, and Jefferson. "Subclinical compromise in cardiac strain relates to lower cognitive performances in older adults." *Journal of the American Heart Association*, 2018. https://www.ncbi.nlm.nih.gov/pmc/articles/PMC5850190/

562   Dominy, Lynch, Ermini, Benedyk, Marczyk, Konradi, Nguyen, Haditsch, Raha, Griffin, Holsinger, Arastu-Kapur, Kaba, Lee, Ryder, Potempa, Mydel, Hellvard, Adamowicz, Hasturk, Walker, Reynolds, Faull, Curtis, Dragunow, and Potempa. "*Porphyromonas gingivalis* in Alzheimer's disease brains: evidence for disease causation and treatment with small-molecule inhibitors." *Science Advances*, 2019. https://www.ncbi.nlm.nih.gov/pmc/articles/PMC6357742/

563   Nicolini, Ciulla, Malfatto, Abbate, Mari, Rossi, Pettenuzzo, Magrini, Consonni, and Lombardi. "Autonomic dysfunction in mild cognitive impairment: evidence from power spectral analysis of heart rate variability in a cross-sectional case-control study." *PLOS One*, 2014. https://journals.plos.org/plosone/article?id=10.1371/journal.pone.0096656

564 Werner. "Mild cognitive impairment and caregiver burden: a critical review and research agenda." *Public Health Reviews*, 2012. https://publichealthreviews.biomedcentral.com/articles/10.1007/BF03391684

565 Abulafia, Fiorentini, Loewenstein, Curiel-Cid, Sevlever, Nemeroff, Villarreal, Vigo, and Guinjoan. "Executive functioning in cognitively normal middle-aged offspring of late-onset Alzheimer's disease patients." *Journal of Psychiatric Research*, 2019. https://doi.org/10.1016/j.jpsychires.2019.02.016

566 Abulafia, Duarte-Abritta, Villarreal, Ladrón-de-Guevara, García, Sequeyra, Sevlever, Fiorentini, Bär, Gustafson, Vigo, and Guinjoan. "Relationship between cognitive and sleep-wake variables in asymptomatic offspring of patients with late-onset Alzheimer's disease." *Frontiers in Aging Neuroscience*, 2017. https://www.frontiersin.org/articles/10.3389/fnagi.2017.00093/full

567 Abulafia, Loewenstein, Curiel-Cid, Duarte-Abritta, Sánchez, Vigo, Castro, Drucaroff, Vázquez, Sevlever, Nemeroff, Guinjoan, and Villarreal. "Brain structural and amyloid correlates of recovery from semantic interference in cognitively normal individuals with or without family history of late-onset Alzheimer's disease." *Journal of Neuropsychiatry and Clinical Neuroscience*, 2019. https://doi.org/10.1176/appi.neuropsych.17120355

568 Duarte-Abritta, Villarreal, Abulafia, Loewenstein, Curiel Cid, Castro, Surace, Sánchez, Vigo, Vázquez, Nemeroff, Sevlever, and Guinjoan. "Cortical thickness, brain metabolic activity, and in vivo amyloid deposition in asymptomatic, middle-aged offspring of patients with late-onset Alzheimer's disease." *Journal of Psychiatric Research*, 2018. https://doi.org/10.1016/j.jpsychires.2018.10.008

569 Wilson, Abulafia, Loewenstein, Vigo, Sevlever, Nemeroff, Villarreal, and Guinjoan. "Individual cognitive and depressive traits associated with maternal versus paternal family history of late-onset Alzheimer's disease: proactive semantic interference versus standard neuropsychological assessments." *Personalized Medicine in Psychiatry*, 2018. https://doi.org/10.1016/j.pmip.2018.09.002

570 Pugh, Jaramillo, Eapen, Roman, and Kent. "The nexus of traumatic brain injury and mild cognitive impairment. *Neurology*, 2013. https://n.neurology.org/content/80/7_Supplement/P03.102

571 LoBue, Denney, Hynan, Rossetti, Lacritz, Hart, Womack, Woon, and Cullum. "Self-reported traumatic brain injury and mild cognitive impairment: increased risk and earlier age of diagnosis." *Journal of Alzheimer's Disease*, 2016. https://www.ncbi.nlm.nih.gov/pmc/articles/PMC4853649/

572 Hu, Zhang, Li, Tan, Li, Xu, and Chen. "Sleep disturbance in mild cognitive impairment: a systematic review of objective measures." *Neurological Sciences*, 2017. https://pubmed.ncbi.nlm.nih.gov/28455768/

573 Westerberg, Mander, Florczak, Weintraub, Mesulam, Zee, and Paller. "Concurrent impairments in sleep and memory in amnestic mild cognitive impairment." *Journal of the International Neuropsychological Society*, 2012. https://www.ncbi.nlm.nih.gov/pmc/articles/PMC3468412/

574 Cai, Li, Zhang, Shi, Liao, Li, Cheng, Tan, and Rong. "Characteristics of sleep structure assessed by objective measurements in patients with amnestic mild cognitive impairment: a meta-analysis." *Frontiers in Neurology*, 2020. https://www.ncbi.nlm.nih.gov/pmc/articles/PMC7689212/

575 Sjögren, Hellström, Jonsson, Runnerstam, Silander, and Ben-Menachem. "Cognition-enhancing effect of vagus nerve stimulation in patients with Alzheimer's disease: a pilot study." *Journal of Clinical Psychiatry*, 2002. https://pubmed.ncbi.nlm.nih.gov/16965193/

576   Merrill, Jonsson, Minthon, Ejnell, Silander, Blennow, Karlsson, Nordlund, Rolstad, Warkentin, Ben-Menachem, and Sjögren. "Vagus nerve stimulation in patients with Alzheimer's disease: additional follow-up results of a pilot study through 1 year." *Journal of Clinical Psychiatry*, 2006. https://pubmed.ncbi.nlm.nih.gov/16965193/

577   Broncel, Bocian, Kłos-Wojtczak, Kulbat-Warycha, and Konopacki. "Vagal nerve stimulation as a promising tool in the improvement of cognitive disorders." *Brain Research Bulletin*, 2020. https://doi.org/10.1016/j.brainresbull.2019.11.011

578   Vargas-Caballero, Warming, Walker, Holmes, Cruickshank, and Patel. "Vagus nerve stimulation as a potential therapy in early Alzheimer's disease: a review." *Frontiers in Human Neuroscience*, 2022. https://www.ncbi.nlm.nih.gov/pmc/articles/PMC9098960/

579   Rangon, Krantic, Moyse, and Fougère. "The vagal autonomic pathway of COVID-19 at the crossroad of Alzheimer's disease and aging: a review of knowledge." *Journal of Alzheimer's Disease Reports* 4, 2020. https://www.ncbi.nlm.nih.gov/pmc/articles/PMC7835993/

580   Rangon, Krantic, Moyse, and Fougere. "The vagal autonomic pathway of COVID-19 at the crossroad of Alzheimer's disease and aging: a review of knowledge." *Journal of Alzheimer's Disease Reports* 4, 2020. https://www.ncbi.nlm.nih.gov/pmc/articles/PMC7835993/

581   Chang, Koo, Yu, Kan, Chu, Hsu, and Chen. "The effect of t'ai chi exercise on autonomic nervous function of patients with coronary artery disease." *Journal of Alternative and Complementary Medicine*, 2008. https://doi.org/10.1089/acm.2008.0166

582   Goldbeck, Xie, Hautzinger, Fallgatter, Sudeck, and Ehlis. "Relaxation or regulation: the acute effect of mind-body exercise on heart rate variability and subjective state in experienced qi gong practitioners." *Evidence-Based Complementary and Alternative Medicine*, 2021. https://www.ncbi.nlm.nih.gov/pmc/articles/PMC8208883/

583   Damerla, Goldstein, Wolf, Madhavan, and Patterson. "Novice meditators of an easily learnable audible mantram sound self-induce an increase in vagal tone during short-term practice: a preliminary study." *Integrative Medicine: A Clinician's Journal*, 2018. https://www.ncbi.nlm.nih.gov/pmc/articles/PMC6469452/

584   Manjunath and Telles. "Effects of sirsasana (headstand) practice on autonomic and respiratory variables." *Indian Journal of Physiology and Pharmacology*, 2003. https://pubmed.ncbi.nlm.nih.gov/12708122/

585   Breit, Kupferberg, Rogler, and Hasler. "Vagus nerve as modulator of the brain-gut axis in psychiatric and inflammatory disorders." *Frontiers in Psychiatry*, 2018. https://www.frontiersin.org/articles/10.3389/fpsyt.2018.00044/full

586   Vásquez-Trincado, Garcia-Carvajal, Pennanen, Parra, Hill, Rothermel, and Lavandero. "Mitochondrial dynamics, mitophagy and cardiovascular disease." *Journal of Physiology*, 2016. https://www.ncbi.nlm.nih.gov/pmc/articles/PMC5341713/

587   Nicolini, Mari, Abbate, Inglese, Bertagnoli, Tomasini, Rossi, and Lombardi. "Autonomic function in amnestic and non-amnestic mild cognitive impairment: spectral heart rate variability analysis provides evidence for a brain-heart axis." *Scientific Reports*, 2020. https://doi.org/10.1038/s41598-020-68131-x

588   Esterov and Greenwald. "Autonomic dysfunction after mild traumatic brain injury." *Brain Sciences*, 2017. https://www.mdpi.com/2076-3425/7/8/100

589   Thayer and Lane. "Claude Bernard and the heart-brain connection: further elaboration of a model of neurovisceral integration." *Neuroscience and Behavioral Reviews*, 2009. https://pubmed.ncbi.nlm.nih.gov/18771686/

REFERENCES

590 Elias and Torres. "The renaissance of heart rate variability as a predictor of cognitive functioning." *Maine-Syracuse Longitudinal Papers*, 2017. https://digitalcommons.library. umaine.edu/longitudinal_papers/70/

591 Da Silva, Ramalho Oliveira, Tavares Mello, Moraes, Deslandes, and Laks. "Heart rate variability indexes in dementia: a systematic review with a quantitative analysis." *Current Alzheimer Research*, 2018. https://pubmed.ncbi.nlm.nih.gov/28558638/

592 Elias, Goodell, and Dore. "Hypertension and cognitive functioning: a perspective in historical context." *Hypertension*, 2012. https://www.ahajournals.org/doi/10.1161/ HYPERTENSIONAHA.111.186429

593 Hansen, Johnsen, and Thayer. "Vagal influence on working memory and attention." *International Journal of Psychophysiology*, 2003. https://www.sciencedirect.com/science/ article/abs/pii/S0167876003000734

594 Shah, Su, Veledar, Bremner, Goldstein, Lampert, Goldberg, and Vaccarino. "Is heart rate variability related to memory performance in middle-aged men?" *Psychosomatic Medicine*, 2011. https://doi.org/10.1097/PSY.0b013e3182227d6a

595 Oka. "Heart rate variability and neurological disorders." *Clinical Assessment of the Autonomic Nervous System*, 2016. https://link.springer.com/ chapter/10.1007/978-4-431-56012-8_11

596 Elias and Torres. "The renaissance of heart rate variability as a predictor of cognitive functioning." *American Journal of Hypertension*, 2018. https://academic.oup.com/ajh/ article/31/1/21/4082798

597 Forte, Favieri, and Casagrande. "Heart rate variability and cognitive function: a systematic review." *Frontiers in Neuroscience*, 2019. https://www.frontiersin.org/articles/10.3389/ fnins.2019.00710/full

598 Al Hazzouri, Elfassy, Carnethon, Lloyd-Jones, and Yaffe. "Heart rate variability and cognitive function in middle-age adults: The coronary artery risk development in young adults." *American Journal of Hypertension*, 2018. https://doi.org/10.1093/ajh/hpx125

599 Yoon and Hong. "Heart rate variability to differentiate dementia with Lewy bodies from Alzheimer's disease in patients with mild cognitive impairment." *Movement Disorders*, 2016. https://www.mdsabstracts.org/abstract/heart-rate-variability-to-differenti- ate-dementia-with-lewy-bodies-from-alzheimers-disease-in-patients-with-mild-cogni- tive-impairment/

600 Kim, Yoon, and Hong. "Early differentiation of dementia with Lewy bodies and Alzheimer's disease: Heart rate variability at mild cognitive impairment stage." *Clinical Neurophysiology*, 2018. https://doi.org/10.1016/j.clinph.2018.05.004

601 Kim, Yoon, and Hong. "Early differentiation of dementia with Lewy bodies and Alzheimer's disease: heart rate variability at mild cognitive impairment stage." *Clinical Neurophysiology*, 2018. https://doi.org/10.1016/j.clinph.2018.05.004

602 Yang, Tsai, Hong, Yang, Hsieh, and Liu. "Association between heart rate variability and cognitive function in elderly community-dwelling men without dementia: a preliminary report." *Journal of the American Geriatrics Society*, 2008. https://agsjournals.onlineli- brary.wiley.com/doi/10.1111/j.1532-5415.2008.01662.x

603 Barefoot and Schroll. "Symptoms of depression, acute myocardial infarction, and total mortality in a community sample." *Circulation*, 1996. https://www.ahajournals.org/ doi/10.1161/01.cir.93.11.1976

604 Frasure-Smith, Lespérance, and Talajic. "Depression and 18-month prognosis after myo- cardial infarction." *Circulation*, 1995. https://www.ahajournals.org/doi/10.1161/01. cir.91.4.999

605 Penninx, Beekman, Honig, Deeg, Schoevers, van Eijk, and van Tilburg. "Depression and cardiac mortality: results from a community-based longitudinal study." *Archives of General Psychiatry*, 2001. https://jamanetwork.com/journals/jamapsychiatry/fullarticle/481731

606 Carney and Freedland. "Depression, mortality, and medical morbidity in patients with coronary heart disease." *Biological Psychiatry*, 2003. https://pubmed.ncbi.nlm.nih.gov/12893100/

607 Lett, Blumenthal, Babyak, Sherwood, Strauman, Robins, and Newman. "Depression as a risk factor for coronary artery disease: evidence, mechanisms, and treatment." *Psychosomatic Medicine*, 2004. https://pubmed.ncbi.nlm.nih.gov/15184688/

608 Zellweger, Osterwalder, Langewitz, and Pfisterer. "Coronary artery disease and depression." *European Heart Journal*, 2004. https://academic.oup.com/eurheartj/article/25/1/3/619401

609 Glassman. "Depression and cardiovascular comorbidity." *Dialogues in Clinical Neuroscience*, 2007. https://www.ncbi.nlm.nih.gov/pmc/articles/PMC3181839/

610 Nemeroff and Goldschmidt-Clermont. "Heartache and heartbreak—the link between depression and cardiovascular disease." *Nature Reviews: Cardiology*, 2012. https://www.nature.com/articles/nrcardio.2012.91

611 Kemp and Quintana. "The relationship between mental and physical health: insights from the study of heart rate variability." *International Journal of Psychophysiology*, 2013. https://www.sciencedirect.com/science/article/abs/pii/S016787601300189X

612 Mahinrad, van Heemst, Macfarlane, Stott, Jukema, De Craen, and Sabayan. "Short-term heart rate variability and cognitive function in older subjects at risk of cardiovascular disease." *Journal of Hypertension*, 2015. https://journals.lww.com/jhypertension/Abstract/2015/06001/4C_03__SHORT_TERM_HEART_RATE_VARIABILITY_AND.147.aspx

613 Kim, Lipsitz, Ferrucci, Varadhan, Guralnik, Carlson, Fleisher, Fried, and Chaves. "Association between reduced heart rate variability and cognitive impairment in older disabled women in the community: Women's Health and Aging Study." *Journal of the American Geriatric Society*, 2006. https://www.ncbi.nlm.nih.gov/pmc/articles/PMC2276586/

614 Galluzzi, Nicosia, Geroldi, Alicandri, Bonetti, Romanelli, Zulli, and Frisoni. "Cardiac autonomic dysfunction is associated with white matter lesions in patients with mild cognitive impairment." *Journals of Gerontology Series A: Biological Sciences and Medical Sciences*, 2009. https://doi.org/10.1093/gerona/glp105

615 Breit, Kupferberg, Rogler, and Hasler. "Vagus nerve as modulator of the brain-gut axis in psychiatric and inflammatory disorders." *Frontiers in Psychiatry*, 2018. https://www.frontiersin.org/articles/10.3389/fpsyt.2018.00044/full

616 Frewen, Finucane, Savva, Boyle, Coen, and Kenny. "Cognitive function is associated with impaired heart rate variability in ageing adults: the Irish Longitudinal Study on Ageing wave one results." *Clinical Autonomic Research*, 2013. https://doi.org/10.1007/s10286-013-0214-x

617 Thayer and Sternberg. "Beyond heart rate variability: vagal regulation of allostatic systems." *Annals of the New York Academy of Sciences*, 2006. https://doi.org/10.1196/annals.1366.014

618 Sgoifo, Carnevali, Pico Alfonso, and Amore. "Autonomic dysfunction and heart rate variability in depression." *Stress*, 2015. https://doi.org/10.3109/10253890.2015.1045868

[619] Cukierman-Yaffe, Gerstein, Basile, Bethel, Cardona-Muñoz, Conget, Dagenais, Franek, Hall, Hancu, Jansky, Lakshmanan, Lanas, Leiter, Lopez-Jaramillo, Pirags, Pogosova, Probstfield, Rao-Melacini, Ramasundarahettige, Raubenheimer, Riddle, Rydén, Shaw, Sheu, and Temelkova-Kurktschiev. "Novel indices of Cognitive impairment and incident cardiovascular outcomes in the REWIND trial." *Journal of Clinical Endocrinology & Metabolism*, 2022. https://doi.org/10.1210/clinem/dgac200

[620] Zeki al Hazzouri, Elfassy, Carnethon, Lloyd-Jones, and Yaffe. "Heart rate variability and cognitive function in middle-age adults: the coronary artery risk development in young adults." *American Journal of Hypertension*, 2017. https://doi.org/10.1093/ajh/hpx125

[621] Nicolini, Ciulla, Malfatto, Abbate, Mari, Rossi, Pettenuzzo, Magrini, Consonni, and Lombardi. "Autonomic dysfunction in mild cognitive impairment: evidence from power spectral analysis of heart rate variability in a cross-sectional case control study." *PLOS One*, 2014. https://doi.org/10.1371/journal.pone.0096656

[622] Giblin, de Leon, Smith, Sztynda, and Lal. "Heart rate variability, blood pressure, and cognitive function: assessing age effects." *Journal of Green Engineering*, 2013. https://www.riverpublishers.com/journal/journal_articles/RP_Journal_1904-4720_337.pdf

[623] Gupta, Chandra, Rukmani, and Sathyaprabha. "Autonomic dysfunction in patients with Alzheimer's disease." *Alzheimer's, Dementia, and Cognitive Neurology*, 2017. https://www.researchgate.net/publication/314198031_Autonomic_dysfunction_in_patients_with_Alzheimer's_disease

[624] Keary, Galioto, Hughes, Waechter, Spitznagel, Rosneck, Josephson, and Gunstad. "Reduced heart rate recovery is associated with poorer cognitive function in older adults with cardiovascular disease." Cardiovascular *Psychiatry and Neurology*, 2012. https://www.ncbi.nlm.nih.gov/pmc/articles/PMC3439935/

[625] Qiu, Winblad, Viitanen, and Fratiglioni. "Pulse pressure and risk of Alzheimer disease in persons aged 75 years and older." *Stroke*, 2003. https://doi.org/10.1161/01.str.0000083487.94236.3d

[626] Bhambhani, Maikala, Farag, and Rowland. "Reliability of near infrared spectroscopy measures of cerebral oxygenation and blood volume during handgrip exercise in non-disabled and traumatic brain-injured subjects." *Journal of Rehabilitation Research and Development*, 2006. https://pubmed.ncbi.nlm.nih.gov/17436171/

[627] Sen, Gopinath, and Robertson. "Clinical application of near-infrared spectroscopy in patients with traumatic brain injury: a review of the progress of the field." *Neurophotonics*, 2016. https://doi.org/10.1117/1.NPh.3.3.031409

[628] Bishop and Neary. "Assessing prefrontal cortex oxygenation after sport concussion with near-infrared spectroscopy." *Clinical Physiology and Functional Imaging*, 2017. https://doi.org/10.1111/cpf.12447

[629] Keary, Galioto, Hughes, Waechter, Spitznagel, Rosneck, Josephson, and Gunstad. "Reduced heart rate recovery is associated with poorer cognitive function in older adults with cardiovascular disease." *Cardiovascular Psychiatry and Neurology*, 2012. https://www.ncbi.nlm.nih.gov/pmc/articles/PMC3439935/

[630] Nicolini, Ciulla, Malfatto, Abbate, Mari, Rossi, Pettenuzzo, Magrini, Consonni, and Lombardi. "Autonomic dysfunction in mild cognitive impairment: evidence from power spectral analysis of heart rate variability in a cross-sectional case-control study." *PLOS One*, 2014. https://doi.org/10.1371/journal.pone.0096656

[631] Mellingsæter, Wyller, Ranhoff, Bogdanovic, and Wyller. "Reduced sympathetic response to head-up tilt in subjects with mild cognitive impairment or mild Alzheimer's dementia." *Dementia and Geriatric Cognitive Disorders Extra*, 2015. https://doi.org/10.1159/000375297

632 Allan, Ballard, Allen, Murray, Davidson, McKeith, and Kenny. "Autonomic dysfunction in dementia." *Journal of Neurology, Neurosurgery, and Psychiatry*, 2007. http://dx.doi.org/10.1136/jnnp.2006.102343

633 Zakrzewska-Pniewska, Gawel, Szmidt-Salkowska, Kepczynska, and Nojszewska. "Clinical and functional assessment of dysautonomia and its correlation in Alzheimer's disease." *American Journal of Alzheimer's Disease and Other Dementias*, 2012. https://doi.org/10.1177/1533317512459792

634 Rangon, Krantic, Moyse, and Fougère. "The vagal autonomic pathway of COVID-19 at the crossroad of Alzheimer's disease and aging: a review of knowledge." *Journal of Alzheimer's Disease Reports*, 2020. https://www.ncbi.nlm.nih.gov/pmc/articles/PMC7835993/

635 Silva, Oliveira, Mello, Moraes, Deslandes, and Laks. "Heart rate variability indexes in dementia: a systematic review with quantitative analysis." *Current Alzheimer Research*, 2018. https://www.researchgate.net/publication/317265798

636 Tan, Beilharz, Vollmer-Conna, and Cvejic. "Heart rate variability as a marker of healthy ageing." *International Journal of Cardiology*, 2019. https://doi.org/10.1016/j.ijcard.2018.08.005

637 Thayer. "What the heart says to the brain (and vice versa) and why we should listen." *Psihologijske Teme*, 2007. https://www.researchgate.net/publication/26571590

638 Thayer. "Vagal tone and the inflammatory reflex." *Cleveland Clinic Journal of Medicine*, 2009. https://doi.org/10.3949/ccjm.76.s2.05

639 Jennings, Allen, Gianaros, Thayer, and Manuck. "Focusing neurovisceral integration: cognition, heart rate variability, and cerebral blood flow." *Psychophysiology*, 2015. https://www.ncbi.nlm.nih.gov/pmc/articles/PMC4387874/

640 Wei, Han, Zhang, Hannak, Dai, and Liu. "Affective emotion increases heart rate variability and activates left dorsolateral prefrontal cortex in post-traumatic growth." *Scientific Reports*, 2017. https://www.ncbi.nlm.nih.gov/pmc/articles/PMC5709461/

641 Winkelmann, Grimm, Pohlack, Nees, Cacciaglia, Dinu-Biringer, Steiger, Wicking, Ruttorf, Schad, and Flor. "Brain morphology correlates of interindividual differences in conditioned fear acquisition and extinction learning." *Brain Structure & Function*, 2016. https://doi.org/10.1007/s00429-015-1013-z

642 Yoo, Thayer, Greening, Lee, Ponzio, Min, Sakaki, Nga, Mather, and Koenig. "Brain structural concomitants of resting state heart rate variability in the young and old: evidence from two independent samples." *Brain Structure & Function*, 2018. https://www.ncbi.nlm.nih.gov/pmc/articles/PMC5828882/

643 Koolschijn, van Haren, Lensvelt-Mulders, Hulshoff Pol, and Kahn. "Brain volume abnormalities in major depressive disorder: a meta-analysis of magnetic resonance imaging studies." *Human Brain Mapping*, 2009. https://onlinelibrary.wiley.com/doi/epdf/10.1002/hbm.20801

644 Kempton, Salvador, Munafò, Geddes, Simmons, Frangou, and Williams. "Structural neuroimaging studies in major depressive disorder: meta-analysis and comparison with bipolar disorder." *Archives of General Psychiatry*, 2011. https://jamanetwork.com/journals/jamapsychiatry/fullarticle/1107416

645 Arnone, McIntosh, Ebmeier, Munafò, and Anderson. "Magnetic resonance imaging studies in unipolar depression: systematic review and meta-regression analyses." *European Neuropsychopharmacology*, 2011. https://doi.org/10.1016/j.euroneuro.2011.05.003

646 Bora, Harrison, Davey, Yücel, and Pantelis. "Meta-analysis of volumetric abnormalities in cortico-striatal-pallidal-thalamic circuits in major depressive disorder." *Psychological Medicine*, 2011. https://doi.org/10.1017/S0033291711001668

[647] Zhao, Du, Huang, Lui, Chen, Liu, Luo, Wang, Kemp, and Gong. "Brain grey matter abnormalities in medication-free patients with major depressive disorder: a meta-analysis." *Psychological Medicine*, 2014. https://doi.org/10.1017/S0033291714000518

[648] Koenig, Westlund Schreiner, Klimes-Dougan, Ubani, Mueller, Kaess, and Cullen. "Brain structural thickness and resting state autonomic function in adolescents with major depression." *Social Cognitive and Affective Neuroscience*, 2018. https://doi.org/10.1093/scan/nsy046

[649] Nikolin, Boonstra, Loo, and Martin. "Combined effect of prefrontal transcranial direct current stimulation and a working memory task on heart rate variability." *PLOS One*, 2017. https://doi.org/10.1371/journal.pone.0181833

[650] Kumral, Schaare, Beyer, Reinelt, Uhlig, Liem, Lampe, Babayan, Reiter, Erbey, Roebbig, Loeffler, Schroeter, Husser, Witte, Villringer, and Gaebler. "The age-dependent relationship between resting heart rate variability and functional brain connectivity." *Neuroimage*, 2019. https://doi.org/10.1016/j.neuroimage.2018.10.027

[651] Lane, Reiman, Ahern, and Thayer. "Activity in medial prefrontal cortex correlates with vagal component of heart rate variability during emotion." *Psychosomatic Medicine*, 2000. https://www.researchgate.net/publication/295490318

[652] Marci, Glick, Loh, and Dougherty. "Autonomic and prefrontal cortex responses to autobiographical recall of emotions." *Cognitive, Affective, and Behavioral Neuroscience*, 2007. https://doi.org/10.3758/CABN.7.3.243

[653] Lane, McRae, Reiman, Chen, Ahern, and Thayer. "Neural correlates of heart rate variability during emotion." *Neuroimage*, 2009. https://doi.org/10.1016/j.neuroimage.2008.07.056

[654] Steinfurth, Wendt, Geisler, Hamm, Thayer, and Koenig. "Resting state vagally-mediated heart rate variability is associated with neural activity during explicit emotion regulation." *Frontiers in Neuroscience*, 2018. https://www.ncbi.nlm.nih.gov/pmc/articles/PMC6231057/

[655] Forte, Favieri, and Casagrande. "Heart rate variability and cognitive function: a systematic review." *Frontiers in Neuroscience*, 2019. https://www.frontiersin.org/articles/10.3389/fnins.2019.00710/full

[656] Durantin, Gagnon, Tremblay, and Denais. "Using near infrared spectroscopy and heart rate variability to detect mental overload." *Behavioural Brain Research*, 2014. https://core.ac.uk/reader/33663529

[657] Allen, Jennings, Gianaros, Thayer, and Manuck. "Resting high-frequency heart rate variability is related to resting brain perfusion." *Psychophysiology*, 2015. https://www.ncbi.nlm.nih.gov/pmc/articles/PMC4387872/

[658] Brown and Thore. "Review: Cerebral microvascular pathology in ageing and neurodegeneration." *Neuropathology and Applied Neurobiology*, 2011. https://doi.org/10.1111/j.1365-2990.2010.01139.x

[659] Sierra-Marcos. "Regional cerebral blood flow in mild cognitive impairment and Alzheimer's disease measured with arterial spin labeling magnetic resonance imaging." *International Journal of Alzheimer's Disease*, 2017. https://www.ncbi.nlm.nih.gov/pmc/articles/PMC5442339/

[660] Yoon, Kong, Choi, Baek, Kim, Shin, Ko, Shin, and Shin. "Neural compensatory response during complex cognitive function tasks in mild cognitive impairment: a near-infrared spectroscopy study." *Neural Plasticity*, 2019. https://www.hindawi.com/journals/np/2019/7845104/

661 de la Torre. "Critically attained threshold of cerebral hypoperfusion: the CATCH hypothesis of Alzheimer's pathogenesis." *Neurobiology of Aging*, 2000. https://doi.org/10.1016/S0197-4580(00)00111-1

662 Aharon-Peretz, Harel, Revach, and Ben-Haim. "Increased sympathetic and decreased parasympathetic cardiac innervation in patients with Alzheimer's disease." *Archives of Neurology*, 1992. https://jamanetwork.com/journals/jamaneurology/article-abstract/591875

663 Waki, Suzuki, Tanaka, Tamai, Minakawa, Miyazaki, Yoshida, Uebaba, Imai, and Hisajima. "Effects of electroacupuncture to the trigeminal nerve area on the autonomic nervous system and cerebral blood flow in the prefrontal cortex." *Acupuncture in Medicine*, 2017. https://doi.org/10.1136/acupmed-2016-011247

664 Blanco, Saucedo, and Gonzalez-Lima. "Transcranial infrared laser stimulation improves rule-based, but not information-integration, category learning in humans." *Neurobiology of Learning and Memory*, 2017. https://doi.org/10.1016/j.nlm.2016.12.016

665 de la Torre. "Cardiac dysfunction and cognitive decline." *European Heart Journal*, 2017. https://academic.oup.com/eurheartj/article/38/8/584/2884299

666 Mazza, Marano, Traversi, Bria, and Mazza. "Primary cerebral blood flow deficiency and Alzheimer's disease: shadows and lights." *Journal of Alzheimer's Disease*, 2011. https://content.iospress.com/articles/journal-of-alzheimers-disease/jad090700

667 Serviddio, Romano, Cassano, Bellanti, Altomare, and Vendemiale. "Principles and therapeutic relevance for targeting mitochondria in aging and neurodegenerative diseases." *Current Pharmaceutical Design*, 2011. https://www.researchgate.net/publication/233613157

668 Hirao, Ohnishi, Hirata, Yamashita, Mori, Moriguchi, Matsuda, Nemoto, Imabayashi, Yamada, Iwamoto, Arima, and Asada. "The prediction of rapid conversion to Alzheimer's disease in mild cognitive impairment using regional cerebral blood flow SPECT." *NeuroImage*, 2005. https://doi.org/10.1016/j.neuroimage.2005.06.066

669 Meier, Bellgowan, Signh, Kuplicki, Polanski, and Mayer. "Recovery of cerebral blood flow following sports-related concussion." *JAMA Neurology*, 2015. https://jamanetwork.com/journals/jamaneurology/fullarticle/2173271

670 Rajna, Mattila, Huotari, Tuovinen, Krüger, Holst, Korhonen, Remes, Seppänen, Hennig, Nedergaard, and Kiviniemi. "Cardiovascular brain impulses in Alzheimer's disease." *Brain*, 2021. https://doi.org/10.1093/brain/awab144

671 Mestre, Tithof, Du, Song, Peng, Sweeney, Olveda, Thomas, Nedergaard, and Kelley. "Flow of cerebrospinal fluid is driven by arterial pulsations and is reduced in hypertension." *Nature Communications*, 2018. https://www.nature.com/articles/s41467-018-07318-3

672 Petersen, Dufour, Befroy, Garcia, and Shulman. "Impaired mitochondrial activity in the insulin-resistant offspring of patients with type 2 diabetes." *New England Journal of Medicine*, 2004. https://www.ncbi.nlm.nih.gov/pmc/articles/PMC2995502/

673 de la Torre. "Treating cognitive impairment with transcranial low-level laser therapy." *Journal of Photochemistry and Photobiology B*, 2017. https://www.sciencedirect.com/science/article/abs/pii/S1011134416306765

674 Johnstone, Moro, Stone, Benabid, and Mitrofanis. "Turning on lights to stop neurodegeneration: the potential of near infrared light therapy in Alzheimer's and Parkinson's disease." *Frontiers in Neuroscience*, 2016. https://www.frontiersin.org/articles/10.3389/fnins.2015.00500/full

675 Schon and Przedborski. "Mitochondria: the next (neurode)generation." *Neuron*, 2011. https://www.ncbi.nlm.nih.gov/pmc/articles/PMC3407575/

[676] Kann. "The interneuron energy hypothesis: implications for brain disease." *Neurobiology of Disease*, 2015. https://doi.org/10.1016/j.nbd.2015.08.005

[677] Vásquez-Trincado, Garcia-Carvajal, Pennanen, Parra, Hill, Rothermel, and Lavandero. "Mitochondrial dynamics, mitophagy and cardiovascular disease." *Journal of Physiology*, 2015. https://physoc.onlinelibrary.wiley.com/doi/full/10.1113/JP271301

[678] Picard and McEwen. "Mitochondria impact brain function and cognition." *Proceedings of the National Academy of Sciences*, 2014. https://www.ncbi.nlm.nih.gov/pmc/articles/PMC3890847

[679] Tam, Gruber, Ng, Halliwell, and Gunawan. "Effects of lithium on age-related decline in mitochondrial turnover and function in *Caenorhabditis elegans*." *The Journals of Gerontology: Series A*, 2014. https://academic.oup.com/biomedgerontology/article/69/7/810/662957

[680] Schon and Przedborski. "Mitochondria: the next (neurode)generation." *Neuron*, 2011. https://www.ncbi.nlm.nih.gov/pmc/articles/PMC3407575/

[681] Zhu, Perry, Smith, and Wang. "Abnormal mitochondrial dynamics in the pathogenesis of Alzheimer's disease." *Journal of Alzheimer's Disease*, 2013. https://www.ncbi.nlm.nih.gov/pmc/articles/PMC4097015/

[682] Hirai, Aliev, Nunomura, Fujioka, Russell, Atwood, Johnson, Kress, Vinters, Tabaton, Shimohama, Cash, Siedlak, Harris, Jones, Petersen, Perry, and Smith. "Mitochondrial abnormalities in Alzheimer's disease." *Journal of Neuroscience*, 2001. https://www.ncbi.nlm.nih.gov/pmc/articles/PMC6762571/

[683] Serviddio, Romano, Cassano, Bellanti, Altomare, and Vendemiale. "Principles and therapeutic relevance for targeting mitochondria in aging and neurodegenerative diseases." *Current Pharmaceutical Design*, 2011. https://pubmed.ncbi.nlm.nih.gov/21718251/

[684] Bosetti, Brizzi, Barogi, Mancuso, Siciliano, Tendi, Murri, Rapoport, and Solaini. "Cytochrome c oxidase and mitochondrial F_1F_0-ATPase (ATP synthase) activities in platelets and brain from patients with Alzheimer's disease." *Neurobiology of Aging*, 2002. https://doi.org/10.1016/S0197-4580(01)00314-1

[685] Saucedo, Courtois, Wade, Kelley, Kheradbin, Barrett, and Gonzalez-Lima. "Transcranial laser stimulation: mitochondrial and cerebrovascular effects in younger and older healthy adults." *Brain Stimulation*, 2021. https://doi.org/10.1016/j.brs.2021.02.011

[686] Hroudová, Singh, and Fišar. "Mitochondrial dysfunctions in neurodegenerative diseases: relevance to Alzheimer's disease." *BioMed Research International*, 2014. https://doi.org/10.1155/2014/175062

[687] Romanello. "The interplay between mitochondrial morphology and myomitokines in aging sarcopenia." *International Journal of Molecular Sciences*, 2020. https://doi.org/10.3390/ijms22010091

[688] Paulin and Michelakis. "The metabolic theory of pulmonary arterial hypertension." *Circulation Research*, 2014. https://doi.org/10.1161/CIRCRESAHA.115.301130

[689] Galindo, Solesio, Atienzar-Aroca, Zamora, and Jordán Bueso. "Mitochondrial dynamics and mitophagy in the 6-hydroxydopamine preclinical model of Parkinson's disease." *Parkinson's Disease*, 2012. https://doi.org/10.1155/2012/131058

[690] Galindo, Solesio, Atienzar-Aroca, Zamora, and Jordán Bueso. "Mitochondrial dynamics and mitophagy in the 6-hydroxydopamine preclinical model of Parkinson's disease." *Parkinson's Disease*, 2012. https://doi.org/10.1155/2012/131058

[691] Luo, Hoffer, Hoffer, and Qi. "Mitochondria: a therapeutic target for Parkinson's disease?" *International Journal of Molecular Sciences*, 2015. https://doi.org/10.3390/ijms160920704

692 Onyango, Khan, Miller, Swerdlow, Trimmer, and Bennett. "Mitochondrial genomic contribution to mitochondrial dysfunction in Alzheimer's disease." *Journal of Alzheimer's Disease*, 2006. https://content.iospress.com/articles/journal-of-alzheimers-disease/jad00603

693 Valla, Schneider, Niedzielko, Coon, Caselli, Sabbagh, Ahern, Baxter, Alexander, Walker, and Reiman. "Impaired platelet mitochondrial activity in Alzheimer's disease and mild cognitive impairment." *Mitochondrion*, 2006. https://pubmed.ncbi.nlm.nih.gov/17123871/

694 Silva, Santana, Esteves, Baldeiras, Arduino, Oliveira, and Cardoso. "Prodromal metabolic phenotype in MCI cybrids: implications for Alzheimer's disease." *Current Alzheimer Research*, 2013. https://pubmed.ncbi.nlm.nih.gov/22746213/

695 Caldwell, Yao, and Brinton. "Targeting the prodromal stage of Alzheimer's disease: bioenergetic and mitochondrial opportunities." *Neurotherapeutics*, 2015. https://www.ncbi.nlm.nih.gov/pmc/articles/PMC4322082/

696 Kim, Kim, Hong, Lee, and Jung. "Sex differences in cardiovascular risk factors for dementia." *Biomolecules and Therapeutics*, 2018. https://www.ncbi.nlm.nih.gov/pmc/articles/PMC6254640/

697 Lejri, Grimm, and Eckert. "Mitochondria, estrogen, and female brain aging." *Frontiers in Aging Neuroscience*, 2018. https://www.ncbi.nlm.nih.gov/pmc/articles/PMC5934418/

698 Viña, Gambini, García-García, Rodriguez-Mañas, and Borrás. "Role of oestrogens on oxidative stress and inflammation in ageing." *Hormone Molecular Biology and Clinical Investigation*, 2013. https://doi.org/10.1515/hmbci-2013-0039

699 Lee. "Effect of mitochondrial stress on systemic metabolism." *Annals of the New York Academy of Sciences*, 2015. https://doi.org/10.1111/nyas.12822

700 Cobb, Lee, Xiao, Yen, Wong, Nakamura, Mehta, Gao, Ashur, Huffman, Wan, Muzumdar, Barzilai, and Cohen. "Naturally occurring mitochondrial-derived peptides are age-dependent regulators of apoptosis, insulin sensitivity, and inflammatory markers." *Aging*, 2016. https://www.ncbi.nlm.nih.gov/pmc/articles/PMC4925829/

701 Ito, Ohta, Nishimaki, Kagawa, Soma, Kuno, Komatsuzaki, Mizusawa, and Hayashi. "Functional integrity of mitochondrial genomes in human platelets and autopsied brain tissues from elderly patients with Alzheimer's disease." *Proceedings of the National Academy of Sciences*, 1999. https://www.pnas.org/content/96/5/2099

702 Tyrrell, Bharadwaj, Jorgensen, Register, Shively, Andrews, Neth, Keene, Mintz, Craft, and Molina. "Blood-based bioenergetics profiling reflects differences in brain bioenergetics and metabolism." *Oxidative Medicine and Cellular Longevity*, 2017. https://www.ncbi.nlm.nih.gov/pmc/articles/PMC5643153/

703 Picone, Nuzzo, Caruana, Scafidi, and di Carlo. "Mitochondrial dysfunction: different routes to Alzheimer's disease therapy." *Oxidative Medicine and Cellular Longevity*, 2014. https://www.hindawi.com/journals/omcl/2014/780179/

704 Toth, Tarantini, Csiszar, and Ungvari. "Functional vascular contributions to cognitive impairment and dementia: mechanisms and consequences of cerebral autoregulatory dysfunction, endothelial impairment, and neurovascular uncoupling in aging." *American Journal of Physiology: Heart and Circulatory Physiology*, 2017. https://www.ncbi.nlm.nih.gov/pmc/articles/PMC5283909/

705 Toth, Tarantini, Csiszar, and Ungvari. "Functional vascular contributions to cognitive impairment and dementia: mechanisms and consequences of cerebral autoregulatory

dysfunction, endothelial impairment, and neurovascular uncoupling in aging." *American Journal of Physiology: Heart and Circulatory Physiology*, 2017. https://www.ncbi.nlm.nih. gov/pmc/articles/PMC5283909/

706   de la Torre. "Critically attained threshold of cerebral hypoperfusion: the CATCH hypothesis of Alzheimer's pathogenesis." *Neurobiology of Aging*, 2000. https://doi. org/10.1016/S0197-4580(00)00111-1

707   Maksimovich. "Transcatheter cerebral revascularization in the treatment of athero-sclerotic lesions of the brain." *Brain Disorders & Therapy*, 2016. https://www.walsh-medicalmedia.com/open-access/transcatheter-cerebral-revascularization-in-the-treat-ment-of-atherosclerotic-lesions-of-the-brain-23156.html

708   Snowdon, Greiner, Mortimer, Riley, Greiner, and Markesbery. "Brain infarction and the clinical expression of Alzheimer disease: the Nun Study." *Journal of the American Medical Association*, 1997. https://pubmed.ncbi.nlm.nih.gov/9052711/

709   Hartmann, Hyacinth, Liao, and Shih. "Does pathology of small venules contribute to cerebral microinfarcts and dementia?" *Journal of Neurochemistry*, 2017. https://doi. org/10.1111/jnc.14228

710   Aanerud, Borghammer, Chakravarty, Vang, Rodell, Jónsdottir, Møller, Ashkanian, Vafaee, Iversen, Johannsen, and Gjedde. "Brain energy metabolism and blood flow dif-ferences in healthy aging." *Journal of Cerebral Blood Flow & Metabolism*, 2012. https:// www.ncbi.nlm.nih.gov/pmc/articles/PMC3390816/

711   Luchsinger, Reitz, Honig, Tang, Shea, and Mayeux. "Aggregation of vascular risk factors and risk of incident Alzheimer's disease." *Neurology*, 2005. https://www.ncbi.nlm.nih. gov/pmc/articles/PMC1619350/

712   Tarumi and Zhang. "Cerebral hemodynamics of the aging brain: risk of Alzheimer dis-ease and benefit of aerobic exercise." *Frontiers in Physiology*, 2014. https://www.ncbi. nlm.nih.gov/pmc/articles/PMC3896879/

713   de la Torre. "Alzheimer disease as a vascular disorder: nosological evidence." *Stroke*, 2002. https://doi.org/10.1161/01.STR.0000014421.15948.67

714   Bourassa. "Transcranial low-level laser therapy (tLLLT) in the chiropractic manage-ment of mild traumatic brain injury." Working paper, 2017. https://www.researchgate. net/publication/316145447

715   Albrecht, Isenberg, Stradford, Monreal, Sagare, Pachicano, Sweeney, Toga, Zlokovic, Chui, Joe, Schneider, Conti, Jann, and Pa. "Associations between vascular function and tau PET are associated with global cognition and amyloid." *Journal of Neuroscience*, 2020. https://www.jneurosci.org/content/40/44/8573

716   Shabir, Berwick, and Francis. "Neurovascular dysfunction in vascular dementia, Alzheimer's and atherosclerosis." *BMC Neuroscience*, 2018. https://doi.org/10.1186/ s12868-018-0465-5

717   Rangon, Krantic, Moyse, and Fougère. "The vagal autonomic pathway of COVID-19 at the crossroad of Alzheimer's disease and aging: a review of knowledge." *Journal of Alzheimer's Disease Reports 4*, 2020. https://doi.org/10.3233/ADR-200273

718   Shabir, Berwick, and Francis. "Neurovascular dysfunction in vascular dementia, Alzheimers, and atherosclerosis." *BMC Neuroscience*, 2018. https://doi.org/10.1186/ s12868-018-0465-5

719   Tariq and Barber. "Dementia risk and prevention by targeting modifiable vascular risk factors." *Journal of Neurochemistry*, 2017. https://onlinelibrary.wiley.com/doi/10.1111/ jnc.14132

720   Ardura-Fabregat, Boddeke, Boza-Serrano, Brioschi, Castro-Gomez, Ceyzériat, Dansokho, Dierkes, Gelders, Heneka, Hoeijmakers, Hoffmann, Iaccarino, Jahnert,

Kuhbandner, Landreth, Lonnemann, Löschmann, McManus, Paulus, Reemst, Sanchez-Caro, Tiberi, Van der Perren, Vautheny, Venegas, Webers, Weydt, Wijasa, Xiang, and Yang. "Targeting neuroinflammation to treat Alzheimer's disease." *CNS Drugs*, 2017. https://www.ncbi.nlm.nih.gov/pmc/articles/PMC5747579/

[721] de la Torre. "Cardiovascular risk factors promote brain hypoperfusion leading to cognitive decline and dementia." *Cardiovascular Psychiatry and Neurology*, 2012. https://doi.org/10.1155/2012/367516

[722] Rius-Pérez, Tormos, Pérez, and Taléns-Visconti. "Vascular pathology: cause or effect in Alzheimer disease?" *Neurología*, 2018. https://pubmed.ncbi.nlm.nih.gov/26385017/

[723] Ułamek-Kozioł, Pluta, Bogucka-Kocka, Januszewski, Kocki, and Czuczwar. "Brain ischemia with Alzheimer phenotype dysregulates Alzheimer's disease-related proteins." *Pharmacological Reports*, 2016. https://doi.org/10.1016/j.pharep.2016.01.006

[724] Kato, Miyata, Ando, Matsuoka, Yasuma, Iwamoto, Kawano, Banno, Ozaki, and Noda. "Influence of sleep duration on cortical oxygenation in elderly individuals." *Psychiatry and Clinical Neurosciences*, 2016. https://onlinelibrary.wiley.com/doi/full/10.1111/pcn.12464

[725] Ardura-Fabregat, Boddeke, Boza-Serrano, Brioschi, Castro-Gomez, Ceyzériat, Dansokho, Dierkes, Gelders, Heneka, Hoeijmakers, Hoffmann, Iaccarino, Jahnert, Kuhbandner, Landreth, Lonnemann, Löschmann, McManus, Paulus, Reemst, Sanchez-Caro, Tiberi, Van der Perren, Vautheny, Venegas, Webers, Weydt, Wijasa, Xiang, and Yang. "Targeting neuroinflammation to treat Alzheimer's disease." *CNS Drugs*, 2017. https://www.ncbi.nlm.nih.gov/pmc/articles/PMC5747579/

[726] Bishop, Dech, Guzik, and Neary. "Heart rate variability and implication for sport concussion." *Clinical Physiology and Functional Imaging*, 2018. https://doi.org/10.1111/cpf.12487

[727] Miller-Hodges and Dhaun. "Pulse-wave velocity is associated with cognitive impairment in haemodialysis patients." *Clinical Science* (London), 2017. https://www.ncbi.nlm.nih.gov/pmc/articles/PMC5869851/

[728] Iulita, Noriega de la Colina, and Girouard. "Arterial stiffness, cognitive impairment, and dementia: confounding factor or real risk?" *Journal of Neurochemistry*, 2018. https://onlinelibrary.wiley.com/doi/10.1111/jnc.14235

[729] Pasha, Rutjes, Tomoto, Tarumi, Stowe, Claassen, Cullum, Zhu, and Zhang. "Carotid stiffness is associated with brain amyloid-ß burden in amnestic mild cognitive impairment." *Journal of Alzheimer's Disease*, 2020. https://doi.org/10.3233/JAD-191073

[730] Scuteri and Wang. "Pulse wave velocity as a marker of cognitive impairment in the elderly." *Journal of Alzheimer's Disease*, 2014. https://doi.org/10.3233/JAD-141416

[731] Claassen and Zhang. "Cerebral autoregulation in Alzheimer's disease." *Journal of Cerebral Blood Flow & Metabolism*, 2011. https://www.ncbi.nlm.nih.gov/pmc/articles/PMC3137479/

[732] Tarumi, Dunsky, Khan, Liu, Hill, Armstrong, Martin-Cook, Cullum, and Zhang. "Dynamic cerebral autoregulation and tissue oxygenation in amnestic mild cognitive impairment." *Journal of Alzheimer's Disease*, 2014. https://doi.org/10.3233/jad-132018

[733] Phillips, Chan, Zheng, Krassioukov, and Ainslie. "Neurovascular coupling in humans: physiology, methodological advances, and clinical implications." *Journal of Cerebral Blood Flow & Metabolism*, 2016. https://www.ncbi.nlm.nih.gov/pmc/articles/PMC4821024/

[734] Purkayastha and Sorond. "Cerebral hemodynamics and the aging brain." *International Journal of Clinical Neurosciences and Mental Health*, 2014. https://www.researchgate.net/publication/299570633

735 Zhang, Pasha, Liu, Xing, Cardim, Tarumi, Womack, Hynan, Cullum, and Zhang. "Steady-state cerebral autoregulation in older adults with amnestic mild cognitive impairment: linear mixed model analysis." *Journal of Applied Physiology*, 2020. https://www.ncbi.nlm.nih.gov/pmc/articles/PMC7473943/

736 Zhang, Liu, Khan, Tseng, Tarumi, Armstrong, Hill, Martin-Cook, Weiner, and Cullum. "Brain hypoperfusion and neurovascular decoupling in amnestic mild cognitive impairment." *Alzheimer's Association International Conference*, 2013. https://doi.org/10.1016/j.jalz.2013.05.1583

737 Li, Kitamura, Beverley, Koudelka, Duncombe, Lennen, Jansen, Marshall, Platt, Wiegand, Cárare, Kalaria, Iliff, and Horsburgh. "Impaired glymphatic function and pulsation alterations in a mouse model of vascular cognitive impairment." *Frontiers in Aging Neuroscience*, 2022. https://doi.org/10.3389/fnagi.2021.788519

738 Tin, Bressler, Simino, Sullivan, Mei, Windham, Griswold, Gottesman, Boerwinkle, Fornage, and Mosley. "Genetic risk, midlife Life's Simple 7, and incident dementia in the Atherosclerosis Risk in Communities Study." *Neurology*, 2022. https://doi.org/10.1212/WNL.0000000000200520

739 de la Torre. "Alzheimer disease as a vascular disorder: nosological evidence." *Stroke*, 2002. https://doi.org/10.1161/01.STR.0000014421.15948.67

740 Bu, Huo, Xu, Liu, Li, Fan, and Li. "Alteration in brain functional and effective connectivity in subjects with hypertension." *Frontiers in Physiology*, 2018. https://www.frontiersin.org/articles/10.3389/fphys.2018.00669/full

741 Meltzer, Cantwell, Greer, Ben-Eliezer, Smith, Frank, Kaye, Houck, and Price. "Does cerebral blood flow decline in healthy aging? A PET study with partial-volume correction." *Journal of Nuclear Medicine*, 2000. https://jnm.snmjournals.org/content/41/11/1842.long

742 de la Torre. "Cerebral perfusion enhancing interventions: a new strategy for the prevention of Alzheimer's dementia." *Brain Pathology*, 2016. https://www.ncbi.nlm.nih.gov/pmc/articles/PMC8029146/

743 Saucedo, Courtois, Wade, Kelley, Kheradbin, Barrett, and Gonzalez-Lima. "Transcranial laser stimulation: mitochondrial and cerebrovascular effects in younger and older healthy adults." *Brain Stimulation*, 2021. https://doi.org/10.1016/j.brs.2021.02.011

744 Uozumi, Nawashiro, Sato, Kawauchi, Shima, and Kikuchi. "Targeted increase in cerebral blood flow by transcranial near-infrared laser irradiation." *Lasers in Surgery and Medicine*, 2010. https://doi.org/10.1002/lsm.20938

745 Maegawa, Itoh, Hosokawa, Yaegashi, and Nishi. "Effects of near-infrared low-level laser irradiation on microcirculation." *Lasers in Surgery and Medicine*, 2000. https://doi.org/10.1002/1096-9101(2000)27:5<427::AID-LSM1004>3.0.CO;2-A

746 Dmochowski, Shereen, Berisha, and Dmochowski. "Near-infrared light increases functional connectivity with a non-thermal mechanism." *Cerebral Cortex Communications*, 2020. https://academic.oup.com/cercorcomms/article/1/1/tgaa004/5809511

747 Tian, Hase, Gonzalez-Lima, and Liu. "Transcranial laser stimulation improves human cerebral oxygenation." *Lasers in Surgery and Medicine*, 2016. https://www.ncbi.nlm.nih.gov/pmc/articles/PMC5066697/

748 Litscher. "Brain photobiomodulation: preliminary results from regional cerebral oximetry and thermal imaging." *Medicines*, 2019. https://www.ncbi.nlm.nih.gov/pmc/articles/PMC6473852/

749 Linares, Beltrame, Ferraresi, Galdino, and Catai. "Photobiomodulation effect on local hemoglobin concentration assessed by near-infrared spectroscopy in humans." *Lasers in Medical Science*, 2019. https://doi.org/10.1007/s10103-019-02861-x

750   Holmes, Barrett, Saucedo, O'Connor, Liu, and Gonzalez-Lima. "Cognitive enhancement by transcranial photobiomodulation is associated with cerebrovascular oxygenation of the prefrontal cortex." *Frontiers in Neuroscience*, 2019. https://www.ncbi.nlm.nih.gov/pmc/articles/PMC6813459/

751   Nawashiro, Wada, Nakai, and Sato. "Focal increase in cerebral blood flow after treatment with near-infrared light to the forehead in a patient in a persistent vegetative state." *Photomedicine and Laser Surgery*, 2012. https://doi.org/10.1089/pho.2011.3044

752   Salgado, Zângaro, Parreira, and Kerppers. "The effects of transcranial LED therapy (TCLT) on cerebral blood flow in the elderly women." *Lasers in Medical Science*, 2015. https://doi.org/10.1007/s10103-014-1669-2

753   Maksimovich. "Laser technologies as a new direction in transcatheter interventions." *Photobiomodulation, Photomedicine, and Laser Surgery*, 2019.https://doi.org/10.1089/photob.2019.4631

754   Maksimovich. "Endovascular application of low-energy laser in the treatment of dyscirculatory angiopathy of Alzheimer's type." *Journal of Behavioral and Brain Science*, 2012. https://www.researchgate.net/publication/266488712

755   DiDuro, Salehpour, Wang, and Kokos. "Acute effects of intranasal photobiomodulation on blood flow and cerebral oxygen delivery." Abstract presented at the *Photobiomodulation, Photomedicine, and Laser Surgery* Photobiomodulation Virtual Summit, 2021.

756   Dmochowski, Shereen, Berisha, and Dmochowski. "Near-infrared light increases functional connectivity with a non-thermal mechanism." *Cerebral Cortex Communications*, 2020. https://academic.oup.com/cercorcomms/article/1/1/tgaa004/5809511

757   Johnstone, Mitrofanis, and Stone. "Targeting the body to protect the brain: inducing neuroprotection with remotely-applied near infrared light." *Neural Regeneration Research*, 2015. https://www.ncbi.nlm.nih.gov/pmc/articles/PMC4396086/

758   Matsushita, Kibayashi, Katayama, Yamashita, Suzuki, Kawamata, Honmou, Minami, and Shimohama. "Mesenchymal stem cells transmigrate across brain microvascular endothelial cell monolayers through transiently formed inter-endothelial gaps." *Neuroscience Letters*, 2011. https://doi.org/10.1016/j.neulet.2011.07.021

759   Farfara, Tuby, Trudler, Doron-Mandel, Maltz, Vassar, Frenkel, and Oron. "Low-level laser therapy ameliorates disease progression in a mouse model of Alzheimer's disease." *Journal of Molecular Neuroscience*, 2015. https://doi.org/10.1007/s12031-014-0354-z

760   Salehpour, Khademi, Bragin, and DiDuro. "Photobiomodulation therapy and the glymphatic system: promising applications for augmenting the brain lymphatic drainage system." *International Journal of Molecular Sciences*, 2022. https://www.ncbi.nlm.nih.gov/pmc/articles/PMC8950470/

761   Gordon and Johnstone. "Remote photobiomodulation research: an emerging strategy for neuroprotection." *Neural Regeneration Research*, 2019. https://doi.org/10.4103/1673-5374.262573

762   Caldieraro, Salehpour, and Cassano. "Transcranial and systemic photobiomodulation for the enhancement of mitochondrial metabolism in depression." *Clinical Bioenergetics*, 2021. https://doi.org/10.1016/B978-0-12-819621-2.00028-0

763   Farfara, Tuby, Trudler, Doron-Mandel, Maltz, Vassar, Frenkel, and Oron. "Low-level laser therapy ameliorates disease progression in a mouse model of Alzheimer's disease." *Journal of Molecular Neuroscience*, 2015. https://doi.org/10.1007/s12031-014-0354-z

764   Blivet, Meunier, Roman, and Touchon. "Neuroprotective effect of a new photobiomodulation technique against $A\beta_{25-35}$ peptide-induced toxicity in mice: novel hypothesis for therapeutic approach of Alzheimer's disease suggested." *Alzheimer's & Dementia*, 2018. https://www.ncbi.nlm.nih.gov/pmc/articles/PMC6021268/

[765] Kim, Mitrofanis, Stone, and Johnstone. "Remote tissue conditioning is neuroprotective against MPTP insult in mice." *IBRO Reports*, 2018. https://www.ncbi.nlm.nih.gov/pmc/articles/PMC6084900/

[766] Johnstone, el Massri, Moro, Spana, Wang, Torres, Chabrol, De Jaeger, Reinhart, Purushothuman, Benabid, Stone, and Mitrofanis. "Indirect application of near infrared light induces neuroprotection in a mouse model of parkinsonism: an abscopal neuroprotective effect." *Neuroscience*, 2014. https://doi.org/10.1016/j.neuroscience.2014.05.023

[767] Ganeshan, Skladnev, Kim, Mitrofanis, Stone, and Johnstone. "Pre-conditioning with remote photobiomodulation modulates the brian transcriptome and protects against MPTP insult in mice." *Neuroscience*, 2019. https://doi.org/10.1016/j.neuroscience.2018.12.050

[768] Liu, Cheng, Su, Zhang, Shi, Liu, Zhang, and Qian. "Randomized, double-blind, and placebo-controlled clinic report of intranasal low-intensity laser therapy on vascular diseases." *International Journal of Photoenergy*, 2012. https://www.hindawi.com/journals/ijp/2012/489713/

[769] Elwood, Pickering, and Gallacher. "Cognitive function and blood rheology: results from the Caerphilly cohort of older men." *Age and Ageing*, 2001. https://doi.org/10.1093/ageing/30.2.135

[770] Li. "The relationship between hemorheological changes and the anxiety and depression symptoms in schizophrenia." *Chinese Journal of Hemorheology*, 2004. https://www.semanticscholar.org/paper/The-Relationship-between-Hemorheological-Changes-in-Li/4dd89afbe5bc234fa62ae34c77467c1cd23cfc6f#related-papers

[771] Chakraborty, Davis, and Muthuchamy. "Emerging trends in the pathophysiology of lymphatic contractile function." *Seminars in Cell & Developmental Biology*, 2015. https://www.ncbi.nlm.nih.gov/pmc/articles/PMC4397138/

[772] Salehpour, Gholipour-Khalili, Farajdokht, Kamari, Walski, Hamblin, DiDuro, and Cassano. "Therapeutic potential of intranasal photobiomodulation therapy for neurological and neuropsychiatric disorders: a narrative review." *Reviews in the Neurosciences*, 2019. https://doi.org/10.1515/revneuro-2019-0063

[773] Salehpour, Gholipour-Khalili, Farajdokht, Kamari, Walski, Hamblin, DiDuro, and Cassano. "Therapeutic potential of intranasal photobiomodulation therapy for neurological and neuropsychiatric disorders: a narrative review." *Reviews in the Neurosciences*, 2019. https://doi.org/10.1515/revneuro-2019-0063

[774] Attwell, Buchan, Charpak, Lauritzen, Macvicar, and Newman. "Glial and neuronal control of brain blood flow." *Nature*, 2010. https://pubmed.ncbi.nlm.nih.gov/21068832/

[775] Quirk and Whelan. "What lies at the heart of photobiomodulation: light, cytochrome c oxidase, and nitric oxide—review of the evidence." *Photobiomodulation, Photomedicine, and Laser Surgery*, 2020. https://doi.org/10.1089/photob.2020.4905

[776] Zhao. "Interplay among nitric oxide and reactive oxygen species: a complex network determining cell survival or death." *Plant Signaling & Behavior*, 2007. https://www.ncbi.nlm.nih.gov/pmc/articles/PMC2634364/

[777] Litscher, Min, Passegger, Litscher, Li, Wang, Ghaffari-Tabrizi-Wiszy, Stelzer, Feigl, Gaischek, Wang, Sadjak, and Bahr. "Transcranial yellow, red, and infrared laser and LED stimulation: changes of vascular parameters in a chick embryo model." *Integrative Medicine International*, 2015. https://www.karger.com/Article/Fulltext/431176

[778] Mitchell and Mack. "Low-level laser treatment with near-infrared light increases venous nitric oxide levels acutely: a single-blind, randomized clinical trial of efficacy." *American Journal of Physical Medicine & Rehabilitation*, 2013. https://doi.org/10.1097/PHM.0b013e318269d70a

779   Weihrauch, Keszler, Lindemer, Krolikowski, and Lohr. "Red light stimulates vasodila-
      tion through extracellular vesicle trafficking." *Journal of Photochemistry and Photobiology
      (Biology)*, 2021. https://doi.org/10.1016/j.jphotobiol.2021.112212
780   Maegawa, Itoh, Hosokawa, Yaegashi, and Nishi. "Effects of near-infrared low-level laser
      irradiation on microcirculation." *Lasers in Surgery and Medicine*, 2000. https://doi.
      org/10.1002/1096-9101(2000)27:5<427::AID-LSM1004>3.0.CO;2-A
781   Naeser, Zafonte, Krengel, Martin, Frazier, Hamblin, Knight, Meehan, and Baker.
      "Significant improvements in cognitive performance post-transcranial red/near-infrared
      light-emitting diode treatments in chronic, mild traumatic brain injury: open-protocol
      study." *Journal of Neurotrauma*, 2014. https://doi.org/10.1089/neu.2013.3244
782   Venturelli, Pedrinolla, Galazzo, Fonte, Smania, Tamburin, Muti, Crispoltoni, Stabile,
      Pistilli, Rende, Pizzini, and Schena. "Impact of nitric oxide bioavailability on the pro-
      gressive cerebral and peripheral circulatory impairments during aging and Alzheimer's
      disease." *Frontiers in Physiology*, 2018. https://doi.org/10.3389/fphys.2018.00169
783   Caldieraro, Salehpour, and Cassano. "Transcranial and systemic photobiomodulation
      for the enhancement of mitochondrial metabolism in depression." *Clinical Bioenergetics*,
      2021. https://doi.org/10.1016/B978-0-12-819621-2.00028-0
784   Wang, Tian, Reddy, Nalawade, Barrett, Gonzalez-Lima, and Liu. "Up-regulation of
      cerebral cytochrome-c-oxidase and hemodynamics by transcranial infrared laser stimu-
      lation: a broadband near-infrared spectroscopy study." *Journal of Cerebral Blood Flow &
      Metabolism*, 2017. https://doi.org/10.1177/0271678X17691783
785   Pruitt, Wang, Wu, Kallioniemi, Husain, and Liu. "Transcranial photobiomodulation
      (tPBM) with 1,064-nm laser to improve cerebral metabolism of the human brain in
      vivo." *Lasers in Surgery and Medicine*, 2020. https://doi.org/10.1002/lsm.23232
786   Ahluwalia and Tarnawski. "Critical role of hypoxia sensor HIF-1⊠ in VEGF gene
      activation: implications for angiogenesis and tissue injury healing." *Current Medicinal
      Chemistry*, 2012. https://doi.org/10.2174/092986712803413944
787   Purushothuman, Johnstone, Nandasena, Mitrofanis, and Stone. "Photobiomodulation
      with near infrared light mitigates Alzheimer's disease-related pathology in cerebral cor-
      tex – evidence from two transgenic mouse models." *Alzheimer's Research & Therapy*,
      2014. https://www.ncbi.nlm.nih.gov/pmc/articles/PMC3978916/
788   Purushothuman, Johnston, Nandasena, van Eersel, Ittner, Mitrofanis, and Stone. "Near
      infrared light mitigates cerebellar pathology in transgenic mouse models of dementia."
      Neuroscience Letters, 2015. https://doi.org/10.1016/j.neulet.2015.02.037
789   Eltchechem, Salgado, Zângaro, Pereira, Kerppers, da Silva, and Parreira. "Transcranial
      LED therapy on amyloid-ß toxin 25-35 in the hippocampal region of rats." *Lasers in
      Medical Science*, 2017. https://link.springer.com/article/10.1007/s10103-017-2156-3
790   Zinchenko, Navolokin, Shirokov, Khlebtsov, Dubrovsky, Saranceva, Abdurashitov,
      Khorovodov, Terskov, Mamedova, Klimova, Agranovich, Martinov, Tuchin,
      Semyachkina-Glushkovskaya, and Kurts. "Pilot study of transcranial photobiomodula-
      tion of lymphatic clearance of beta-amyloid from the mouse brain: breakthrough strat-
      egies for non-pharmacologic therapy of Alzheimer's disease." *Biomedical Optics Express*,
      2019. https://www.ncbi.nlm.nih.gov/pmc/articles/PMC6701516/
791   Zinchenko, Navolokin, Shirokov, Khlebtsov, Dubrovsky, Saranceva, Abdurashitov,
      Khorovodov, Terskov, Mamedova, Klimova, Agranovich, Martinov, Tuchin,
      Semyachkina-Glushkovskaya, and Kurts. "Pilot study of transcranial photobiomodula-
      tion of lymphatic clearance of beta-amyloid from the mouse brain: breakthrough strat-

egies for non-pharmacologic therapy of Alzheimer's disease." *Biomedical Optics Express*, 2019. https://www.ncbi.nlm.nih.gov/pmc/articles/PMC6701516/

792   De Taboada, Yu, El-Amouri, Gattoni-Celli, Richieri, McCarthy, Streeter, and Kindy. "Transcranial laser therapy attenuates amyloid-ß peptide neuropathology in amyloid-ß protein precursor transgenic mice." *Journal of Alzheimer's Disease*, 2011. https://doi.org/10.3233/JAD-2010-100894

793   Semyachkina-Glushkovskaya, Klimova, Iskra, Bragin, Abdurashitov, Dubrovsky, Khorovodov, Terskov, Blokhina, Lezhnev, Vinnik, Agranovich, Mamedova, Shirokov, Navolokin, Khlebsov, Tuchin, and Kurths. "Transcranial photobiomodulation of clearance of beta-amyloid from the mouse brain: effects on the meningeal lymphatic drainage and blood oxygen saturation of the brain." *Advances in Experimental Medicine and Biology*, 2021. https://link.springer.com/chapter/10.1007/978-3-030-48238-1_9

794   Yue, Mei, Zhang, Tong, Cui, Yang, Wang, Wang, Fei, Ai, Di, Luo, Li, Luo, Lu, Li, Duan, Gao, Yang, Sun, He, Song, Han, and Tong. "New insight into Alzheimer's disease: light reverses Aß-obstructed interstitial fluid flow and ameliorates memory decline in APP/PS1 mice." *Alzheimer's & Dementia*, 2019. https://www.ncbi.nlm.nih.gov/pmc/articles/PMC6838540/

795   Li, Liu, Yu, Liu, Sun, Bragin, Navolokin, Kurths, Glushkovskaya-Semyachkina, and Zhu. "Photostimulation of lymphatic clearance of red blood cells from the mouse brain after intraventricular hemorrhage." *bioRxiv*, 2020. https://doi.org/10.1101/2020.11.16.384149

796   Zinchenko, Klimova, Mamedova, Agranovich, Blokhina, Antonova, Terskov, Shirokov, Navolokin, Morgun, Osipova, Boytsova, Yu, Zhu, Kurths, and Semyachkina-Glushkovskaya. "Photostimulation of extravasation of beta-amyloid through the model of blood-brain barrier." *Electronics*, 2020. https://www.mdpi.com/2079-9292/9/6/1056/htm

797   Semyachkina-Glushkovskaya, Abdurashitov, Dubrovsky, Klimova, Agranovich, Terskov, Shirokov, Vinnik, Kuzmina, Lezhnev, Blokhina, Shnitenkova, Tuchin, Rafailov, and Kurths. "Photobiomodulation of lymphatic drainage and clearance: prospective strategy for augmentation of meningeal lymphatic functions." *Biomedical Optics Express*, 2020. https://www.ncbi.nlm.nih.gov/pmc/articles/PMC7041454/

798   Lim. "Intranasal photobiomodulation improves cognitive and memory performance of Alzheimer's disease patients in case studies." *Proceedings of the NAALT/WALT Conference*, 2014.

799   Saltmarche, Naeser, Ho, Hamblin, and Lim. "Significant improvement in cognition in mild to moderately severe dementia cases treated with transcranial plus intranasal photobiomodulation: case series report." *Photomedicine and Laser Surgery*, 2017. https://www.ncbi.nlm.nih.gov/pmc/articles/PMC5568598/

800   Chao. "Effects of home photobiomodulation treatments on cognitive and behavioral function, cerebral perfusion, and resting-state functional connectivity in patients with dementia: a pilot trial." *Photobiomodulation, Photomedicine, and Laser Surgery*, 2019. https://doi.org/10.1089/photob.2018.4555

801   Zomorrodi, Saltmarche, Loheswarran, Ho, and Lim. "Complementary EEG evidence for a significantly improved Alzheimer's disease case after photobiomodulation treatment." *Alzheimer's Association International Conference*, 2017. https://doi.org/10.1016/j.jalz.2017.06.691

802   Peci, Giannelli, Pica, Salvo, Ivic, and Peci. "A pilot study of photobiomodulation therapy using NIR: pre and post 810 nm stimulation in patients affected by neurological diseases." *EC Neurology*, 2020. https://www.researchgate.net/publication/340454403

803 Arakelyan. "Treatment of Alzheimer's disease with a combination of laser, magnetic field, and chromo light (colour) therapies: a double-blind controlled trial based on a review and overview of the etiological pathophysiology of Alzheimer's disease." *Laser Therapy*, 2005. https://doi.org/10.5978/islsm.14.19

804 Berman, Halper, Nichols, Jarrett, Lundy, and Huang. "Photobiomodulation with near infrared light helmet in a pilot, placebo controlled clinical trial in dementia patients testing memory and cognition." *Journal of Neurology and Neuroscience*, 2017. https://www.ncbi.nlm.nih.gov/pmc/articles/PMC5459322/

805 Salehpour, Hamblin, and DiDuro. "Rapid reversal of cognitive decline, olfactory dysfunction, and quality of life using multi-modality photobiomodulation therapy: case report." *Photobiomodulation, Photomedicine, and Laser Surgery*, 2019. https://doi.org/10.1089/photob.2018.4569

806 Salehpour, Ahmadian, Rasta, Farhoudi, Karimi, and Sadigh-Eteghad. "Transcranial low-level laser therapy improves brain mitochondrial function and cognitive impairment in D-galactose-induced aging mice." *Neurobiology of Aging*, 2017. https://doi.org/10.1016/j.neurobiolaging.2017.06.025

807 Eltchechem, Salgado, Zângaro, Pereira, Kerppers, da Silva, and Parreira. "Transcranial LED therapy on amyloid-ß toxin 25-35 in the hippocampal region of rats." *Lasers in Medical Science*, 2017. https://link.springer.com/article/10.1007/s10103-017-2156-3

808 Zinchenko, Klimova, Mamedova, Agranovich, Blokhina, Antonova, Terskov, Shirokov, Navolokin, Morgun, Osipova, Boytsova, Yu, Zhu, Kurths, and Semyachkina-Glushkovskaya. "Photostimulation of extravasation of beta-amyloid through the model of blood-brain barrier." *Electronics*, 2020. https://www.mdpi.com/2079-9292/9/6/1056/htm

809 Semyachkina-Glushkovskaya, Abdurashitov, Klimova, Dubrovsky, Shirokov, Fomin, Terskov, Agranovich, Mamedova, Khorovodov, Vinnik, Blokhina, Lezhnev, Shareef, Kuzmina, Sokolovski, Tuchin, Rafailov, and Kurths. "Photostimulation of cerebral and peripheral lymphatic functions." *Translational Biophotonics*, 2020. https://onlinelibrary.wiley.com/doi/full/10.1002/tbio.201900036

810 Albrecht and Ripperger. "Circadian clocks and sleep: impact of rhythmic metabolism and waste clearance on the brain." *Trends in Neurosciences*, 2018. https://doi.org/10.1016/j.tins.2018.07.007

811 Yassine, Self, Kerman, Santoni, Shanmugam, Abdullah, Golden, Fonteh, Harrington, Gräff, Gibson, Kalaria, Luchsinger, Feldman, Swerdlow, Johnson, Albensi, Zlokovic, Tanzi, Cunnane, Samieri, Scarmeas, and Bowman. "Nutritional metabolism and cerebral bioenergetics in Alzheimer's disease and related dementias." *Alzheimer's & Dementia*, 2022. https://alz-journals.onlinelibrary.wiley.com/doi/full/10.1002/alz.12845?utm_source=google&utm_medium=paidsearch&utm_campaign=R3MR425&utm_content=Medicine

812 Dos Santos, Paiva, and Teixeira. "Transcranial light-emitting diode therapy for neuropsychological improvement after traumatic brain injury: a new perspective for diffuse axonal lesion management." *Medical Devices: Evidence and Research*, 2018. https://www.ncbi.nlm.nih.gov/pmc/articles/PMC5927185/

813 Salehpour, Khademi, Bragin, and DiDuro. "Photobiomodulation therapy and the glymphatic system: promising applications for augmenting the brain lymphatic drainage system." *International Journal of Molecular Sciences*, 2022. https://www.ncbi.nlm.nih.gov/pmc/articles/PMC8950470/

814 Lee, Lee, Kim, Kim, Park, Choi, Shin, and Shin. "Pretreatment with light-emitting diode therapy reduces ischemic brain injury in mice through endothelial nitric oxide

synthase-dependent mechanisms." *Biochemical and Biophysical Research Communications*, 2017. https://doi.org/10.1016/j.bbrc.2017.03.131

[815] Pruitt, Wang, Wu, Kallioniemi, Husain, and Liu. "Transcranial photobiomodulation (tPBM) with 1,064-nm laser to improve cerebral metabolism of the human brain in vivo." *Lasers in Surgery and Medicine*, 2020. https://doi.org/10.1002/lsm.23232

[816] Mikhaylov. "The use of intravenous laser blood irradiation (ILBI) at 630-640 nm to prevent vascular diseases and to increase life expectancy." *Laser Therapy*, 2015. https://www.ncbi.nlm.nih.gov/pmc/articles/PMC4416141/

[817] Yan, Liu, Zhang, Li, Sun, Zhao, Dong, Qian, and Sun. "Low-level laser irradiation modulates brain-derived neurotrophic factor mRNA transcription through calcium-dependent activation of the ERK/CREB pathway." *Lasers in Medical Science*, 2016. https://doi.org/10.1007/s10103-016-2099-0

[818] Meng, He, and Xing. "Low-level laser therapy rescues dendrite atrophy via upregulating BDNF expression: implications for Alzheimer's disease." *Journal of Neuroscience*, 2013. https://www.ncbi.nlm.nih.gov/pmc/articles/PMC6705158/

[819] Johnstone, Moro, Stone, Benabid, and Mitrofanis. "Turning on lights to stop neurodegeneration: the potential of near infrared light therapy in Alzheimer's and Parkinson's disease." *Frontiers in Neuroscience*, 2016. https://www.frontiersin.org/articles/10.3389/fnins.2015.00500/full

[820] Liebert, Bicknell, Laakso, Heller, Jalilitabaei, Tilley, Mitrofanis, and Kiat. "Improvements in clinical signs of Parkinson's disease using photobiomodulation: a prospective proof-of-concept study." *BMC Neurology*, 2021. https://doi.org/10.1186/s12883-021-02248-y

[821] Johnstone, Hamilton, Gordon, Moro, Torres, Nicklason, Stone, Benabid, and Mitrofanis. "Exploring the use of intracranial and extracranial (remote) photobiomodulation devices in Parkinson's disease: a comparison of direct and indirect systemic stimulations." *Journal of Alzheimer's Disease*, 2021. https://doi.org/10.3233/JAD-210052

[822] Ying, Liang, Whelan, Eells, and Wong-Riley. "Pretreatment with near-infrared light via light-emitting diode provides added benefit against rotenone- and MPP+-induced neurotoxicity." *Brain Research*, 2008. https://doi.org/10.1016/j.brainres.2008.09.057

[823] Bikmulina, Kosheleva, Shpichka, Timashev, Yusupov, Maximchik, Gogvadze, and Rochev. "Photobiomodulation enhances mitochondrial respiration in an *in vitro* rotenone model of Parkinson's disease." *Optical Engineering*, 2020. https://doi.org/10.1117/1.OE.59.6.061620

[824] de la Torre, Olmo, and Valles. "Can mild cognitive impairment be stabilized by showering brain mitochondria with laser photons?" *Neuropharmacology*, 2019. https://doi.org/10.1016/j.neuropharm.2019.107841

[825] Chen and Zhong. "Oxidative stress in Alzheimer's disease." *Neuroscience Bulletin*, 2014. https://www.ncbi.nlm.nih.gov/pmc/articles/PMC5562667/

[826] Cardoso, Mansur, Araújo, Gonzalez-Lima, and Gomes da Silva. "Photobiomodulation improves the inflammatory response and intracellular signaling proteins linked to vascular function and cell survival in the brain of aged rats." *Molecular Neurobiology*, 2022. https://doi.org/10.1007/s12035-021-02606-4

[827] Lu, Wang, Dong Tucker, Zhao, Ahmed, Zhu, Liu, Cohen, and Zhang. "Low-level laser therapy for beta amyloid toxicity in rat hippocampus." *Neurobiology of Aging*, 2017. https://www.ncbi.nlm.nih.gov/pmc/articles/PMC5458630/

[828] Comerota, Krishnan, and Taglialatela. "Near infrared light decreases synaptic vulnerability to amyloid beta oligomers." *Scientific Reports*, 2017. https://www.ncbi.nlm.nih.gov/pmc/articles/PMC5678170/

829 Comerota, Tumurbaatar, Krishnan, Kayed, and Taglialatela. "Near infrared light treatment reduces synaptic levels of toxic tau oligomers in two transgenic mouse models of human tauopathies." *Molecular Neurobiology*, 2019. https://www.ncbi.nlm.nih.gov/pmc/articles/PMC6476871/

830 Stepanov, Golovynska, Zhang, Golovynskyi, Stepanova, Gorbach, Dobvynchuk, Garmanchuk, Ohulchanskyy, and Qu. "Near-infrared light reduces ß-amyloid-stimulated microglial toxicity and enhances survival of neurons: mechanisms of light therapy for Alzheimer's disease." *Alzheimer's Research & Therapy*, 2022. https://www.ncbi.nlm.nih.gov/pmc/articles/PMC9206341/

831 Blivet, Meunier, Roman, and Touchon. "Neuroprotective effect of a new photobiomodulation technique against $Aß_{25-35}$ peptide-induced toxicity in mice: novel hypothesis for therapeutic approach of Alzheimer's disease suggested." *Alzheimer's & Dementia*, 2018. https://www.ncbi.nlm.nih.gov/pmc/articles/PMC6021268/

832 Grillo, Duggett, Ennaceur, and Chazot. "Non-invasive infra-red therapy (1072 nm) reduces ß-amyloid protein levels in the brain of an Alzheimer's disease mouse model, TASTPM." *Journal of Photochemistry and Photobiology B*, 2013. https://doi.org/10.1016/j.jphotobiol.2013.02.015

833 Soto. "Unfolding the role of protein misfolding in neurodegenerative diseases." *Nature Reviews Neuroscience*, 2003. https://www.nature.com/articles/nrn1007

834 Mitrofanis and Jeffery. "Does photobiomodulation influence ageing?" *Aging*, 2018. https://www.ncbi.nlm.nih.gov/pmc/articles/PMC6188498/

835 Sommer, Bieschke, Friedrich, Zhu, Wanker, Fecht, Mereles, and Hunstein. "670 nm laser light and EGCG complementarily reduce amyloid-ß aggregates in human neuroblastoma cells: basis for treatment of Alzheimer's disease?" *Photomedicine and Laser Surgery*, 2012. https://doi.org/10.1089/pho.2011.3073

836 Yang, Askarova, Sheng, Chen, Sun, Sun, Yao, and Lee. "Low energy laser light (632.8 nm) suppresses amyloid-ß peptide-induced oxidative and inflammatory responses in astrocytes." *Neuroscience*, 2010. https://doi.org/10.1016/j.neuroscience.2010.09.025

837 Rojas, Bruchey, and Gonzalez-Lima. "Low-level light therapy improves cortical metabolic capacity and memory retention." *Journal of Alzheimer's Disease*, 2012. https://doi.org/10.3233/JAD-2012-120817

838 Saucedo, Courtois, Wade, Kelley, Kheradbin, Barrett, and Gonzalez-Lima. "Transcranial laser stimulation: mitochondrial and cerebrovascular effects in younger and older healthy adults." *Brain Stimulation*, 2021. https://doi.org/10.1016/j.brs.2021.02.011

839 Hamblin. "Photobiomodulation for Alzheimer's disease: Has the light dawned?" *Photonics*, 2019. https://www.ncbi.nlm.nih.gov/pmc/articles/PMC6664299/

840 Huang, Nagata, Tedford, McCarthy, and Hamblin. "Low-level laser therapy (LLLT) reduces oxidative stress in primary cortical neurons *in vitro*." *Journal of Biophotonics*, 2013. https://www.ncbi.nlm.nih.gov/pmc/articles/PMC3651776/

841 Sharma, Kharkwal, Sajo, Huang, de Taboada, McCarthy, and Hamblin. "Dose response effects of 810 nm laser light on mouse primary cortical neurons." *Lasers in Surgery and Medicine*, 2011. https://doi.org/10.1002/lsm.21100

842 Huang, Nagata, Tedford, and Hamblin. "Low-level laser therapy (810 nm) protects primary cortical neurons against excitotoxicity *in vitro*." *Journal of Biophotonics*, 2014. https://www.ncbi.nlm.nih.gov/pmc/articles/PMC4057365/

843 Yang, Youngblood, Wu, and Zhang. "Mitochondria as a target for neuroprotection: role of methylene blue and photobiomodulation." *Translational Neurodegeneration*, 2020. https://doi.org/10.1186/s40035-020-00197-z

REFERENCES

[844] Barrett and Gonzalez-Lima. "Transcranial infrared laser stimulation produces beneficial cognitive and emotional effects in humans." *Neuroscience*, 2013. https://doi.org/10.1016/j.neuroscience.2012.11.016

[845] Gonzalez-Lima and Barrett. "Augmentation of cognitive brain functions with transcranial lasers." *Frontiers in Systems Neuroscience*, 2014. https://www.ncbi.nlm.nih.gov/pmc/articles/PMC3953713/

[846] Jahan, Nazari, Mahmoudi, Salehpour, and Salimi. "Transcranial near-infrared photobiomodulation could modulate brain electrophysiological features and attentional performance in healthy young adults." *Lasers in Medical Science*, 2019. https://www.researchgate.net/publication/332565401

[847] Dougal, Ennaceur, and Chazot. "Effect of transcranial near-infrared light 1,068 nm upon memory performance in aging healthy individuals: a pilot study." *Photobiomodulation, Photomedicine, and Laser Surgery*, 2021. https://doi.org/10.1089/photob.2020.4956

[848] Michalikova, Ennaceur, van Rensburg, and Chazot. "Emotional responses and memory performance of middle-aged CD1 mice in a 3D maze: effects of low infrared light." *Neurobiology of Learning and Memory*, 2007. https://doi.org/10.1016/j.nlm.2007.07.014

[849] Chan, Lee, Yeung, and Hamblin. "Photobiomodulation improves the frontal cognitive function of older adults." *International Journal of Geriatric Psychiatry*, 2019. https://www.ncbi.nlm.nih.gov/pmc/articles/PMC6333495/

[850] Blanco, Maddox, and Gonzalez-Lima. "Improving executive function using transcranial infrared laser stimulation." *Journal of Neuropsychology*, 2017. https://www.ncbi.nlm.nih.gov/pmc/articles/PMC4662930/

[851] Vargas, Barrett, Saucedo, Huang, Abraham, Tanaka, Haley, and Gonzalez-Lima. "Beneficial neurocognitive effects of transcranial laser in older adults." *Lasers in Medical Science*, 2017. https://www.ncbi.nlm.nih.gov/pmc/articles/PMC6802936/

[852] Chan, Lee, Sze, and Hamblin. "Photobiomodulation improves memory in mild cognitive impairment: three case reports." *Alzheimer's Disease & Dementia*, 2021. https://scholars.direct/Articles/alzheimers-disease-and-dementia/add-5-018.php?jid=alzheimers-disease-and-dementia

[853] Chan, Lee, Hamblin, and Cheung. "Photobiomodulation enhances memory processing in older adults with mild cognitive impairment: a functional near-infrared spectroscopy study." *Journal of Alzheimer's Disease*, 2021. https://doi.org/10.3233/jad-201600

[854] Blanco, Saucedo, and Gonzalez-Lima. "Transcranial infrared laser stimulation improves rule-based, but not information-integration, category learning in humans." *Neurobiology of Learning and Memory*, 2017. https://doi.org/10.1016/j.nlm.2016.12.016

[855] Liu, Gong, Xia, Wang, Peng, Shen, and Liu. "Light therapy: a new option for neurodegenerative diseases." *Chinese Medical Journal*, 2021. https://www.ncbi.nlm.nih.gov/pmc/articles/PMC7990011/

[856] Spera, Sitnikova, Ward, Farzam, Hughes, Gazecki, Bui, Maiello, de Taboada, Hamblin, Franceschini, and Cassano. "Pilot study on dose-dependent effects of transcranial photobiomodulation on brain electrical oscillations: a potential therapeutic target in Alzheimer's disease." *Journal of Alzheimer's Disease*, 2021. https://doi.org/10.3233/jad-210058

[857] Urquhart, Wanniarachchi, Wang, Gonzalez-Lima, Alexandrakis, and Liu. "Transcranial photobiomodulation-induced changes in human brain functional connectivity and network metrics mapped by whole-head functional near-infrared spectroscopy *in vivo*." *Biomedical Optics Express*, 2020. https://www.ncbi.nlm.nih.gov/pmc/articles/PMC7587286/

[858] Chan, Lee, Hamblin, and Cheung. "Photoneuromodulation makes a difficult cognitive task less arduous." *Scientific Reports*, 2021. https://www.researchgate.net/publication/352900690

[859] de la Torre. "Detection, prevention, and pre-clinical treatment of Alzheimer's disease." *Journal of Alzheimer's Disease*, 2014. https://doi.org/10.3233/JAD-141800

[860] Cassano. "Photomedicine and pharmaceuticals: a brain new deal." *Photobiomodulation, Photomedicine, and Laser Surgery*, 2019. https://doi.org/10.1089/photob.2019.4733

[861] Bradford, Kunik, Schulz, Williams, and Singh. "Missed and delayed diagnosis of dementia in primary care: prevalence and contributing factors." *Alzheimer Disease and Associated Disorders*, 2009. https://www.ncbi.nlm.nih.gov/pmc/articles/PMC2787842/

[862] Stephan and Brayne. "Risk factors and screening methods for detecting dementia: a narrative review." *Journal of Alzheimer's Disease*, 2014. https://doi.org/10.3233/JAD-141413

[863] Anstey, Eramudugolla, and Dixon. "Contributions of a risk assessment approach to the prevention of Alzheimer's disease and dementia." *Journal of Alzheimer's Disease*, 2014. https://doi.org/10.3233/JAD-141248

[864] Alderman, Olson, and Brush. "Using event-related potentials to study the effects of chronic exercise on cognitive function." *International Journal of Sport and Exercise Psychology*, 2016. https://doi.org/10.1080/1612197X.2016.1223419

[865] Van Praag, Christie, Sejnowski, and Gage. "Running enhances neurogenesis, learning, and long-term potentiation in mice." *Proceedings of the National Academy of Sciences*, 1999. https://www.pnas.org/doi/10.1073/pnas.96.23.13427

[866] Erickson, Voss, Prakash, Basak, Szabo, Chaddock, Kim, Heo, Alves, White, Wojcicki, Mailey, Vieira, Martin, Pence, Woods, McAuley, and Kramer. "Exercise training increases size of hippocampus and improves memory." *Proceedings of the National Academy of Sciences*, 2011. https://www.pnas.org/doi/10.1073/pnas.1015950108

[867] Thomas, Tarumi, Sheng, Tseng, Womack, Cullum, Rypma, Zhang, and Lu. "Brain perfusion change in patients with mild cognitive impairment after 12 months of aerobic exercise training." *Journal of Alzheimer's Disease*, 2020. https://doi.org/10.3233/JAD-190977

[868] Cruz, Ahmadi, Naismith, and Stamatakis. "Association of daily step count and intensity with incident dementia in 78430 adults living in the UK." *JAMA Neurology*, 2022. https://jamanetwork.com/journals/jamaneurology/fullarticle/2795819

[869] Tarumi, Gonzales, Fallow, Nualnim, Pyron, Tanaka, and Haley. "Central artery stiffness, neuropsychological function, and cerebral perfusion in sedentary and endurance-trained middle-aged adults." *Journal of Hypertension*, 2013. https://doi.org/10.1097/HJH.0b013e328364decc

[870] Tomoto, Tarumi, Chen, Hynan, Cullum, and Zhang. "One-year aerobic exercise altered cerebral vasomotor reactivity in mild cognitive impairment." *Journal of Applied Physiology*, 2021. https://doi.org/10.1152/japplphysiol.00158.2021

[871] Wrann, White, Salogiannis, Laznik-Bogoslavski, Wu, Ma, Lin, Greenberg, and Spiegelman. "Exercise induces hippocampal BDNF through a PGC-1α/FNDC5 pathway." *Cell Metabolism*, 2013. https://www.ncbi.nlm.nih.gov/pmc/articles/PMC3980968/

[872] Trezza, Baarendse, and Vanderschuren. "The pleasures of play: pharmacological insights into social reward mechanisms." *Trends in Pharmacological Sciences*, 2010. https://www.ncbi.nlm.nih.gov/pmc/articles/PMC2946511/

[873] Yorgason, Johnson, Hill, and Selland. "Marital benefits of daily individual and conjoint exercise among older couples." *Family Relations*, 2018. https://doi.org/10.1111/fare.12307

[874] Patrick and Ames. "Vitamin D and the omega-3 fatty acids control serotonin synthesis and action, part 2: relevance for ADHD, bipolar, schizophrenia, and impulsive behavior." *FASEB Journal*, 2015. https://doi.org/10.1096/fj.14-268342

[875] Geda, Roberts, Knopman, Christianson, Pankratz, Ivnik, Boeve, Tangalos, Petersen, and Rocca. "Physical exercise, aging, and mild cognitive impairment: a population-based study." *Archives of Neurology*, 2010. https://doi.org/10.1001/archneurol.2009.297

[876] Andel, Crowe, Pedersen, Fratiglioni, Johansson, and Gatz. "Physical exercise at midlife and risk of dementia three decades later: a population-based study of Swedish twins." *Journals of Gerontology Series A: Biological Sciences and Medical Sciences*, 2008. https://doi.org/10.1093/gerona/63.1.62

[877] Laurin, Verreault, Lindsay, MacPherson, and Rockwood. "Physical activity and risk of cognitive impairment and dementia in elderly persons." *Archives of Neurology*, 2001. https://doi.org/10.1001/archneur.58.3.498

[878] Hamer and Chida. "Physical activity and risk of neurodegenerative disease: a systematic review of prospective evidence." *Psychological Medicine*, 2009. https://doi.org/10.1017/S0033291708003681

[879] Hill and Gammie. "Alzheimer's disease large-scale gene expression portrait identifies exercise as the top theoretical treatment." *Scientific Reports*, 2022. https://www.nature.com/articles/s41598-022-22179-z

[880] Baker, Frank, Foster-Schubert, Green, Wilkinson, McTiernan, Plymate, Fishel, Watson, Cholerton, Duncan, Mehta, and Craft. "Effects of aerobic exercise on mild cognitive impairment: a controlled trial." *Archives of Neurology*, 2010. https://www.ncbi.nlm.nih.gov/pmc/articles/PMC3056436/

[881] Stuckenschneider, Askew, Rüdiger, Polidori, Abeln, Vogt, Krome, Olde Rikkert, Lawlor, Schneider, and NeuroExercise Study Group. "Cardiorespiratory fitness and cognitive function are positively related among participants with mild and subjective cognitive impairment." *Journal of Alzheimer's Disease*, 2018. https://doi.org/10.3233/JAD-170996

[882] Lautenschlager, Cox, Flicker, Foster, van Bockxmeer, Xiao, Greenop, and Almeida. "Effect of physical activity on cognitive function in older adults at risk for Alzheimer disease: a randomized trial." *Journal of the American Medical Association*, 2008. https://doi.org/10.1001/jama.300.9.1027

[883] Öhman, Savikko, Strandberg, and Pitkälä. "Effect of physical exercise on cognitive performance in older adults with mild cognitive impairment or dementia: a systematic review." *Dementia and Geriatric Cognitive Disorders*, 2014. https://doi.org/10.1159/000365388

[884] Nagamatsu, Handy, Hsu, Voss, and Liu-Ambrose. "Resistance training promotes cognitive and functional brain plasticity in seniors with probable mild cognitive impairment: a 6-month randomized controlled trial." *Archives of Internal Medicine*, 2012. https://www.ncbi.nlm.nih.gov/pmc/articles/PMC3514552/

[885] Nagamatsu, Chan, Davis, Beattie, Graf, Voss, Sharma, and Liu-Ambrose. "Physical activity improves verbal and spatial memory in older adults with probable mild cognitive impairment: a 6-month randomized controlled trial." *Journal of Aging Research*, 2013. https://www.ncbi.nlm.nih.gov/pmc/articles/PMC3595715/

[886] Amjad, Toor, Niazi, Afzal, Jochumsen, Shafique, Allen, Haavik, and Ahmed. "Therapeutic effects of aerobic exercise on EEG parameters and higher cognitive functions in mild cognitive impairment patients." *International Journal of Neuroscience*, 2019. https://doi.org/10.1080/00207454.2018.1551894

887 Krell-Roesch, Feder, Roberts, Mielke, Christianson, Knopman, Petersen, and Geda. "Leisure-time physical activity and the risk of incident dementia: the Mayo Clinic Study of Aging." *Journal of Alzheimer's Disease*, 2018. https://www.ncbi.nlm.nih.gov/pmc/articles/PMC5900557/

888 Tomoto, Tarumi, Chen, Hynan, Cullum, and Zhang. "One-year aerobic exercise altered cerebral vasomotor reactivity in mild cognitive impairment." *Journal of Applied Physiology*, 2021. https://doi.org/10.1152/japplphysiol.00158.2021

889 Bherer, Erickson, and Liu-Ambrose. "A review of the effects of physical activity and exercise on cognitive and brain functions in older adults." *Journal of Aging Research*, 2013. https://doi.org/10.1155/2013/657508

890 Gons, Tuladhar, de Laat, van Norden, van Dijk, Norris, Zwiers, and de Leeuw. "Physical activity is related to the structural integrity of cerebral white matter." *Neurology*, 2013. https://doi.org/10.1212/WNL.0b013e3182a43e33

891 Tseng, Gundapuneedi, Khan, Diaz-Arrastia, Levine, Lu, Huang, and Zhang. "White matter integrity in physically fit older adults." *NeuroImage*, 2013. https://www.ncbi.nlm.nih.gov/pmc/articles/PMC3759589/

892 Pereira, Huddleston, Brickman, Sosunov, Hen, McKhann, Sloan, Gage, Brown, and Small. "An *in vivo* correlate of exercise-induced neurogenesis in the adult dentate gyrus." *Proceedings of the National Academy of Sciences*, 2007. https://www.ncbi.nlm.nih.gov/pmc/articles/PMC1838482/

893 He, Liu, Zhang, Liang, Dai, Zeng, Pei, Xu, and Lan. "Voluntary exercise promotes glymphatic clearance of amyloid beta and reduces the activation of astrocytes and microglia in aged mice." *Frontiers in Molecular Neuroscience*, 2017. https://www.ncbi.nlm.nih.gov/pmc/articles/PMC5437122/

894 von Holstein-Rathlou, Petersen, and Nedergaard. "Voluntary running enhances glymphatic influx in awake behaving, young mice." *Neuroscience Letters*, 2018. https://www.ncbi.nlm.nih.gov/pmc/articles/PMC5696653/

895 Head, Bugg, Goate, Fagan, Mintun, Benzinger, Holtzman, and Morris. "Exercise engagement as a moderator of APOE effects on amyloid deposition." *Archives of Neurology*, 2013. https://www.ncbi.nlm.nih.gov/pmc/articles/PMC3583203/

896 Seals, DeSouza, Donato, and Tanaka. "Habitual exercise and arterial aging." *Journal of Applied Physiology*, 2008. https://www.ncbi.nlm.nih.gov/pmc/articles/PMC2576026/

897 Pedrinolla, Venturelli, Fonte, Tamburin, Di Baldassarre, Naro, Varalta, Giuriato, Ghinassi, Muti, Smania, and Schena. "Exercise training improves vascular function in patients with Alzheimer's disease." *European Journal of Applied Physiology*, 2020. https://www.ncbi.nlm.nih.gov/pmc/articles/PMC7502067/

898 Tarumi, Gonzales, Fallow, Nualnim, Lee, Pyron, Tanaka, and Haley. "Cerebral/peripheral vascular reactivity and neurocognition in middle-age athletes." *Medicine & Science in Sports & Exercise*, 2015. https://www.ncbi.nlm.nih.gov/pmc/articles/PMC4644461/

899 Rikli and Edwards. "Effects of a three-year exercise program on motor function and cognitive processing speed in older women." *Research Quarterly for Exercise and Sport*, 1991. https://doi.org/10.1080/02701367.1991.10607519

900 Gronek, Haas, Czarny, Podstawski, Delabary, Clark, Boraczyński, Tarnas, Wycichowska, Pawlaczyk, and Gronek. "The mechanism of physical activity-induced amelioration of Parkinson's disease: a narrative review." *Aging and Disease*, 2021. https://doi.org/10.14336/AD.2020.0407

901 Casaletto, Lindbergh, VandeBunte, Neuhaus, Schneider, Buchman, Honer, and Bennett. "Microglial correlates of late life physical activity: relationship with synaptic and cog-

nitive aging in older adults." *Journal of Neuroscience*, 2022. https://www.jneurosci.org/content/42/2/288

902 Tarumi and Zhang. "Cerebral hemodynamics of the aging brain: risk of Alzheimer disease and benefit of aerobic exercise." *Frontiers in Physiology*, 2014. https://www.frontiersin.org/articles/10.3389/fphys.2014.00006/full

903 Sorriento, Di Vaiai, and Iaccarino. "Physical exercise: a novel tool to protect mitochondrial health." *Frontiers in Physiology*, 2021. www.frontiersin.org/articles/10.3389/fphys.2021.660068/full

904 Jensen, Bahl, Østergaard, Høgh, Wermuth, Heslegrave, Zetterberg, Heegaard, Hasselbalch, and Simonsen. "Exercise as a potential modulator of inflammation in patients with Alzheimer's disease measured in cerebrospinal fluid and plasma." *Experimental Gerontology*, 2019. https://doi.org/10.1016/j.exger.2019.04.003

905 Dolezal, Neufeld. Boland, Martin, and Cooper. "Interrelationship between sleep and exercise: A systematic review." *Advances in Preventive Medicine*, 2017. https://www.ncbi.nlm.nih.gov/pmc/articles/PMC5385214/

906 Kline. "The bidirectional relationship between exercise and sleep: Implications for exercise adherence and sleep improvement." *American Journal of Lifestyle Medicine*, 2014. https://www.ncbi.nlm.nih.gov/pmc/articles/PMC4341978/

907 Monda, Villano, Messina, Valenzano, Esposito, Moscatelli, Viggiano, Cibelli, Chieffi, Monda, and Messina. "Exercise modifies the gut microbiota with positive health effects." *Oxidative Medicine and Cellular Longevity*, 2017. https://www.ncbi.nlm.nih.gov/pmc/articles/PMC5357536/

908 Estaki, Pither, Baumeister, Little, Gill, Ghosh, Ahmadi-Vand, Marsden, and Gibson. "Cardiorespiratory fitness as a predictor of intestinal microbial diversity and distinct metagenomic functions." *Microbiome*, 2016. https://doi.org/10.1186/s40168-016-0189-7

909 Bherer, Erickson, and Liu-Ambrose. "A review of the effects of physical activity and exercise on cognitive and brain functions in older adults." *Journal of Aging Research*, 2013. https://doi.org/10.1155/2013/657508

910 Bherer, Erickson, and Liu-Ambrose. "A review of the effects of physical activity and exercise on cognitive and brain functions in older adults." *Journal of Aging Research*, 2013. https://doi.org/10.1155/2013/657508

911 Fiatarone Singh, Gates, Saigal, Wilson, Meiklejohn, Brodaty, Wen, Singh, Baune, Suo, Baker, Foroughi, Wang, Sachdev, and Valenzuela. "The Study of Mental and Resistance Training (SMART) Study—resistance training and/or cognitive training in mild cognitive impairment: a randomized, double-blind, double-sham controlled trial." *Journal of the American Medical Directors Association*, 2014. https://doi.org/10.1016/j.jamda.2014.09.010

912 Figueroa, Kingsley, McMillan, and Panton. "Resistance exercise training improves heart rate variability in women with fibromyalgia." *Clinical Physiology and Functional Imaging*, 2008. https://doi.org/10.1111/j.1475-097X.2007.00776.x

913 Fiatarone Singh, Gates, Saigal, Wilson, Meiklejohn, Brodaty, Wen, Singh, Baune, Suo, Baker, Foroughi, Wang, Sachdev, and Valenzuela. "The Study of Mental and Resistance Training (SMART) Study—resistance training and/or cognitive training in mild cognitive impairment; a randomized, double-blind, double-sham controlled trial." *Journal of the American Medical Directors Association*, 2014. https://doi.org/10.1016/j.jamda.2014.09.010

914 Northey, Cherbuin, Pumpa, Smee, and Rattray. "Exercise interventions for cognitive function in adults older than 50: a systematic review with meta-analysis." *British Journal of Sports Medicine*, 2018. http://dx.doi.org/10.1136/bjsports-2016-096587

915 Hurley and Roth. "Strength training in the elderly: effects on risk factors for age-related diseases." *Sports Medicine*, 2000. https://doi.org/10.2165/00007256-200030040-00002

916 Morrison, Colberg, Mariano, Parson, and Vinik. "Balance training reduces falls risk in older individuals with type 2 diabetes." *Diabetes Care*, 2010. https://diabetesjournals.org/care/article/33/4/748/26925

917 De la Rosa, Olaso-Gonzalez, Arc-Chagnaud, Millan, Salvador-Pascual, García-Lucerga, Blasco-Lafarga, Garcia-Dominguez, Carretero, Correas, Viña, and Gomez-Cabrera. "Physical exercise in the prevention and treatment of Alzheimer's disease." *Journal of Sport and Health Science*, 2020. https://www.ncbi.nlm.nih.gov/pmc/articles/PMC7498620/

918 Pesta, Hoppel, Macek, Messner, Faulhaber, Kobel, Parson, Burtscher, Schocke, and Gnaiger. "Similar qualitative and quantitative changes of mitochondrial respiration following strength and endurance training in normoxia and hypoxia in sedentary humans." *American Journal of Physiology: Regulatory, Integrative, and Comparative Physiology*, 2011. https://journals.physiology.org/doi/full/10.1152/ajpregu.00285.2011

919 Torma, Gombos, Jokai, Takeda, Mimura, and Radak. "High intensity interval training and molecular adaptive response of skeletal muscle." *Sports Medicine and Health Science*, 2019. https://www.ncbi.nlm.nih.gov/pmc/articles/PMC9219277/

920 Chang and Namkung. "Effects of exercise intervention on mitochondrial stress biomarkers in metabolic syndrome patients: a randomized controlled trial." *International Journal of Environmental Research and Public Health*, 2021. https://www.ncbi.nlm.nih.gov/pmc/articles/PMC7956208/

921 Dao, Hsiung, and Liu-Ambrose. "The role of exercise in mitigating subcortical ischemic vascular cognitive impairment." *Journal of Neurochemistry*, 2018. https://onlinelibrary.wiley.com/doi/10.1111/jnc.14153

922 Heijnen, Hommel, Kibele, and Colzato. "Neuromodulation of aerobic exercise—a review." *Frontiers in Psychology*, 2016. https://www.frontiersin.org/articles/10.3389/fpsyg.2015.01890/full

923 Dang, Castrellon, Perkins, Le, Cowan, Zaid, and Samanez-Larkin. "Reduced effects of age on dopamine D2 receptor levels in physically active adults." *NeuroImage*, 2017. https://www.ncbi.nlm.nih.gov/pmc/articles/PMC5344739/

924 Schmitt, Upadhyay, Martin, Rojas, Strüder, and Boecker. "Modulation of distinct intrinsic resting state brain networks by acute exercise bouts of differing intensity." *Brain Plasticity*, 2019. https://content.iospress.com/articles/brain-plasticity/bpl190081

925 Trejo, Carro, and Torres-Alemán. "Circulating insulin-like growth factor I mediates exercise-induced increases in the number of new neurons in the adult hippocampus." *Journal of Neuroscience*, 2001. https://www.jneurosci.org/content/21/5/1628

926 Lee, Duan, and Mattson. "Evidence that brain-derived neurotrophic factor is required for basal neurogenesis and mediates, in part, the enhancement of neurogenesis by dietary restriction in the hippocampus of adult mice." *Journal of Neurochemistry*, 2002. https://onlinelibrary.wiley.com/doi/full/10.1046/j.1471-4159.2002.01085.x

927 Fabel, Fabel, Tam, Kaufer, Baiker, Simmons, Kuo, and Palmer. "VEGF is necessary for exercise-induced adult hippocampal neurogenesis." *European Journal of Neuroscience*, 2003. https://doi.org/10.1111/j.1460-9568.2003.03041.x

928 Lopez-Lopez, LeRoith, and Torres-Alemán. "Insulin-like growth factor I is required for vessel remodeling in the adult brain." *Proceedings of the National Academy of Sciences*, 2004. https://doi.org/10.1073/pnas.0400337101

REFERENCES

929 Caldieraro, Salehpour, and Cassano. "Transcranial and systemic photobiomodulation for the enhancement of mitochondrial metabolism in depression." *Clinical Bioenergetics*, 2021. https://doi.org/10.1016/B978-0-12-819621-2.00028-0

930 Bathini, Raghushaker, and Mahato. "The molecular mechanisms of action of photobiomodulation against neurodegenerative diseases: a systematic review." *Cellular and Molecular Neurobiology*, 2022. https://link.springer.com/article/10.1007/s10571-020-01016-9

931 Hansen, Johnsen, Sollers, Stenvik, and Thayer. "Heart rate variability and its relation to prefrontal cognitive function: the effects of training and detraining." *European Journal of Applied Physiology*, 2004. https://doi.org/10.1007/s00421-004-1208-0

932 Shastry, Mirajkar, Moodithaya, and Halahalli. "Resting heart rate variability and cardiorespiratory fitness in healthy young adults." *Indian Journal of Medical Specialties*, 2017. https://doi.org/10.1016/j.injms.2016.11.004

933 Memmini, La Fountaine, Broglio, and Moore. "Long-term influence of concussion on cardio-autonomic function in adolescent hockey players." *Journal of Athletic Training*, 2021. https://meridian.allenpress.com/jat/article/56/2/141/450235/

934 Abaji, Curnier, Moore, and Ellemberg. "Persisting effects of concussion on heart rate variability during physical exertion." *Journal of Neurotrauma*, 2016. https://doi.org/10.1089/neu.2015.3989

935 Luque-Casado, Zabala, Morales, Mateo-March, and Sanabria. "Cognitive performance and heart rate variability: the influence of fitness level." *PLOS One*, 2013. https://journals.plos.org/plosone/article?id=10.1371/journal.pone.0056935

936 Lyytikäinen, Toivonen, Hynynen, Lindholm, and Kyröläinen. "Recovery of rescuers from a 24-h shift and its association with aerobic fitness." *International Journal of Occupational Medicine and Environmental Health*, 2017. https://doi.org/10.13075/ijomeh.1896.00720

937 Albinet, Boucard, Bouquet, and Audiffren. "Increased heart rate variability and executive performance after aerobic training in the elderly." *European Journal of Applied Physiology*, 2010. https://doi.org/10.1007/s00421-010-1393-y

938 Fortes, Ferreira, Paes, Costa, Lima-Júnior, Costa, and Cyrino. "Effect of resistance training volume on heart rate variability in young adults." *Isokinetics and Exercise Science*, 2019. https://doi.org/10.3233/IES-182207

939 Prasad, Sinha, Ghate, and Sinha. "Resting and post exercise heart rate variability in preobese individuals: a comparative study." *Asian Journal of Medical Sciences*, 2018. https://www.researchgate.net/publication/326131119

940 Toni, Murri, Piepoli, Zanetidou, Cabassi, Squatrito, Bagnoli, Piras, Musssi, Senaldi, Menchetti, Zocchi, Ermini, Ceresini, Tripi, Rucci, Alexopoulos, and Amore. "Physical exercise for late-life depression: effects on heart rate variability." *American Journal of Geriatric Psychiatry*, 2016. https://doi.org/10.1016/j.jagp.2016.08.005

941 Murad, Brubaker, Fitzgerald, Morgan, Goff, Soliman, Eggebeen, and Kitzman. "Exercise training improves heart rate variability in older patients with heart failure: a randomized, controlled, single-blinded trial." *Congestive Heart Failure*, 2012. https://doi.org/10.1111/j.1751-7133.2011.00282.x

942 Meyer, Gayda, Juneau, and Nigam. "High-intensity aerobic interval exercise in chronic heart failure." *Current Heart Failure Reports*, 2013. https://doi.org/10.1007/s11897-013-0130-3

943 Sandercock, Bromley, and Brodie. "Effects of exercise on heart rate variability: inferences from meta-analysis." *Medicine & Science in Sports & Exercise*, 2005. https://doi.org/10.1249/01.MSS.0000155388.39002.9D

[944] Little, Safdar, Bishop, Tarnopolsky, and Gibala. "An acute bout of high-intensity interval training increases the nuclear abundance of PGC-1α and activates mitochondrial biogenesis in human skeletal muscle." *American Journal of Physiology: Regulatory, Integrative, and Comparative Physiology*, 2011. https://journals.physiology.org/doi/full/10.1152/ajpregu.00538.2010

[945] Hwang, Castelli, and Gonzalez-Lima. "Cognitive enhancement by transcranial laser stimulation and acute aerobic exercise." *Lasers in Medical Science*, 2016. https://doi.org/10.1007/s10103-016-1962-3

[946] Dellagrana, Rossato, Sakugawa, Baroni, and Diefenthaeler. "Photobiomodulation therapy on physiological and performance parameters during running tests: dose-response effects." *Journal of Strength and Conditioning Research*, 2018. https://doi.org/10.1519/JSC.0000000000002488

[947] Aver Vanin, De Marchi, Tomazoni, Tairova, Leão Casalechi, de Tarso Camillo de Carvalho, Bjordal, and Leal-Junior. "Pre-exercise infrared low-level laser therapy (810 nm) in skeletal muscle performance and postexercise recovery in humans, What is the optimal dose? A randomized, double-blind, placebo-controlled clinical trial." *Photomedicine and Laser Surgery*, 2016. https://doi.org/10.1089/pho.2015.3992

[948] Lanferdini, Bini, Baroni, Klein, Carpes, and Vaz. "Improvement of performance and reduction of fatigue with low-level laser therapy in competitive cyclists." *International Journal of Sports Physiology and Performance*, 2018. https://doi.org/10.1123/ijspp.2016-0187

[949] Ferraresi, de Brito Oliveira, de Oliveira Zafalon, Bezerra de Menezes Reiff, Baldissera, de Andrade Perez, Matheucci Júnior, and Parizotto. "Effects of low level laser therapy (808 nm) on physical strength training in humans." *Lasers in Medical Science*, 2011. https://doi.org/10.1007/s10103-010-0855-0

[950] Baroni, Rodrigues, Freire, Franke, Geremia, and Vaz. "Effect of low-level laser therapy on muscle adaptation to knee extensor eccentric training." *European Journal of Applied Physiology*, 2015. https://doi.org/10.1007/s00421-014-3055-y

[951] Vanin, Miranda, Machado, de Paiva, Albuquerque-Pontes, Casalechi, Camillo de Carvalho, and Leal-Junior. "What is the best moment to apply phototherapy when associated to a strength training program? A randomized, double-blinded, placebo-controlled trial: phototherapy in association to strength training." *Lasers in Medical Science*, 2016. https://doi.org/10.1007/s10103-016-2015-7

[952] da Silva Alves, Pinfildi, Neto, Lourenço, de Azevedo, and Dourado. "Acute effects of low-level laser therapy on physiologic and electromyographic responses to the cardiopulmonary exercise testing in healthy untrained adults." *Lasers in Medical Science*, 2014. https://doi.org/10.1007/s10103-014-1595-3

[953] Antonialli, De Marchi, Tomazoni, Vanin, dos Santos Grandinetti, de Paiva, Pinto, Miranda, de Tarso Camillo de Carvalho, and Leal-Junior. "Phototherapy in skeletal muscle performance and recovery after exercise: effect of combination of super-pulsed laser and light-emitting diodes." *Lasers in Medical Science*, 2014. https://doi.org/10.1007/s10103-014-1611-7

[954] Vanin, Verhagen, Barboza, Costa, and Leal-Junior. "Photobiomodulation therapy for the improvement of muscular performance and reduction of muscular fatigue associated with exercise in healthy people: a systematic review and meta-analysis." *Lasers in Medical Science*, 2018. https://doi.org/10.1007/s10103-017-2368-6

[955] Toma, Tucci, Antunes, Pedroni, de Oliveira, Buck, Ferreira, Vassão, and Renno. "Effect of 808 nm low-level laser therapy in exercise-induced skeletal muscle fatigue in elderly women." *Lasers in Medical Science*, 2013. https://doi.org/10.1007/s10103-012-1246-5

[956] Molina Correa, Padoin, Varoni, Demarchi, Flores, Nampo, and de Paula Ramos. "Ergogenic effects of photobiomodulation on performance in the 30-second Wingate test: a randomized, double-blind, placebo-controlled, crossover study." *Journal of Strength & Conditioning Research*, 2020. https://doi.org/10.1519/JSC.0000000000003734

[957] Patrocinio, Sardim, Assis, Fernandes, Rodrigues, and Renno. "Effect of low-level laser therapy (808 nm) in skeletal muscle after resistance exercise training in rats." *Photomedicine and Laser Surgery*, 2013. https://doi.org/10.1089/pho.2013.3540

[958] Toma, Oliveira, Renno, and Laakso. "Photobiomodulation (PBM) therapy at 904 nm mitigates effects of exercise-induced skeletal muscle fatigue in young women." *Lasers in Medical Science*, 2018. https://doi.org/10.1007/s10103-018-2454-4

[959] Leal Junior, Lopes-Martins, Dalan, Ferrari, Sbabo, Generosi, Baroni, Penna, Iversen, and Bjordal. "Effect of 655-nm low-level laser therapy on exercise-induced skeletal muscle fatigue in humans." *Photomedicine and Laser Surgery*, 2008. https://doi.org/10.1089/pho.2007.2160

[960] Machado, Peserico, Mezzaroba, Manoel, and da Silva. "Light-emitting diode (LED) therapy applied between two running time trials has a moderate effect on attenuating delayed onset muscle soreness but does not change recovery markers and running performance." *Science & Sports*, 2017. https://doi.org/10.1016/j.scispo.2016.06.010

[961] De Marchi, Schmitt, Danúbia da Silva Fabro, da Silva, Sene, Tairova, and Salvador. "Phototherapy for improvement of performance and exercise recovery: comparison of 3 commercially available devices." *Journal of Athletic Training*, 2017. https://www.ncbi.nlm.nih.gov/pmc/articles/PMC5455246/

[962] Ferraresi, Bertucci, Schiavinato, Reiff, Araújo, Panepucci, Matheucci, Cunha, Arakelian, Hamblin, Parizotto, and Bagnato. "Effects of light-emitting diode therapy on muscle hypertrophy, gene expression, performance, damage, and delayed-onset muscle soreness: case-control study with a pair of identical twins." *American Journal of Physical Medicine & Rehabilitation*, 2016. https://www.ncbi.nlm.nih.gov/pmc/articles/PMC5026559/

[963] Francisco, Beltrame, Hughson, Milan-Mattos, Ferroli-Fabricio, Benze, Ferraresi, Parizotto, Bagnato, Borghi-Silva, Porta, and Catai. "Effects of light-emitting diode therapy on cardiopulmonary and hemodynamic adjustments during aerobic exercise and glucose levels in patients with diabetes mellitus: a randomized, crossover, double-blind and placebo-controlled clinical trial." *Complementary Therapies in Medicine*, 2018. https://doi.org/10.1016/j.ctim.2018.11.015

[964] Nagy, Ali, Behiry, Naguib, and Elsayed. "Impact of combined photobiomodulation and aerobic exercise on cognitive function and quality of life in elderly Alzheimer patients with anemia: a randomized clinical trial." *International Journal of General Medicine*, 2021. https://www.ncbi.nlm.nih.gov/pmc/articles/PMC7813463/

[965] Fritsch, Dornelles, Teodoro, da Silva, Vaz, Pinto, Cadore, and Baroni. "Effects of photobiomodulation therapy associated with resistance training in elderly men: a randomized double-blinded placebo-controlled trial." *European Journal of Applied Physiology*, 2019. https://doi.org/10.1007/s00421-018-4023-8

[966] Leal-Junior, Vanin, Miranda, Tarso, de Carvalho, Dal Corso, and Bjordal. "Effect of phototherapy (low-level laser therapy and light-emitting diode therapy) on exercise performance and markers of exercise recovery: a systematic review with meta-analysis." *Lasers in Medical Science*, 2013. https://doi.org/10.1007/s10103-013-1465-4

[967] Ferraresi, Hamblin, and Parizotto. "Low-level laser (light) therapy (LLLT) on muscle tissue: performance, fatigue and repair benefited by the power of light." *Photonics & Lasers in Medicine*, 2012. https://www.degruyter.com/document/doi/10.1515/plm-2012-0032/html

968 Alves, Fernandes, Deana, Bussadori, and Mesquita-Ferrari. "Effects of low-level laser therapy on skeletal muscle repair." *American Journal of Physical Medicine & Rehabilitation*, 2014. https://doi.org/10.1097/PHM.0000000000000158

969 Gupta, Avci, Sadasivam, Chandran, Parizotto, Vecchio, de Melo, Dai, Chiang, and Hamblin. "Shining light on nanotechnology to help repair and regeneration." *Biotechnology Advances*, 2013. https://doi.org/10.1016/j.biotechadv.2012.08.003

970 Naterstad, Rossi, Marcos, Parizotto, Frigo, Joensen, Leonardo, Bjordal, and Lopes-Martins. "Comparison of photobiomodulation and anti-inflammatory drugs on tissue repair on collagenase-induced Achilles tendon inflammation in rats." *Photomedicine and Laser Surgery*, 2017. http://dx.doi.org/10.1089/pho.2017.4364

971 Paolillo, Arena, Dutra, de Cassia Marqueti Durigan, de Araujo, de Souza, Parizotto, Cipriano, Chiappa, and Borghi-Silva. "Low-level laser therapy associated with high intensity resistance training on cardiac autonomic control of heart rate and skeletal muscle remodeling in Wistar rats." *Lasers in Surgery and Medicine*, 2014. https://doi.org/10.1002/lsm.22298

972 Park, Song, Oh, Miyazaki, and Son. "Comparison of physiological and psychological relaxation using measurements of heart rate variability, prefrontal cortex activity, and subjective indexes after completing tasks with and without foliage plants." *International Journal of Environmental Research and Public Health*, 2017. https://www.ncbi.nlm.nih.gov/pmc/articles/PMC5615624/

973 Ritchie, Tucker-Drob, Cox, Dickie, Valdés Hernández, Corley, Royle, Redmond, Muños Maniega, Pattie, Aribisala, Taylor, Clarke, Gow, Starr, Bastin, Wardlaw, and Deary. "Risk and protective factors for structural brain ageing in the eighth decade of life." *Brain Structure & Function*, 2017. https://www.ncbi.nlm.nih.gov/pmc/articles/PMC5676817/

974 Booth, Royle, Corley, Gow, Valdés Hernández, Muños Maniega, Ritchie, Bastin, Starr, Wardlaw, and Deary. "Association of allostatic load with brain structure and cognitive ability in later life." *Neurobiology of Aging*, 2015. https://www.ncbi.nlm.nih.gov/pmc/articles/PMC4353502/

975 Sigrist, Mürner-Lavanchy, Peschel, Schmidt, Kaess, and Koenig. "Early life maltreatment and resting-state heart rate variability: a systematic review and meta-analysis." *Neuroscience and Biobehavioral Reviews*, 2021. https://doi.org/10.1016/j.neubiorev.2020.10.026

976 Thayer, Åhs, Fredrikson, Sollers, and Wager. "A meta-analysis of heart rate variability and neuroimaging studies: implications for heart rate variability as a marker of stress and health." *Neuroscience & Biobehavioral Reviews*, 2012. https://doi.org/10.1016/j.neubiorev.2011.11.009

977 De Peuter, Lemaigre, Van Diest, and Van den Bergh. "Illness-specific catastrophic thinking and overperception in asthma." *Health Psychology*, 2008. https://doi.org/10.1037/0278-6133.27.1.93

978 Williams, Feeling, Hill, Spangler, Koenig, and Thayer. "Resting heart rate variability, facets of rumination, and trait anxiety: implications for the perseverative cognition hypothesis." *Frontiers in Human Neuroscience*, 2017. https://www.frontiersin.org/articles/10.3389/fnhum.2017.00520/full

979 Carnevali, Thayer, Brosschot, and Ottaviani. "Heart rate variability mediates the link between rumination and depressive symptoms: a longitudinal study." *International Journal of Psychophysiology*, 2018. https://doi.org/10.1016/j.ijpsycho.2017.11.002

[980] Shahane, LeRoy, Denny, and Fagundes. "Connecting cognition, cardiology, and chromosomes: cognitive reappraisal impacts the relationship between heart rate variability and telomere length in CD8+CD28- cells." *Psychoneuroendocrinology*, 2020. https://doi.org/10.1016/j.psyneuen.2019.104517

[981] Davidson, Kabat-Zinn, Schumacher, Rosenkranz, Muller, Santorelli, Urbanowski, Harrington, Bonus, and Sheridan. "Alterations in brain and immune function produced by mindfulness meditation." *Psychosomatic Medicine*, 2003. https://doi.org/10.1097/01.PSY.0000077505.67574.E3

[982] Creswell, Myers, Cole, and Irwin. "Mindfulness meditation training effects on CD4+ T lymphocytes in HIV-1 infected adults: a small randomized controlled trial." *Brain, Behavior, and Immunity*, 2009. https://www.ncbi.nlm.nih.gov/pmc/articles/PMC2725018/

[983] van der Zwan, de Vente, Huizink, Bögels, and de Bruin. "Physical activity, mindfulness meditation, or heart rate variability biofeedback for stress reduction: a randomized controlled trial." *Applied Psychophysiology and Biofeedback*, 2015. https://www.ncbi.nlm.nih.gov/pmc/articles/PMC4648965/

[984] Zaccaro, Piarulli, Laurino, Garbella, Menicucci, Neri, and Gemignani. "How breath-control can change your life: a systematic review on psycho-physiological correlates of slow breathing." *Frontiers in Human Neuroscience*, 2018. https://www.ncbi.nlm.nih.gov/pmc/articles/PMC6137615/

[985] Sharma, Dinesh, Rajajeyakumar, Grrishma, and Bhavanani. "Impact of fast and slow pranayam on cardiovascular autonomic function among healthy young volunteers: randomized controlled study." *Alternative and Integrative Medicine*, 2018. https://doi.org/10.4172/2327-5162.1000265

[986] Sheiko and Feketa. "Dynamics of heart rate variability under the influence of course yoga breathing exercises on healthy young people." *Wiadomości Lekarskie*, 2019. https://pubmed.ncbi.nlm.nih.gov/31055542/

[987] Field, Hernandez-Reif, Diego, Schanberg, and Kuhn. "Cortisol decreases and serotonin and dopamine increase following massage therapy." *International Journal of Neuroscience*, 2005. https://pubmed.ncbi.nlm.nih.gov/16162447/

[988] Bayo-Tallón, Esquirol-Caussa, Pàmias-Massana, Planells-Keller, and Palao-Vidal. "Effects of manual cranial therapy on heart rate variability in children without associated disorders: translation to clinical practice." *Complementary Therapies in Clinical Practice*, 2019. https://doi.org/10.1016/j.ctcp.2019.06.008

[989] Chung, Yan, and Zhang. "Effect of acupuncture on heart rate variability: a systematic review." *Evidence-Based Complementary and Alternative Medicine*, 2014. https://doi.org/10.1155/2014/819871

[990] Henley, Ivins, Mills, Wen, and Benjamin. "Osteopathic manipulative treatment and its relationship to autonomic nervous system activity as demonstrated by heart rate variability: a repeated measures study." *Osteopathic Medicine and Primary Care*, 2008. https://om-pc.biomedcentral.com/articles/10.1186/1750-4732-2-7

[991] Amoroso Borges, Bortolazzo, and Neto. "Effects of spinal manipulation and myofascial techniques on heart rate variability: a systematic review." *Journal of Bodywork and Movement Therapies*, 2018. https://doi.org/10.1016/j.jbmt.2017.09.025

[992] Yeater, Clark, Hoyos, Valdes-Hernandez, Peraza, Allen, and Cruz-Almeida. "Chronic pain is associated with reduced sympathetic nervous system reactivity during simple and complex walking tasks: potential cerebral mechanisms." *Chronic Stress*, 2021. https://journals.sagepub.com/doi/full/10.1177/24705470211030273

[993] Sabia, Fayosse, Dumurgier, van Hees, Paquet, Sommerlad, Kivimäki, Dugravot, and Singh-Manoux. "Association of sleep duration in middle and old age with incidence of dementia." *Nature Communications*, 2021. https://www.nature.com/articles/s41467-021-22354-2

[994] Tononi and Cirelli. "Sleep and synaptic homeostasis: a hypothesis." *Brain Research Bulletin*, 2003. https://doi.org/10.1016/j.brainresbull.2003.09.004

[995] Ako, Kawara, Uchida, Miyazaki, Nishihara, Mukai, Hirao, Ako, and Okubo. "Correlation between electroencephalography and heart rate variability during sleep." *Psychiatry and Clinical Neurosciences*, 2003. https://onlinelibrary.wiley.com/doi/full/10.1046/j.1440-1819.2003.01080.x

[996] Ren, Covassin, Zhang, Lei, Yang, Zhou, Tan, Li, Li, Shi, Lu, Somers, and Tang. "Interaction between slow wave sleep and obstructive sleep apnea in prevalent hypertension." *Hypertension*, 2020. https://doi.org/10.1161/HYPERTENSIONAHA.119.13720

[997] Vanoli, Adamson, Ba-Lin, Pinna, Lazzara, and Orr. "Heart rate variability during specific sleep stages: a comparison of healthy subjects with patients after myocardial infarction." *Circulation*, 1995. https://www.ahajournals.org/doi/10.1161/01.CIR.91.7.1918

[998] Buratti, Cruciani, Pulcini, Rocchi, Totaro, Lattanzi, Viticchi, Falsetti, and Silvestrini. "Lacunar stroke and heart rate variability during sleep." *Sleep Medicine*, 2020. https://doi.org/10.1016/j.sleep.2020.04.005

[999] Kato, Miyata, Ando, Matsuoka, Yasuma, Iwamoto, Kawano, Banno, Ozaki, and Noda. "Influence of sleep duration on cortical oxygenation in elderly individuals." *Psychiatry and Clinical Neurosciences*, 2016. https://onlinelibrary.wiley.com/doi/10.1111/pcn.12464

[1000] Rafalson, Donahue, Stranges, LaMonte, Dmochowski, Dorn, and Trevisan. "Short sleep duration is associated with the development of impaired fasting glucose: The Western New York Health Study." *Annals of Epidemiology*, 2010. https://www.ncbi.nlm.nih.gov/pmc/articles/PMC2962429/

[1001] Sabia, Fayosse, Dumurgier, van Hees, Paquet, Sommerlad, Kivimäki, Dugravot, and Singh-Manoux. "Association of sleep duration in middle and old age with incidence of dementia." *Nature Communications*, 2021. https://www.nature.com/articles/s41467-021-22354-2

[1002] Kong, Hoyos, Phillips, McKinnon, Lin, Duffy, Mowszowski, LaMonica, Grunstein, Naismith, and Gordon. "Altered heart rate variability during sleep in mild cognitive impairment." *Sleep*, 2021. https://doi.org/10.1093/sleep/zsaa232

[1003] Pallayova, Donic, Gresova, Peregrim, and Tomori. "Do differences in sleep architecture exist between persons with type 2 diabetes and nondiabetic controls?" *Journal of Diabetes Science and Technology*, 2010. https://www.ncbi.nlm.nih.gov/pmc/articles/PMC2864170/

[1004] Ngo, Martinetz, Born, and Mölle. "Auditory closed-loop stimulation of the sleep slow oscillation enhances memory." *Neuron*, 2013. https://www.cell.com/neuron/fulltext/S0896-6273(13)00230-4

[1005] Prehn-Kristensen, Munz, Göder, Wilhelm, Korr, Vahl, Wiesner, and Baving. "Transcranial oscillatory direct current stimulation during sleep improves declarative memory consolidation in children with attention-deficit/hyperactivity disorder to a level comparable to healthy controls." *Brain Stimulation*, 2014. https://www.brainstim-jrnl.com/article/S1935-861X(14)00265-4/fulltext

[1006] Ladenbauer, Külzow, Passmann, Antonenko, Grittner, Tamm, and Flöel. "Brain stimulation during an afternoon nap boosts slow oscillatory activity and memory consolidation in older adults." *NeuroImage*, 2016. https://doi.org/10.1016/j.neuroimage.2016.06.057

REFERENCES

1007 Lee, Gerashchenko, Timofeev, Bacskai, and Kastanenka. "Slow wave sleep is a promising intervention target for Alzheimer's disease." *Frontiers in Neuroscience*, 2020. https://www.ncbi.nlm.nih.gov/pmc/articles/PMC7340158/

1008 Rüger, Gordijn, Beersma, de Vries, and Daan. "Time-of-day-dependent effects of bright light exposure on human psychophysiology: comparison of daytime and nighttime exposure." *American Journal of Physiology: Regulatory, Integrative and Comparative Physiology*, 2006. https://journals.physiology.org/doi/full/10.1152/ajpregu.00121.2005

1009 Luo, Sandhu, Rungratanawanich, Williams, Akbar, Zhou, Song, and Wang. "Melatonin and autophagy in aging-related neurodegenerative diseases." *International Journal of Molecular Sciences*, 2020. https://www.ncbi.nlm.nih.gov/pmc/articles/PMC7584015/

1010 Goel and Mangel. "Dopamine-mediated circadian and light/dark-adaptive modulation of chemical and electrical synapses in the outer retina." *Frontiers in Cellular Neuroscience*, 2021. https://www.frontiersin.org/articles/10.3389/fncel.2021.647541/full

1011 Campbell and Murphy. "Extraocular circadian phototransduction in humans." *Science*, 1998. https://www.science.org/doi/10.1126/science.279.5349.396

1012 Jurvelin. "Transcranial bright light: the effect on human psychophysiology." Doctoral dissertation, University of Oulu, 2018. http://jultika.oulu.fi/files/isbn9789526218113.pdf

1013 Lee, Xie, Yu, Kang, Feng, Deane, Logan, Nedergaard, and Benveniste. "The effect of body posture on brain glymphatic transport." *Journal of Neuroscience*, 2015. https://www.ncbi.nlm.nih.gov/pmc/articles/PMC4524974/

1014 McConnell, Froeliger, Garland, Ives, and Sforzo. "Auditory driving of the autonomic nervous system: listening to theta-frequency binaural beats post-exercise increases parasympathetic activation and sympathetic withdrawal." *Frontiers in Psychology*, 2014. https://www.ncbi.nlm.nih.gov/pmc/articles/PMC4231835/

1015 Papillon-Ferland and Mallet. "Should melatonin be used as a sleeping aid for elderly people?" *Canadian Journal of Hospital Pharmacy*, 2019. https://www.ncbi.nlm.nih.gov/pmc/articles/PMC6699865/

1016 Shell, Bullias, Charuvastra, May, and Silver. "A randomized, placebo-controlled trial of an amino acid preparation on timing and quality of sleep." *American Journal of Therapeutics*, 2010. https://doi.org/10.1097/MJT.0b013e31819e9eab

1017 Hong, Park, and Suh. "Sleep-promoting effects of a GABA/5-HTP mixture: behavioral changes and neuromodulation in an invertebrate model." *Life Sciences*, 2016. https://doi.org/10.1016/j.lfs.2016.02.086

1018 Hong, Park, and Suh. "Sleep-promoting effects of the GABA/5-HTP mixture in vertebrate models." *Behavioural Brain Research*, 2016. https://doi.org/10.1016/j.bbr.2016.04.049

1019 Shinjyo, Waddell, and Green. "Valerian root in treating sleep problems and associated disorders—a systematic review and meta-analysis." *Journal of Evidence-Based Integrative Medicine*, 2020. https://www.ncbi.nlm.nih.gov/pmc/articles/PMC7585905/

1020 Hidese, Ogawa, Ota, Ishida, Yasukawa, Ozeki, and Kunugi. "Effects of L-theanine administration on stress-related symptoms and cognitive functions in healthy adults: a randomized controlled trial." *Nutrients*, 2019. https://www.ncbi.nlm.nih.gov/pmc/articles/PMC6836118/

1021 Kim, Jo, Hong, Han, and Suh. "GABA and L-theanine mixture decreases sleep latency and improves NREM sleep." *Pharmaceutical Biology*, 2019. https://www.ncbi.nlm.nih.gov/pmc/articles/PMC6366437/

1022 Durlach, Pagès, Bac, Bara, and Guiet-Bara. "Biorhythms and possible central regulation of magnesium status, phototherapy, darkness therapy, and chronopathological forms of magnesium depletion." *Magnesium Research*, 2002. https://pubmed.ncbi.nlm.nih.gov/12030424/

[1023] Poleszak. "Benzodiazepine/GABA(A) receptors are involved in magnesium-induced anxiolytic-like behavior in mice." *Pharmacological Reports*, 2008. https://pubmed.ncbi.nlm.nih.gov/18799816/

[1024] Farina, Dittoni, Colicchio, Testani, Losurdo, Gnoni, Di Blasi, Brunetti, Contardi, Mazza, and Della Marca. "Heart rate and heart rate variability modification in chronic insomnia patients." *Behavioral Sleep Medicine*, 2014. https://doi.org/10.1080/15402002.2013.801346

[1025] Naeser, Saltmarche, Krengel, Hamblin, and Knight. "Improved cognitive function after transcranial, light-emitting diode treatments in chronic, traumatic brain injury: two case reports." *Photomedicine and Laser Surgery*, 2011. https://doi.org/10.1089/pho.2010.2814

[1026] Zhao, Tian, Nie, Xu, and Liu. "Red light and the sleep quality and endurance performance of Chinese female basketball players." *Journal of Athletic Training*, 2012. https://www.ncbi.nlm.nih.gov/pmc/articles/PMC3499892/

[1027] Bogdanova, Martin, Ho, Krengel, Ho, Yee, Knight, Hamblin, and Naeser. "LED therapy improves sleep and cognition in chronic moderate TBI: pilot case studies." *Archives of Physical Medicine & Rehabilitation*, 2014. https://doi.org/10.1016/j.apmr.2014.07.247

[1028] Naeser, Martin, Ho, Krengel, Bogdanova, Knight, Yee, Zafonte, Frazier, Hamblin, and Koo. "Transcranial, red/near-infrared light-emitting diode therapy to improve cognition in chronic traumatic brain injury." *Photomedicine and Laser Surgery*, 2016. https://doi.org/10.1089/pho.2015.4037

[1029] Bogdanova, Martin, Ho, Krengel, Ho, Yee, Knight, Hamblin, and Naeser. "LED therapy improves sleep and cognition in chronic moderate TBI: pilot case studies." *Archives of Physical Medicine & Rehabilitation*, 2014. https://doi.org/10.1016/j.apmr.2014.07.247

[1030] Chao. "Improvements in Gulf War Illness symptoms after near-infrared transcranial and intranasal photobiomodulation: two case reports." *Military Medicine*, 2019. https://pubmed.ncbi.nlm.nih.gov/30916762/

[1031] Martin, Chao, Krengel, Ho, Yee, Lew, Knight, Hamblin, and Naeser. "Transcranial photobiomodulation to improve cognition in Gulf War Illness." *Frontiers in Neurology*, 2020. https://www.ncbi.nlm.nih.gov/pmc/articles/PMC7859640/

[1032] Nizamutdinov, Qi, Berman, Dougal, Dayawansa, Wu, Yi, Stevens, and Huang. "Transcranial near infrared light stimulations improve cognition in patients with dementia." *Aging and Disease*, 2021. https://www.ncbi.nlm.nih.gov/pmc/articles/PMC8219492/

[1033] Zhao, Du, Jiang, and Han. "Brain photobiomodulation improves sleep quality in subjective cognitive decline: a randomized, sham-controlled study." *Journal of Alzheimer's Disease*, 2022. https://doi.org/10.3233/JAD215715

[1034] Zhao, Tian, Nie, Xu, and Liu. "Red light and the sleep quality and endurance performance of Chinese female basketball players." *Journal of Athletic Training*, 2012. https://www.ncbi.nlm.nih.gov/pmc/articles/PMC3499892/

[1035] Flyktman. "Effects of transcranial light on molecules regulating circadian rhythm." Doctoral dissertation, University of Oulu, 2018. http://jultika.oulu.fi/files/isbn9789526219592.pdf

[1036] Ferris. "Rethinking the conditions and mechanism for glymphatic clearance." *Frontiers in Neuroscience*, 2021. https://www.frontiersin.org/articles/10.3389/fnins.2021.624690/full

[1037] Salehpour, Farajdokht, Erfani, Sadigh-Eteghad, Shotorbani, Hamblin, Karimi, Rasta, and Mahmoudi. "Transcranial near-infrared photobiomodulation attenuates memory impairment and hippocampal oxidative stress in sleep-deprived mice." *Brain Research*, 2018. https://doi.org/10.1016/j.brainres.2017.12.040

[1038] Many articles have been written about this study and these findings over the years. For more about the influence of relationships on health, you may enjoy this 2015 TED Talk by the study director, Robert Waldinger: https://www.youtube.com/watch?v=8KkKuTCFvzI

[1039] Waldinger, Cohen, Schulz, and Crowell. "Security of attachment to spouses in late life: concurrent and prospective links with cognitive and emotional well-being." *Clinical Psychological Science*, 2015. https://www.ncbi.nlm.nih.gov/pmc/articles/PMC4579537/

[1040] Novotney. "The risks of social isolation." American Psychological Association blog article, 2019. https://www.apa.org/monitor/2019/05/ce-corner-isolation

[1041] McPherson, Smith-Lovin, and Brashears. "Social isolation in America: changes in core discussion networks over two decades." *American Sociological Review*, 2006. https://doi.org/10.1177/000312240607100301

[1042] Salinas, Beiser, Samra, O'Donnell, DeCarli, Gonzales, Aparicio, and Seshadri. "Association of loneliness with 10-year dementia risk and early markers of vulnerability for neurocognitive decline." *Neurology*, 2022. https://n.neurology.org/content/98/13/e1337

[1043] Alcaraz, Eddens, Blase, Diver, Patel, Teras, Stevens, Jacobs, and Gapstur. "Social isolation and mortality in US Black and white men and women." *American Journal of Epidemiology*, 2019. https://academic.oup.com/aje/article/188/1/102/5133254

[1044] Holt-Lunstad, Smith, Baker, Harris, and Stephenson. "Loneliness and social isolation as risk factors for mortality: a meta-analytic review." *Perspectives on Psychological Science*, 2015. https://doi.org/10.1177/1745691614568352

[1045] Hawkley and Capitanio. "Perceived social isolation, evolutionary fitness and health outcomes: a lifespan approach." *Philosophical Transactions of the Royal Society B*, 2015. https://royalsocietypublishing.org/doi/10.1098/rstb.2014.0114

[1046] Williams, Pang, Delgado, Kocherginsky, Tretiakova, Krausz, Pan, He, McClintock, and Conzen. "A model of gene-environment interaction reveals altered mammary gland gene expression and increased tumor growth following social isolation." *Cancer Prevention Research*, 2009. https://www.ncbi.nlm.nih.gov/pmc/articles/PMC4707045/

[1047] Volden, Wonder, Skor, Carmean, Patel, Ye, Kocherginsky, McClintock, Brady, and Conzen. "Chronic social isolation is associated with metabolic gene expression changes specific to mammary adipose tissue." *Cancer Prevention Research*, 2013. https://www.ncbi.nlm.nih.gov/pmc/articles/PMC3881320/

[1048] Kok, Coffey, Cohn, Catalino Vacharkulsemsuk, Algoe, Brantley, and Fredrickson. "How positive emotions build physical health: perceived positive social connections account for the upward spiral between positive emotions and vagal tone." *Psychological Science*, 2013. https://doi.org/10.1177/0956797612470827

[1049] Smith, Cribbet, Nealey-Moore, Uchino, Williams, MacKenzie, and Thayer. "Matters of the variable heart: respiratory sinus arrhythmia response to marital interaction and associations with marital quality." *Journal of Personality and Social Psychology*, 2011. https://doi.org/10.1037/a0021136

[1050] Johnson, Stewart, Acree, Nápoles, Flatt, Max, and Gregorich. "A community choir intervention to promote well-being among diverse older adults: results from the Community of Voices Trial." *The Journals of Gerontology: Series B*, 2020. https://academic.oup.com/psychsocgerontology/article/75/3/549/5165411

1051 Steffens, Cruwys, Haslam, Jetten, and Haslam. "Social group memberships in retirement are associated with reduced risk of premature death: evidence from a longitudinal cohort study." *British Medical Journal*, 2016. https://bmjopen.bmj.com/content/6/2/e010164

1052 Kok, Coffey, Cohn, Catalino, Vacharkulksemsuk, Algoe, Brantley, and Fredrickson. "How positive emotions build physical health: perceived positive social connections account for the upward spiral between positive emotions and vagal tone." *Psychological Science*, 2013. https://doi.org/10.1177/0956797612470827

1053 Arzate-Mejía, Lottenbach, Schindler, Jawaid, and Mansuy. "Long-term impact of social isolation and molecular underpinnings." *Frontiers in Genetics*, 2020. https://www.frontiersin.org/articles/10.3389/fgene.2020.589621/full

1054 Pishbin, Firoozabadi, Dabanloo, Mohammadi, and Koozehgari. "Effect of physical contact (hand-holding) on heart rate variability." *International Journal of Biomedical and Biological Engineering*, 2010. doi.org/10.5281/zenodo.1334031

1055 Edwards, Young, Curtis, and Johnston. "The immediate effect of therapeutic touch and deep touch pressure on range of motion, interoceptive accuracy and heart rate variability: a randomized controlled trial with moderation analysis." *Frontiers in Integrative Neuroscience*, 2018. https://www.ncbi.nlm.nih.gov/pmc/articles/PMC6160827/

1056 Eckstein, Mamaev, Ditzen, and Sailer. "Calming effects of touch in human, animal, and robotic interaction—scientific state-of-the-art and technical advances." *Frontiers in Psychiatry*, 2020. https://www.ncbi.nlm.nih.gov/pmc/articles/PMC7672023/

1057 Zak, Stanton, and Ahmadi. "Oxytocin increases generosity in humans." *PLOS One*, 2007. https://journals.plos.org/plosone/article?id=10.1371/journal.pone.0001128

1058 Mills, Redwine, Wilson, Pung, Chinh, Greenberg, Lunde, Maisel, Raisinghani, Wood, and Chopra. "The role of gratitude in spiritual well-being in asymptomatic heart failure patients." *Spirituality in Clinical Practice*, 2015. https://doi.org/10.1037/scp0000050

1059 Li, Stampfer, Williams, and VanderWeele. "Association of religious service attendance with mortality among women." *JAMA Internal Medicine*, 2016. https://jamanetwork.com/journals/jamainternalmedicine/fullarticle/2521827

1060 Wallace, Anthony, End, and Way. "Does religion stave off the grave? Religious affiliation in one's obituary and longevity." *Social Psychological and Personality Science*, 2019. https://journals.sagepub.com/doi/full/10.1177/1948550618779820

1061 Bruce, Martins, Duru, Beech, Sims, Harawa, Vargas, Kermah, Nicholas, Brown, and Norris. "Church attendance, allostatic load, and mortality in middle aged adults." *PLOS One*, 2017. https://journals.plos.org/plosone/article?id=10.1371/journal.pone.0177618

1062 Maselko, Kubzansky, Kawachi, Seeman, and Berkman. "Religious service attendance and allostatic load among high-functioning elderly." *Psychosomatic Medicine*, 2007. https://doi.org/10.1097/PSY.0b013e31806c7c57

1063 Morales-Jinez, Gallegos Cabriales, D'Alonzo, Ugarte-Esquivel, López-Rincón, and Salazar-González. "Social factors contributing to the development of allostatic load in older adults: a correlational-predictive study." *Aquichan*, 2018. https://doi.org/10.5294/aqui.2018.18.3.5

1064 Suh, Hill, and Koenig. "Religious attendance and biological risk: a national longitudinal study of older adults." *Journal of Religion and Health*, 2019. https://doi.org/10.1007/s10943-018-0721-0

1065 Manning. "Spirituality as a lived experience: exploring the essence of spirituality for women in late life." *International Journal of Aging and Human Development*, 2012. https://doi.org/10.2190/AG.75.2.a

REFERENCES

1066 Redwine, Henry, Pung, Wilson, Chinh, Knight, Jain, Rutledge, Greenberg, Maisel, and Mills. "Pilot randomized study of a gratitude journaling intervention on heart rate variability and inflammatory biomarkers in patients with Stage B heart failure." *Psychosomatic Medicine*, 2016. https://doi.org/10.1097/PSY.0000000000000316

1067 Jackowska, Brown, Ronaldson, and Steptoe. "The impact of a brief gratitude intervention in subjective well-being, biology and sleep." *Journal of Health Psychology*, 2016. https://doi.org/10.1177/1359105315572455

1068 Southwell and Gould. "A randomised wait list-controlled pre-post-follow-up trial of a gratitude diary with a distressed sample." *Journal of Positive Psychology*, 2017. https://doi.org/10.1080/17439760.2016.1221127

1069 Digdon and Koble. "Effects of constructive worry, imagery distraction, and gratitude interventions on sleep quality: a pilot trial." *Applied Psychology: Health and Well-Being*, 2011. https://doi.org/10.1111/j.1758-0854.2011.01049.x

1070 Jans-Beken, Jacobs, Janssens, Peeters, Reijnders, Lechner, and Lataster. "Gratitude and health: an updated review." *Journal of Positive Psychology*, 2020. https://doi.org/10.1080/17439760.2019.1651888

1071 Wachholtz and Sambamthoori. "National trends in prayer use as a coping mechanism for depression: changes from 2002 to 2007." *Journal of Religion and Health*, 2012. https://doi.org/10.1007/s10943-012-9649-y

1072 Johnson. "Prayer: a helpful aid in recovery from depression." *Journal of Religion and Health*, 2018. https://doi.org/10.1007/s10943-018-0564-8

1073 Wyatt. "Spirituality may help blood pressure." Presentation at American Society of Hypertension annual meeting, 2006. https://www.webmd.com/hypertension-high-blood-pressure/news/20060518/spirituality-may-help-blood-pressure

1074 Paul-Labrador, Polk, Dwyer, Velasquez, Nidich, Rainforth, Schneider, and Merz. "Effects of a randomized controlled trial of transcendental meditation on components of the metabolic syndrome in subjects with coronary heart disease." *Archives of Internal Medicine*, 2006. https://doi.org/10.1001/archinte.166.11.1218

1075 Creswell, Myers, Cole, and Irwin. "Mindfulness meditation training effects on CD4+ T lymphocytes in HIV-1 infected adults: a small randomized controlled trial." *Brain, Behavior, and Immunity*, 2009. https://www.ncbi.nlm.nih.gov/pmc/articles/PMC2725018/

1076 McMahon and Biggs. "Examining spirituality and intrinsic religious orientation as a means of coping with exam anxiety." *Society, Health & Vulnerability*, 2012. https://www.tandfonline.com/doi/full/10.3402/vgi.v3i0.14918

1077 Wang, Davis, Volkow, Berger, Kaelber, and Xu. "Association of COVID-19 with new-onset Alzheimer's disease." *Journal of Alzheimer's Disease*, 2022. https://content.iospress.com/articles/journal-of-alzheimers-disease/jad220717

1078 Rangon, Krantic, Moyse, and Fougère. "The vagal autonomic pathway of COVID-19 at the crossroad of Alzheimer's disease and aging: a review of knowledge." *Journal of Alzheimer's Disease Reports*, 2020. https://www.ncbi.nlm.nih.gov/pmc/articles/PMC7835993/

1079 Woo, Malsy, Pöttgen, Seddiq Zai, Ufer, Hadjilaou, Schmiedel, Addo, Gerloff, Heesen, Schulze Zur Wiesch, and Friese. "Frequent neurocognitive deficits after recovery from mild COVID-19." *Brain Communications*, 2020. https://doi.org/10.1093/braincomms/fcaa205

1080 Pirker-Kees, Platho-Elwischger, Hafner, Redlich, and Baumgartner. "Hyposmia is associated with reduced cognitive function in COVID-19: first preliminary results."

Dementia and Geriatric Cognitive Disorders, 2021. https://www.ncbi.nlm.nih.gov/pmc/articles/PMC8089429/

[1081] Del Brutto, Wu, Mera, Costa, Recalde, and Issa. "Cognitive decline among individuals with history of mild symptomatic SARS-CoV-2 infection: a longitudinal prospective study nested to a population cohort." *European Journal of Neurology*, 2021. https://doi.org/10.1111/ene.14775

[1082] Amalakanti, Arepalli, and Jillella. "Cognitive assessment in asymptomatic COVID-19 subjects." *VirusDisease*, 2021. https://doi.org/10.1007/s13337-021-00663-w

[1083] Liebert, Bicknell, Markman, and Kiat. "A potential role for photobiomodulation therapy in disease treatment and prevention in the era of COVID-19." *Aging and Disease*, 2020. https://doi.org/10.14336/AD.2020.0901

[1084] Moskvin, Askhadulin, and Kochetkov. "Low-level laser therapy in prevention of the development of endothelial dysfunction and clinical experience of treatment and rehabilitation of COVID-19 patients." *Rehabilitation Research and Practice*, 2021. https://www.ncbi.nlm.nih.gov/pmc/articles/PMC7841445/

[1085] Fekrazad and Fekrazad. "The potential role of photobiomodulation in long COVID-19 patients rehabilitation." *Photobiomodulation, Photomedicine, and Laser Surgery*, 2021. https://doi.org/10.1089/photob.2020.4984

[1086] Hanna, Dalvi, Sălăgean, Pop, Bordea, and Benedicenti. "Understanding COVID-19 pandemic: molecular mechanisms and potential therapeutic strategies. An evidence-based review." *Journal of Inflammation Research*, 2021. https://www.ncbi.nlm.nih.gov/pmc/articles/PMC7802346/

[1087] Mehani. "Immunomodulatory effects of two different physical therapy modalities in patients with chronic obstructive pulmonary disease." *Journal of Physical Therapy Science*, 2017. https://www.ncbi.nlm.nih.gov/pmc/articles/PMC5599814/

[1088] Liu, Zeng, Jiao, and Liu. "The mechanism of low-intensity laser irradiation effects on virus." *Proceedings of the Third International Conference on Photonics and Imaging in Biology and Medicine*, 2003. https://doi.org/10.1117/12.546134

[1089] Colombo, Signore, Aicardi, Zekiy, Utyuzh, Benedicenti, and Amaroli. "Experimental and clinical applications of red and near-infrared photobiomodulation on endothelial dysfunction: a review." *Biomedicines*, 2021. https://www.ncbi.nlm.nih.gov/pmc/articles/PMC7998572/

[1090] Oliveira, Greiffo, Rigonato-Oliveira, Custódio, Silva, Damaceno-Rodrigues, Almeida, Albertini, Lopes-Martins, de Oliveira, de Carvalho, de Oliveira, Leal Junior, and Vieira. "Low level laser therapy reduces acute lung inflammation in a model of pulmonary and extrapulmonary LPS-induced ARDS." *Journal of Photochemistry and Photobiology B*, 2014. https://doi.org/10.1016/j.jphotobiol.2014.03.021

[1091] Ajaz, McPhail, Singh, Mujib, Trovato, Napoli, and Agarwal. "Mitochondrial metabolic manipulation by SARS-CoV-2 in peripheral blood mononuclear cells of patients with COVID-19." *American Journal of Physiology: Cell Physiology*, 2021. https://journals.physiology.org/doi/full/10.1152/ajpcell.00426.2020

[1092] Ryback. "How mitochondria protect us from COVID-19." *Psychology Today* online, 2021. https://www.psychologytoday.com/us/blog/the-truisms-wellness/202101/how-mitochondria-protects-us-covid-19

[1093] Johnson. "A new mitochondrial enhancer is being trialed in long COVID." Health Rising blog, 2021. https://www.healthrising.org/blog/2021/11/05/axa1125-mitochondrial-enhancer-long-covid/

REFERENCES

1094 Johnson. "Long-COVID exercise study points to mitochondrial dysfunction and twitchy muscles." Health Rising blog, 2022. https://www.healthrising.org/blog/2022/05/18/long-covid-exercise-cpet-mitochondria/

1095 Belman. "New findings help explain how COVID-19 overpowers the immune system." USC Leonard Davis School of Gerontology blog article, 2021. https://gero.usc.edu/2021/01/08/covid-19-immune-system-mitochondria/

1096 Ailioaie and Litscher. "Probiotics, photobiomodulation, and disease management: controversies and challenges." International Journal of Molecular Sciences, 2021. https://www.ncbi.nlm.nih.gov/pmc/articles/PMC8124384/

1097 Nejatifard, Asefi, Jamali, Hamblin, and Fekrazad. "Probable positive effects of the photobiomodulation as an adjunctive treatment in COVID-19: a systematic review." Cytokine, 2021. https://www.ncbi.nlm.nih.gov/pmc/articles/PMC7550078/

1098 Bjornevik, Cortese, Healy, Kuhle, Mina, Leng, Elledge, Niebuhr, Scher, Munger, and Ascherio. "Longitudinal analysis reveals high prevalence of Epstein-Barr virus associated with multiple sclerosis." Science, 2022. https://www.science.org/doi/10.1126/science.abj8222

1099 Hunskar, Rortveit, Litleskare, Eide, Hanevik, Langeland, and Wensaas. "Prevalence of fibromyalgia 10 years after infection with Giardia lamblia: a controlled prospective cohort study." Scandinavian Journal of Pain, 2021. https://www.degruyter.com/document/doi/10.1515/sjpain-2021-0122/html

1100 Cairns, Itzhaki, and Kaplan. "Potential involvement of varicella zoster virus in Alzheimer's disease via reactivation of quiescent herpes simplex virus type 1." Journal of Alzheimer's Disease, 2022. https://doi.org/10.3233/JAD-220287

Questionnaires

ASSESS YOUR BRAIN HEALTH HISTORY

This questionnaire is meant to jog your memory about serious incidents that may have affected your brain health for a short or long time afterward. Remember, healing is possible—that's what this entire book is about! Becoming aware of how our life experiences may have lasting emotional and cognitive impacts can help us understand the importance of implementing the information in this book so our brains and bodies can heal. Remember that the recommendations in this book are not a substitute for treatment by a medical professional; rather, they are lifestyle suggestions designed to set you up for optimal healing in combination with medical treatment.

1. How many times have you suffered a blow to the head (e.g., while playing sports, falling off a bike or a horse, falling off of playground equipment, slipping and falling on ice, or running into a wall, tree, or other object)? Write out the details of each incident. At what age did it occur? What symptoms did you have as a result (e.g., concussion, loss of consciousness, confusion or altered mental state, headaches, dizziness, fatigue, problems with memory or concentration, sensitivity to light or sound, trouble with emotional regulation)?

2. Have you ever been in any car accidents? Write down the details of each one. How old were you when it happened? Were you wearing a seatbelt or car seat restraint? Did you sustain a concussion or any other injuries? Did you notice any changes in emotion or cognition afterward?

3. Have you ever experienced whiplash from a car accident or for any other reason? If so, write down the details of each incident.

4. Have you experienced a head injury as a result of assault or violence (e.g., domestic abuse, fights, firearm injury)? If so, note the dates and details of each incident.

5. Have you ever been nearby when an explosion or a blast occurred? If so, write down the details (date, intensity/magnitude, symptoms experienced).

6. Have you ever experienced anoxia (loss of oxygen to the brain, e.g., due to a near drowning or suffocating experience)? If so, write down the details (date, duration, symptoms experienced).

7. Have you ever experienced a seizure or a stroke? If so, note the date(s) and details.

8. Have you ever experienced a drug overdose? If so, note the date(s) and details.

9. Have you experienced meningitis, encephalitis, a sustained high fever, or a brain tumor? If so, note the date(s) and details.

10. Have you received medical treatment for any other injury to your head or neck? If so, note the date(s) and details.

LEARN YOUR ACES SCORE

Answer each question in reference to events that happened before your eighteenth birthday.

1. Did you experience physical abuse?
2. Did you experience verbal/emotional abuse?
3. Did you experience sexual abuse?
4. Did you witness physical, verbal/emotional, or sexual abuse in your home?
5. Were you neglected (physically or emotionally) by your parent(s) or caregiver(s)?
6. Did your parents or caregivers separate or divorce?
7. Did a parent or caregiver pass away?
8. Was a parent or caregiver addicted to drugs or alcohol, or did they engage in substance abuse?
9. Was a parent or caregiver incarcerated?
10. Did a parent or caregiver attempt suicide or struggle with depression or other mental illnesses?

Remember that your Adverse Child Experiences (ACEs) score is not destiny. A higher ACEs score generally means you are more vulnerable to toxic stress and may have a harder time tapping into resiliency—but this just means it takes work. A relatively high ACEs score can serve as motivation to prioritize your health and work to build resiliency. The power to heal lies within each of us, and understanding our starting point can help us gain a clearer sense of why this work is so important.

For more information and resources, visit acesaware.org.

COMPASSION SATISFACTION AND COMPASSION FATIGUE
(PROQOL) VERSION 5 (2009)

When you [help] people you have direct contact with their lives. As you may have found, your compassion for those you [help] can affect you in positive and negative ways. Below are some-questions about your experiences, both positive and negative, as a [helper]. Consider each of the following questions about you and your current work situation. Select the number that honestly reflects how frequently you experienced these things in the *last 30 days*.

1=Never	2=Rarely	3=Sometimes	4=Often	5=Very Often

_____ 1. I am happy.

_____ 2. I am preoccupied with more than one person I [help].

_____ 3. I get satisfaction from being able to [help] people.

_____ 4. I feel connected to others.

_____ 5. I jump or am startled by unexpected sounds.

_____ 6. I feel invigorated after working with those I [help].

_____ 7. I find it difficult to separate my personal life from my life as a [helper].

_____ 8. I am not as productive at work because I am losing sleep over traumatic experiences of a person I [help].

_____ 9. I think that I might have been affected by the traumatic stress of those I [help].

_____ 10. I feel trapped by my job as a [helper].

_____ 11. Because of my [helping], I have felt "on edge" about various things.

_____ 12. I like my work as a [helper].

_____ 13. I feel depressed because of the traumatic experiences of the people I [help].

_____ 14. I feel as though I am experiencing the trauma of someone I have [helped].

_____ 15. I have beliefs that sustain me.

_____ 16. I am pleased with how I am able to keep up with [helping] techniques and protocols.

_____ 17. I am the person I always wanted to be.

_____ 18. My work makes me feel satisfied.

_____ 19. I feel worn out because of my work as a [helper].

_____ 20. I have happy thoughts and feelings about those I [help] and how I could help them.

_____ 21. I feel overwhelmed because my case [work] load seems endless.

_____ 22. I believe I can make a difference through my work.

_____ 23. I avoid certain activities or situations because they remind me of frightening experiences of the people I [help].

_____ 24. I am proud of what I can do to [help].

_____ 25. As a result of my [helping], I have intrusive, frightening thoughts.

_____ 26. I feel "bogged down" by the system.

_____ 27. I have thoughts that I am a "success" as a [helper].

_____ 28. I can't recall important parts of my work with trauma victims.

_____ 29. I am a very caring person.

_____ 30. I am happy that I chose to do this work.

Based on your responses, place your personal scores below. If you have any concerns, you should discuss them with a physical or mental health care professional.

Compassion Satisfaction _____

Compassion satisfaction is about the pleasure you derive from being able to do your work well. For example, you may feel like it is a pleasure to help others through your work. You may feel positively about your colleagues or your ability to contribute to the work setting or even the greater good of society. Higher scores on this scale represent a greater satisfaction related to your ability to be an effective caregiver in your job.

The average score is 50 (SD 10; alpha scale reliability .88). About 25% of people score higher than 57 and about 25% of people score below 43. If you are in the higher range, you probably derive a good deal of professional satisfaction from your position. If your scores are below 40, you may either find problems with your job, or there may be some other reason—for example, you might derive your satisfaction from activities other than your job.

Burnout_____

Most people have an intuitive idea of what burnout is. From the research perspective, burnout is one of the elements of Compassion Fatigue (CF). It is associated with feelings of hopelessness and difficulties in dealing with work or in doing your job effectively. These negative feelings usually have a gradual onset. They can reflect the feeling that your efforts make no difference, or they can be associated with a very high workload or a non-supportive work environment. Higher scores on this scale mean that you are at higher risk for burnout.

The average score on the burnout scale is 50 (SD 10; alpha scale reliability .75). About 25% of people score above 57 and about 25% of people score below 43. If your score is below 43, this probably reflects positive feelings about your ability to be effective in your work. If you score above 57 you may wish to think about what at work makes you feel like you are not effective in your position. Your score may reflect your mood; perhaps you were having a "bad day" or are in need of some time off. If the high score persists or if it is reflective of other worries, it may be a cause for concern.

Secondary Traumatic Stress_____

The second component of Compassion Fatigue (CF) is secondary traumatic stress (STS). It is about your work related, secondary exposure to extremely or traumatically stressful events. Developing problems due to exposure to other's trauma is somewhat rare but does happen to many people who care for those who have experienced extremely or traumatically stressful events. For example, you may repeatedly hear stories about the traumatic things that happen to other people, commonly called Vicarious Traumatization. If your work puts you directly in the path of danger, for example, field work in a war or area of civil violence, this is not secondary exposure; your exposure is primary. However, if you are exposed to others' traumatic events as a result of your work, for example, as a therapist or an emergency worker, this is secondary exposure. The symptoms of STS are usually rapid in onset and associated with a particular event. They may include being afraid, having difficulty sleeping, having images of the upsetting event pop into your mind, or avoiding things that remind you of the event.

The average score on this scale is 50 (SD 10; alpha scale reliability .81). About 25% of people score below 43 and about 25% of people score above 57. If your score is above 57, you may want to take some time to think about what at work may be frightening to you or if there is some other reason for the elevated score. While higher scores do not mean that you do have a problem, they are an indication that you may want to examine how you feel about your work and your work environment. You may wish to discuss this with your supervisor, a colleague, or a health care professional.

2

In this section, you will score your test so you understand the interpretation for you. To find your score on **each section**, total the questions listed on the left and then find your score in the table on the right of the section.

Compassion Satisfaction Scale

Copy your rating on each of these questions on to this table and add them up. When you have added then up you can find your score on the table to the right.

3. ____
6. ____
12. ____
16. ____
18. ____
20. ____
22. ____
24. ____
27. ____
30. ____

Total: ____

The sum of my Compassion Satisfaction questions is	So My Score Equals	And my Compassion Satisfaction level is
22 or less	43 or less	Low
Between 23 and 41	Around 50	Average
42 or more	57 or more	High

Burnout Scale

On the burnout scale you will need to take an extra step. Starred items are "reverse scored." If you scored the item 1, write a 5 beside it. The reason we ask you to reverse the scores is because scientifically the measure works better when these questions are asked in a positive way though they can tell us more about their negative form. For example, question 1. "I am happy" tells us more about the effects of helping when you are *not* happy so you reverse the score

You Wrote	Change to
	5
2	4
3	3
4	2
5	1

*1. ____ = ____
*4. ____ = ____
8. ____
10. ____
*15. ____ = ____
*17. ____ = ____
19. ____
21. ____
26. ____
*29. ____ = ____

Total: ____

The sum of my Burnout Questions is	So my score equals	And my Burnout level is
22 or less	43 or less	Low
Between 23 and 41	Around 50	Average
42 or more	57 or more	High

Secondary Traumatic Stress Scale

Just like you did on Compassion Satisfaction, copy your rating on each of these questions on to this table and add them up. When you have added then up you can find your score on the table to the right.

2. ____
5. ____
7. ____
9. ____
11. ____
13. ____
14. ____
23. ____
25. ____
28. ____

Total: ____

The sum of my Secondary Trauma questions is	So My Score Equals	And my Secondary Traumatic Stress level is
22 or less	43 or less	Low
Between 23 and 41	Around 50	Average
42 or more	57 or more	High

3

Find Resources to Build Your Brain Power at ProNeuroLight.com

If you've read this book, you know exactly how photobiomodulation works to help boost the energy systems of your body and brain. Visit my website, ProNeuroLight.com, to find red and near-infrared light devices that are guaranteed to be safe and effective. We offer body pads as well as intranasal and transcranial photobiomodulation devices for sale, and we are available for consultations to advise you on how to use the light devices.

On our website, you can also schedule a free consultation with our coaching team. Using the **PRONEURO** approach, our coaches have helped people increase their heart rate variability, decrease their resting heart rate, and improve their sleep quality as measured by the percentage of deep sleep and REM sleep relative to light sleep. If you choose to enroll as a client, you will receive weekly coaching calls (recorded for your reference) with assignments, tips, and resources shared with you by our coaches, depending on your needs. You'll have access to a private Slack channel for tracking your materials and communicating with our team, and you'll also get access to our proprietary dashboard that integrates biodata insights from various trackers and devices.

At the very least, you'll want to be sure to visit ProNeuroLight.com to sign up for our email list. This way you'll be notified of discounts on our devices and programming as well as upcoming events like the virtual summits on brain health and healing we regularly organize.

ACKNOWLEDGMENTS

Dr. Joe DiDuro:

This book began when a young undergrad at Hobart College called me up to interview me for our local paper. Russell Payne was doing an internship at the *Finger Lakes Times*, and his assignment was to write a feel-good story about a local boy who returned to town as a now published Alzheimer's scientist with all sorts of new technologies. If I had to put a pin in the moment that this book began, it was then. The book you hold in your hands represents the connection of personal and professional events moving both forward and backward in time from that moment, which provided the spark to catalyze this project.

While Russell was the one who listened and created an outline, legions of people along the way have taught me, guided me, and supported me—both before and after. Some of my professional mentors and personal influences are named in this book, but just as important are all the patients and clients who have shared teaching moments with me.

My deepest appreciation goes to my editor and coauthor, Elizabeth G. Her skill as a talented writer was duly matched by her scientific mind. For our work together, I supplied raw, rough (and heavy) logs, which she honed into furniture that was not only functional but elegant and aesthetically pleasing. I'd say she went above and beyond, finishing it and arranging it into the tastefully decorated house you see here as the final product.

As for the personal influences, to acknowledge one person and leave out another would be unkind. This is especially likely for this book since it describes my journey to recover from acquired brain injuries. (I was that guy who would call all the people around me "buddy" or "sweetie" because I couldn't remember their names.) If you are reading this book and you recall some past interaction with me, you can trust that *you* had an influence on the content written in this book.

I would also like to provide a different kind of acknowledgment—to the people who were affected by the personality changes I suffered due to my acquired brain injuries. This type of injury is often called a "silent pathology" because it's on the inside—but the effects are very real, and I would like to acknowledge the impact my injuries had on my coworkers, my friends, and most of all my family.

Elizabeth Gudrais:

I first want to thank Dr. Joe DiDuro for trusting me to help you bring your life's work into book form. Thank you for trusting in the process even when the timeframe and direction were unclear! Writing a book takes brain power, and I've been putting the **PRONEURO** method into practice throughout this entire journey, so thank you for that, too! Your unwavering passion for bringing this method to more people has been an inspiration for me.

I extend deep gratitude to Amanda Johnson of Awaken Village Press. I am forever in awe of the way your intuition guides you to the perfect clients and projects for me, for you, and for the company as a whole. This book was the right project at the right time to help me grow as a writer and heal as a person. God's timing is always impeccable, and your guidance has been pivotal in helping me learn to trust that.

Thanks to Larry Tye for nurturing my interest in health and medical reporting way back when, to John Rosenberg for your mentorship and guidance as I navigated the learning curve of asking Harvard professors to encapsulate a lifetime of research into a thirty-minute interview and make it accessible to a novice, and to my editors at the *Providence Journal*—Carol Young, Karen Maguire, Tim Murphy—for teaching me there's no such thing as a stupid question.

Thanks to the copy editors who have imparted grammatical lessons along the way (including, most recently, Jean Martin and Marianne Johnson). I still hear your voices whispering over my shoulder while I am writing and editing.

Thanks to my parents for believing in me no matter what. Thanks to all the friends and relatives who have continued to express interest in this book even as it stretched on far past the original anticipated completion date. (I suspect you are in disbelief that it actually got published, and I feel a bit that way myself.)

Last but not least, thank you to Sean, my husband, for your constant support and encouragement. Although we've been staying home a lot anyway these past three years, I appreciate the patience you've shown with this book taking up the bulk of my weekends (as well as with my newfound interest in the red and near-infrared light devices that are now plugged in all throughout our house). As always, we are better together.

ABOUT THE AUTHORS

Dr. Joe DiDuro is dedicated to helping people live a more fulfilling life. His passion is to help people by teaching them how they can create neuroregeneration and healing in their own lives. He is the president and founder of the Neuropathy Treatment Centers of America, a 501(c)3 nonprofit organization. He is also president of ProNeuroLIGHT LLC, a medical technologies company, and the moderator of the tPBMT Brain Research Consortium.

In his thirty-two years of clinical experience, Dr. Joe came to understand the very low quality of life people affected by neurodegenerative diseases experience and observed that their disability touches every aspect of a person's existence—on a personal level, on a family level, and on a social level. Dr. Joe has made it his life's work to help end this suffering, initiate his clients' recovery, and restore their humanity.

Dr. Joe earned his bachelor of arts degree from the State University of New York at Buffalo in 1983 and his doctoral degree from Palmer College of Chiropractic in Davenport, Iowa, in 1986. He lived and practiced in Vicenza, Italy, for ten years. While there, he completed further specialized training in Amsterdam for the American Chiropractic Neurology Board and attained diplomate status in chiropractic neurology in 2000. After returning to the U.S., Dr. Joe obtained a master's degree in clinical research from Palmer College in 2006 in a program supported by the National Institutes of Health.

In recent years, he has dedicated his efforts to research and technological innovation that helps people create more brain power. Since creating the **PRONEURO** approach, he has become a highly sought-after cognitive neurotherapist and brain fitness coach. He currently divides his time between Arizona, Italy, and Costa Rica.

Elizabeth Gudrais has two decades of experience in magazine and newspaper journalism and, more recently, book editing and ghostwriting. She shares her love of the craft of writing with others in her role as the facilitator of a group program that supports authors in completing their manuscripts as well as her one-on-one book coaching and editing work. She holds a bachelor's degree in literature, with a focus in Russian, from Harvard University. *My Brain Matters* offered a unique opportunity for Elizabeth to combine two of her passions: writing and wellness. Elizabeth is a certified yoga instructor and nutrition guide. She also holds a coaching certification in the Tiny Habits method of behavior change and is an Emotional Freedom Techniques practitioner in training. She lives in Madison, Wisconsin, with her husband.